CanMEDS Teaching and Assessment Tools Guide

D1621061

EDITORS

Susan Glover Takahashi, MA(Ed), PhD

Cynthia Abbott, M.Pl.

Anna Oswald, MD, MMEd, FRCPC

Jason R. Frank, MD, MA(Ed), FRCPC

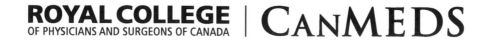

CanMEDS Teaching and Assessment Tools Guide

Royal College of Physicians and Surgeons of Canada
774 Echo Drive
Ottawa, Ontario K1S 5N8 Canada
Telephone: 613-730-8177
Toll-free: 1-800-668-3740
Website: royalcollege.ca
Email: canmeds@royalcollege.ca

©2015 Royal College of Physicians and Surgeons
of Canada. All rights reserved.

All rights reserved. This material may be reproduced for
educational, personal, non-commercial purposes only, with
attribution to the source as noted below or as indicated
on the individual tools. Written permission from the
Royal College is required for all other uses. Permissions
may be sought directly from the CanMEDS and Faculty
Development Unit at canmeds@royalcollege.ca.

Printed in Canada. First printing.

Cover design: ImageStudio Creative Communications Ltd.

ISBN: 978-1-926588-32-2

How to reference this document:
Glover Takahashi S, Abbott C, Oswald A, Frank JR.
CanMEDS Teaching and Assessment Tools Guide. Ottawa:
Royal College of Physicians and Surgeons of Canada; 2015.

Table of contents

© 2015 Royal College of Physicians and Surgeons of Canada

© 2015 Royal College of Physicians and Surgeons of Canada

1. Everything you need to know about the *CanMEDS Tools Guide*

Susan Glover Takahashi, Cynthia Abbott, Anna Oswald and Jason R. Frank

The *CanMEDS Teaching and Assessment Tools Guide (CanMEDS Tools Guide)* is designed as a stand-alone, practical, introductory teaching and assessment resource for competency based residency education. Developed for busy program directors and faculty responsible for implementing the CanMEDS Physician Competency Framework in residency programs, the *CanMEDS Tools Guide* helps clarify important educational concepts in everyday language and provides a selection of teaching and assessment tips and tools that you can use and modify according to your needs.

This resource was inspired by a desire to enhance residency education in Canada and support the implementation of the CanMEDS 2015 Framework. Since CanMEDS was first created in the 1990s, we have received thousands of requests for practical resources that help practical-minded, busy educators incorporate the CanMEDS Framework into their training activities. The *CanMEDS Tools Guide* is our answer to these requests and signals our continued commitment to support ongoing innovation across the continuum of medical education.

This resource is designed to support learning, teaching, and assessment of the core skills and competencies of the CanMEDS Framework as part of everyday resident work. Our work-based approach is designed to help your learners appreciate the relevance of these competencies to the care that they provide and reinforce their commitment to developing the full spectrum of competencies as described in the CanMEDS Framework.

What you will find in the *CanMEDS Tools Guide*

The *CanMEDS Tools Guide* provides ready-to-use resources that have a new and purposeful emphasis on learning, teaching, assessing, and providing feedback in the workplace. This resource was designed for the busy physician who will pick and choose relevant content on a just-in-time basis.

This book dedicates a chapter to each of the seven CanMEDS Roles. If you like you can read it from cover to cover, but we envision that most of you will refer to this guide on an as needed basis (i.e. when you're developing your teaching and assessment plans or when you have a particular problem or question that requires a practical answer). We also hope that the simplicity of the examples and templates will encourage you to create your own tools that you can share with your colleagues.

In the *CanMEDS Tools Guide* you will find many tips and tools that you can use in your programs immediately. It is designed as a reference guide that you will come back to again and again. It is not intended to be a systematic review of its topic areas. Rather, it is meant to serve as a high-level resource that will help you raise the bar when it comes to residency education and more specifically teaching and assessing CanMEDS in your program. The *CanMEDS Tools Guide* has been developed with the expertise and experience of 50 contributors. We hope it becomes a go-to resource for your residency program.

What you will NOT find in the *CanMEDS Tools Guide*

This resource focuses on residency education, that critical phase of medical education that prepares physicians for independent practice in a specific discipline. If your context is different, these tools may be adaptable. In addition, the *CanMEDS Tools Guide* emphasizes training tips that are pragmatic and practical. We left an in-depth review of medical education techniques and theories to others.

Using the *CanMEDS Tools Guide*

This book includes chapters for each of the CanMEDS Roles: Medical Expert, Communicator, Collaborator, Leader, Health Advocate, Scholar and Professional. Each chapter begins with answers to practical questions and then moves on to a series of tips that will prepare you to teach and assess the Roles. You will also find a short list of annotated resources and recommended reading. Each chapter ends with a series of tools designed for teaching and assessing the Role.

The tools in this guide are samples that you can use as is (i.e. photocopied from a hard copy or printed from an electronic format) or you can adapt them to reflect your content area, discipline or context of practice. Electronic versions of many of the tools in this guide are available on the Royal College website. When you do reproduce and modify the tools, please maintain the footer that acknowledges the source of the materials.

The authors and contributors have done an outstanding job in bringing these resources together in an accessible manner, and we trust that you will find the *CanMEDS Teaching and Assessment Tools Guide* both useful and time-effective. We welcome comments and suggestions for future editions. Please contact us at <u>canmeds@royalcollege.ca</u>

And, finally, we thank Tammy Hesson, Megan McComb, Caroline Clouston, Kristopher Tharris and the CanMEDS Team for their dedication to the success of this project.

© 2015 Royal College of Physicians and Surgeons of Canada

TABLE 1: CHAPTER ANATOMY

Icon	Section	Content (This section....)	Notes
	1. Why the Role matters	• Provides a short, high-level overview outlining the key features of the Role and the impact or outcomes of competence in this area	• We believe this is as an ideal starting point for introducing the Role to learners, faculty or other team members. • These talking points can be particularly useful when dealing with people who struggle to appreciate the 'value' of the Role.
	2. What the Role looks like in daily practice	• Helps describe the things that make this Role unique • Presents a set of "Trigger" words, which can help people make the connection between the Role and their daily practice • Includes the Role definition, description and key competencies from the CanMEDS 2015 Physician Competency Framework • Describes key technical terms that learners and teachers should master to understand the evidence that underpins the Role	• Great physicians seem to effortlessly integrate all seven CanMEDS Roles into their practice. This section of the chapter breaks things down to help learners differentiate each Role. • It is important for learners to understand the building blocks of a Role and its relationship with the other CanMEDS Roles so that one day, as their competence progresses, they too can knit the seven Roles together with ease.
	3. Preparing to teach the Role	• Functions as a plain language primer on the fundamentals of the Role • Starts by describing some common misconceptions about the Role and is designed to 'set the record straight' • Addresses content that was introduced in the CanMEDS 2015 version of the Framework • Describes key and important topics including frameworks and models from the literature • Introduces content that is important to all specialties	• This content is designed as a primer that can be used by both learners and teachers. • The content should serve as a starting point. We hope you will add a layer by accounting for your local, specialty specific or program needs and resources.
	4. Hints, tips, and tools for teaching the Role	• Presents practical tips from physicians on how they teach the Role • Emphasizes workplace teaching and ways to include CanMEDS teaching in day-to-day practice • Provides a list of 'ready to use' or easy to modify sample teaching tools • Includes a URL to direct you to easy-to-customize (free) electronic versions of some of the teaching tools for the Role (i.e. in .doc, .ppt and .pdf formats) • Includes workshop materials for an academic half day (i.e. PowerPoint for the Role, small group activities) as well as workplace teaching tools (i.e. case reports) • Features a 'Role Summary Sheet', which is best described as a two page summary of the Role	• The teaching tips and tools in this section are designed to support you to teach the Role. • We encourage you to use these tools to help spark ideas on how to develop your own tools. • Many of the teaching tools can be adapted easily for self-directed learning. • The summary sheets can be used as a handy cheat sheet for teachers and learners.
	5. Hints, tips, and tools for assessing the Role	• Features practical tips from physicians on how to assess the Role • Addresses some common barriers to performance and includes strategies for improvement • Emphasizes the importance of feedback and coaching for improvement • Provides a list of ready-to-use or easy-to-customize sample assessment tools • Includes a URL to direct you to free and easy-to-customize electronic versions of some of the assessment tools for the Role (i.e. in .doc and .pdf formats)	• While learning is often associated most with teaching, there is a growing trend toward seeing assessment as a valuable tool for learning. To this end, we provide tips and tools to encourage workplace assessments that encourage learning and progression of competence.

© 2015 Royal College of Physicians and Surgeons of Canada

Icon	Section	Content (This section....)	Notes
	6. Suggested resources	• Features a short list of the hand-picked important, resources that have been annotated for your convenience • May also include relevant sample videos (i.e. YouTube)	• We know how busy you are so we curated a short list of important resources that will help with understanding the Role as well as teaching and assessing it.
	7. Other resources	• Lists of other important favourite articles, books, websites etc. suggested by authors	• If you have the time to go through a longer list of resources, this section includes other highly recommended resources that you will find useful.
	8. Sample tools	• Teaching tools – features ready-to-use, easy-to-customize tools for the Role. Often includes notes to learners • Assessment tools – includes ready-to-use, easy-to-customize tools for the Role. Includes answer keys where appropriate	• Many of the Tools in this section of the chapter have been designed so that you can pick-them-up and use them with your learners as-is. For this reason, we opted to remove any instructions for you, the teacher. In these cases, you will find the "teacher" notes at the end of the chapter.

2. The big picture: connecting Competence by Design and CanMEDS 2015

In 2015, the Royal College updated the CanMEDS Physician Competency Framework. You may be wondering how and when CanMEDS 2015 and the Royal College's Competence by Design (CBD) initiative will impact you, your program, and your learners. This section of the *CanMEDS Tools Guide* answers these questions.

CanMEDS and the Competence by Design Initiative

Since the Royal College developed the CanMEDS Physician Competency Framework in the 1990s, CanMEDS has been updated every 10 years. Unlike previous editions, however, work on the CanMEDS 2015 Framework occurred in a special context. It was part of the Royal College's CBD initiative, a major, multi-year project to implement an enhanced model for competency-based medical education (CBME) in residency training and specialty practice in Canada. The aim of the CBD project is to improve the fundamental building blocks of Canadian medical training.

At its core, CBD initiates a transition from the practice of credentialing physicians solely on the basis of time spent on rotations, to the practice of assessing learners' progressive achievement of competence over the course of a program. Designed to integrate competency-based education across all of the Royal College's educational and certification programs and services, CBD is transforming the way specialty medical education is delivered in Canada. In support of a new emphasis on progression toward competence, the CanMEDS 2015 component of the CBD initiative updates the content of the CanMEDS Roles and it provides a set of milestones across the continuum of medical education that can be applied both in curriculum development and in learner assessment. The structured rollout of CBD started in 2014 and will continue for about a decade. CBD will not impact all residency programs at the same time. Plans for CBD include a phased rollout with sustained support for Royal College specialty committees and program directors.

How does the Tools Guide help prepare me for CBD and CBME?

Between 2015 and 2025, there will be a number of major changes to medical education and practice as the Royal College and many of its partners transition to a system that is truly competency based. The transition to CBME will not happen overnight, but it's important for you, your teachers, and your learners to begin to see the connections and feel comfortable with the concepts and their implications for your work.

This guide helps implement the key concepts of competency-based medical education including:

- The idea that a learner's competence will progress over time and the fact that your role as a teacher is to help your learner continue to progress along that continuum,

- The importance of using assessment as a strategy to support and inform further learning,

- The importance of teaching and assessing in the workplace.

© 2015 Royal College of Physicians and Surgeons of Canada

Key terms relevant to CBME, CBD, and CanMEDS 2015

Competence by Design (CBD) is the Royal College's transformational initiative designed to enhance competency-based medical education (CBME) in residency training and specialty practice in Canada. The following definitions of key terms will provide you with a common lexicon for CBME.

Competency-based medical education (CBME)[1] is an outcomes-based approach to the design, implementation, assessment, and evaluation of a medical education program using an organizing framework of competencies. To prepare physicians for practice, CBME is:

- oriented on desired outcomes;

- based on patient needs;

- based on the needs of the learner, with more accountability and flexibility;

- focused on achieving skills; and

- demonstrating performance, instead of tracking time-spent in training.

Until the late 20th century, medical trainees were deemed competent if they passed a series of tests, which 'proved' that they had acquired the prescribed body of knowledge and set of skills; the goal of medical education was to produce physicians who knew certain facts and could perform certain skills. With the advent of CBME, the goal of medical education has been recast; the aim is now to produce physicians who possess the set of multi-faceted abilities (called competencies) they will need to meet the needs of the patients they serve. In CBME, trainees acquire knowledge and skills as a means to an end, not as an end in themselves. Designers of CBME programs first determine which competencies their graduates will need and then create a curriculum that carefully maps teaching, feedback, and coaching opportunities to the desired outcomes and sets up a purposeful and systematic approach to monitoring and assessing each learner's progress over the course of their educational program. As their expertise develops, trainees are given increasing degrees of responsibility by their supervising faculty. For example, for surgical residents, the development process moves from focused skills to simple cases to more complex cases, as efficiency and effectiveness increase.

For medical residents, as patient care competencies are used in progressively complex cases, the physician performs data collection and analysis for diagnosis, and applies synthesis and judgment skills for management, with increasing ease and efficiency.

Competencies[1] are the observable abilities of health care professionals. The key and enabling competencies in the CanMEDS Framework identify the knowledge, skills, and attitudes that physicians require to perform competently.

Competence is the collection of competencies across multiple domains or aspects of physician performance in a certain context.[1] Competence is multi-dimensional and dynamic, and changes with time, experience, and context.[1] If you want to comment on a particular physician's competence, you will need to have specific, detailed understanding of:

- the physician's relevant abilities,

- the context, and

- the physician's stage of training or practice (i.e., where they are on the continuum of training or practice).

Relevant abilities include what potential the physician has (i.e. capability) and what the physician can currently do (i.e. competencies), see Table 1.

Context means the "who" (e.g. types of clients, groups, populations), "what" (e.g. areas of practice, types of service), "where" (e.g. practice settings) and "how" (e.g. professional roles, funding models) of an individual's practice or training milieu.[2]

TABLE 1. MULTI-DIMENSIONAL ELEMENTS OF COMPETENCE[2]

Multi-dimensional elements of competence	Definition
Capability	The physical, mental, and emotional "raw materials" of an individual
Competencies	The desired knowledge, skills, and abilities that the individual is able to demonstrate
Context of practice	The practice environment
Continuum of development	The level of expertise and educational level

© 2015 Royal College of Physicians and Surgeons of Canada

The elements of an individual's context of practice are interrelated and have an impact on competence. Performance expectations vary across practice settings and specialties, and sometimes when an individual performs better (or worse) in one context than in another, it is because their competence is currently a better (or worse) match for that context.

Examples of how context can impact your trainees include:

- Your Anesthesiology trainee may be better with adult patients than with pediatric patients (or vice versa).

- Your Diagnostic Radiology trainee may be better with neurology cases than with musculoskeletal cases.

- Your Cardiology trainee may be better with emergency department cases than with follow-up cases in the clinic.

- Your Anatomical Pathology trainee may be better at providing advice in their written reports than in the operating room or at multidisciplinary Oncology rounds.

Milestones[3] are the expected ability of a health care professional at a stage of development. CanMEDS 2015 Milestones acknowledge that competencies develop with experience and practise over time – organized along a continuum that presents an estimate of the usual sequence of learner progress and development. Generally, milestones are used to monitor progress and offer a structured "alert" system so that learners and faculty can identify when a learner's progress is off course. If a learner is progressing more slowly or at a lower level than anticipated, it is important for faculty to determine the source of the problem.

The milestones can:

- illustrate the developmental nature, features, and progression of the competencies;

- assist learners in monitoring their own developmental progress;

- be used as a reference to monitor individual learner progress;

- inform the development of assessment tools so that they reflect usual developmental progression;

- guide teaching program development;

- assist faculty by providing a model of usual developmental progression; and

- assist in the early identification of learners whose progress is not following the typical development sequence and initiate early intervention if needed to ensure a learner's progress, process, and outcomes.

The CanMEDS 2015 Milestones,[4] a companion resource to the CanMEDS 2015 Framework, provides the competencies expected along the continuum of practice.

Royal College Entrustable Professional Activities (RCEPAs)[3]

RCEPAs are statements describing a task of a discipline or profession that a clinician has been confirmed as trusted to perform. The degree of trust given to the learner to complete the EPA reflects the sophistication of the clinician's learning. EPAs are made up of multiple competencies. RCEPAs are defined as "developing in a given stage of training", so RCEPAs are made up of milestones (statements of abilities at a given stage).

Milestones can assist to structure learning, teaching, and assessment so that learner and teacher have a shared understanding of expectations and likely progress. EPAs can assist to provide an authentic work-based identification of those day-to-day activities of a learner that need particular attention and assessment.

The Competence Continuum: There are four stages of a residency program in the competence continuum diagram (Figure 1):

- Transition to Discipline

- Foundations of Discipline

- Core of Discipline

- Transition to Practice

The figure reflects a change in terminology related to medical education when CBD is implemented. For example, pre-CBD, a physician's progress was identified by the traditional stages of junior resident, senior resident, and practicing physician. In the CBD stages, a physician's progress is identified as transitioning to a discipline, mastering the foundations of their discipline (both of which map to the junior resident stage), mastering the core of their discipline (in which traditional junior resident and senior resident stages can overlap), transitioning to practice (which maps to the pre-certification senior resident stage), and then on to continuing professional development, in which the physician is learning in practice.

Assessment for learning: Increasingly the focus of CBME includes providing learners with regular, work-based assessments and feedback that measure learners' progression toward competence and, by extension, the assessments help direct the residents' learning going forward.

© 2015 Royal College of Physicians and Surgeons of Canada

FIGURE 1.

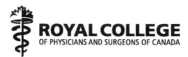

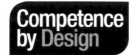

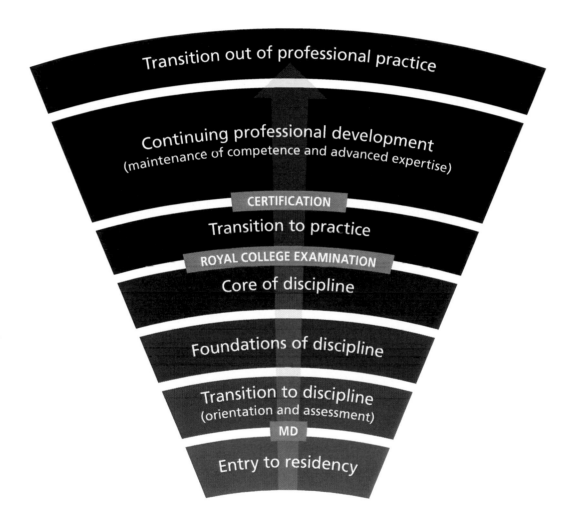

CBD[1,2] Competence Continuum

- Transition out of professional practice
- Continuing professional development (maintenance of competence and advanced expertise)
- **CERTIFICATION**
- Transition to practice
- **ROYAL COLLEGE EXAMINATION**
- Core of discipline
- Foundations of discipline
- Transition to discipline (orientation and assessment)
- **MD**
- Entry to residency

[1] Competence by Design (CBD)
[2] Milestones at each stage describe terminal competencies

© 2015 Royal College of Physicians and Surgeons of Canada

3. Preparing to *teach* and *assess* the CanMEDS Roles

As a medical educator, you are extremely busy. You, your colleagues, and your trainees all feel pressure to meet multiple demands. It can be a struggle to get everything done and to do everything well. The *CanMEDS Tools Guide* acknowledges this reality by providing you with practical, ready-to-use information and tools to help make your job as a Residency educator easier.

To maximize the utility of these tools you will need to:

- clarify the teaching and assessment goals of your specific context,
- select the right tools to match the particular needs and goals of your specific context and
- combine Roles and tools in an effective and efficient manner.

To start we'd like to make a few key points about the teaching and assessment of CanMEDS.

CanMEDS should be integrated into the workplace

A misconception that may be adding unnecessarily to your workload, is the idea that the CanMEDS Roles must be taught in addition to all of the other important content of the discipline. In fact, you do not need to find extra time to teach and assess the CanMEDS Intrinsic Roles if you incorporate it into everyday practice. As much as possible, the learning, teaching, and assessment of the core skills and competencies of the CanMEDS Roles need to be part of everyday resident work.

Of course, you need to dedicate some teaching time to the foundational concepts and skills for the CanMEDS Roles, perhaps by way of academic half-days or journal clubs, for example. However, as learners become more accomplished in, and comfortable with the various CanMEDS Roles, you can begin to leverage a typical patient-care or other practice experience to teach or assess multiple CanMEDS Roles and competencies at once.

A work-based approach is an efficient way to incorporate CanMEDS into your teaching and assessment activities and does not generally require extra time. You're providing the care anyway: the key difference is that you're using it as an opportunity to teach or assess your learners' competence.

Assessing the CanMEDS Roles is not as hard as you might think

There is a widespread misconception that the Royal College expects faculty to assess all seven of the CanMEDS Roles in every assessment activity. You do not need to teach and assess each of the CanMEDS Roles all of the time.

In fact, you won't always be able to judge a learner's competence in all of the Roles based on a single encounter or assessment. For this reason, you'll need to develop a program of assessment that relies on multiple assessment tools and strategies to assess the different competencies in the CanMEDS Framework. Over time, as you collect data informed by multiple tools, multiple circumstances and multiple observers, you will eventually compile an integrated summary of assessment of the learner's competence across all domains of the CanMEDS Framework.

The overall monitoring of the learners' progression towards competence requires sampling throughout residency (e.g. different clinical settings or work locations, different types of patients and clinical problems, different times in residency) and should be informed by multiple assessment tools and a variety of assessors.

Assessments of learning should be complemented by assessments designed for learning

The idea that high-stakes assessments, such as a final exam are the ultimate measure of competence is a long standing misconception. In a competency-based medical education system, frequent assessments, coaching and feedback are important tools to improving competence.

As a teacher, your job is to help your residents learn. While learning has been associated most with teaching, there is a growing trend toward seeing assessment as a valuable tool for learning.

The results of individual assessments can be extremely helpful when shared with the learner in a way that can guide the learner toward further improvement in a specific area. This concept is known as assessment for learning and it is becoming increasingly popular in medical education.

Getting started...

The success of the residency education system relies on the leadership, teaching, and assessment skills of program directors and clinical supervisors like never before. The *CanMEDS Teaching and Assessment Tools Guide* is the first part of a comprehensive plan to support program directors and clinical supervisors in new ways. The future competence of 21st century physicians depends on it.

© 2015 Royal College of Physicians and Surgeons of Canada

References

1. Frank JR, Snell L, ten Cate O, Holmboe ES, Carraccio C, Swing SR, Harris P, Glasgow NJ, Campbell C, Dath D, Harden RM, Iobst W, Long DM, Mungroo R, Richardson DL, Sherbino J, Silver I, Taber S, Talbot M, Harris KA. Competency-based medical education: theory to practice. *Med Teach.* 2010;32(8):638-45.

2. Glover Takahashi S, Martin D, Richardson D. *The CanMEDS Toolkit for Teaching and Assessing the Collaborator Role.* Ottawa: Royal College of Physicians and Surgeons of Canada; 2012.

3. Adapted from Karpinski J's March 27, 2015 webinar entitled Milestones and EPAs in the Royal College CBD Model. http://www.royalcollege.ca/portal/page/portal/rc/resources/cbme/resources/videos_webinars Last retrieved July 31, 2015.

4. canmeds.royalcollege.ca

5. Frank JR, Snell L, Sherbino J, editors. *CanMEDS 2015 Physician Competency Framework.* Ottawa: Royal College of Physicians and Surgeons of Canada; 2015.

© 2015 Royal College of Physicians and Surgeons of Canada

© 2015 Royal College of Physicians and Surgeons of Canada

Assess
Expertise
Therapy MANAGEMENT PLAN
Medical knowledge
DELIBERATE DIAGNOSE
PRACTICE
Clinical skills Best practices
MEDICAL EXPERT
Diagnostic COGNITIVE LOAD
interventions PLAN
Clinical PATIENT-CENTRED CARE
decision-making
HIGH-QUALITY CARE
Help-seeking

Farhan Bhanji

Kenneth Harris

Mark Goldszmidt

Susan Glover Takahashi

Medical Expert

1. Why the Medical Expert Role matters

Medical Expert is the Role that is home to a physician's core clinical expertise. To practise medicine in an expert fashion the clinician must incorporate all of the CanMEDS Roles effectively into his or her professional practice.

As Medical Experts, physicians must be able to collect and interpret clinical information, make appropriate decisions related to clinical care, and carry out diagnostic and therapeutic interventions as required. Effective clinicians integrate the competencies of the Intrinsic CanMEDS Roles as they use their medical knowledge, clinical skills, and professional attitudes to deliver high-quality patient- and family-centred care. The care that physicians provide must be ethical, reflect current best practice, be conducted in partnership with other health care providers, and allocate finite health care resources in an appropriate manner.

When introducing learners to the Medical Expert Role, you may find it helpful to convey these important points:

- Although Medical Expert is one of seven roles in the CanMEDS Framework, it is central to a physician's competence and identity. Medical expertise is one of the main reasons patients come to physicians for care, and essential to physicians' role in society.

- Although the Medical Expert Role is at the centre of medical practice, it is important to note that the competencies of the Role are necessary but not, by themselves, sufficient for the practice of patient-centred care in the 21st century. Medical expertise must be integrated with and incorporate the Intrinsic Roles to optimize patient care.

2. What the Medical Expert Role looks like in daily practice

The Medical Expert Role is perhaps the defining role of physicians. It helps distinguish the work of physicians from that of other colleagues in the health care professions. The ability to integrate the competencies of the Intrinsic Roles while drawing on their individual and specialty specific medical expertise is unique to physicians and the Medical Expert Role.

The Medical Expert competencies allow physicians to appropriately assess, diagnose, and treat patients; to incorporate new medical knowledge and skills into their practice; and to recognize their own limitations. Medical Expert is integral to being a competent specialist and helps focus the physician's work in health care. In Medical Expert, physicians use their specialized skills within the context of generalist medical skills and considering the needs of the **whole** patient.

What Is Uniquely MEDICAL EXPERT?

For many physicians, Medical Expert is the embodiment of their specialized medical knowledge, clinical skills, and professional values used in their provision of high-quality and safe patient-centred care.

In contemporary health care, there are overlapping scopes of practice among specialist physicians, family physicians, and other colleagues in the health care professions. There are also important unique features of professional groups that are meaningful and contribute significantly to patient care. The uniqueness of each group (e.g. profession, specialty, certification) needs to be clearly communicated to your learners as well as to colleagues both inter and intraprofessionally with regard to the what, when, where, why and how your unique expertise helps collaboratively solve and resolve complicated and complex patient problems.

In this Tools Guide you will find a series of trigger words to help orient your learners to each of the CanMEDS Roles (See Table ME-1). These have been included to help your learners orient their daily activities to the specific CanMEDS Roles. Below you will find a list of common actions or processes and topics or content areas related to the Medical Expert Role.

Table ME-2 illustrates how different health care professions that have built their competency frameworks based on CanMEDS have created clarity about the unique aspects to their professional expertise.

TABLE ME-1. TRIGGER WORDS RELATING TO THE PROCESS AND CONTENT OF MEDICAL EXPERT

Trigger words relating to the PROCESS of Medical Expert:	Trigger words relating to the CONTENT of Medical Expert:	
- Assess - Clinical decision-making - Diagnose - Plan - Quality improvement - Treat	- Best practices - Clinical practice - Clinical skills - Diagnostic interventions - High-quality care - Management plan - Medical knowledge	- Patient-centred care - Patient safety at the individual patient level - Professional values - Scope of practice - Therapy

© 2015 Royal College of Physicians and Surgeons of Canada

TABLE ME-2. CENTRAL INTEGRATING ROLE IN THREE HEALTH PROFESSIONS COMPETENCY FRAMEWORKS BASED ON CANMEDS

Health Profession	Title of their central integrating role	Definition of central integrating role
Occupational Therapist[1]	Expert in Enabling Occupation	• Expert in Enabling Occupation is the central role, expertise, and competence of the occupational therapist. • As an Expert in Enabling Occupation, occupational therapists use evidence-based processes that focus on a client's occupations—including self-care, productive pursuits, and leisure—as a medium for action and outcome. • Clients include individuals, families, groups, communities, populations, or organizations.
Physical Therapist[2]	Expert In Function And Mobility	• As experts in function and mobility, physiotherapists integrate all of the Physiotherapist Roles to lead in the promotion, improvement, and maintenance of the mobility, health, and well-being of Canadians.
Physician	Medical Expert	• As Medical Experts, physicians integrate all of the CanMEDS Roles, applying medical knowledge, clinical skills, and professional values in their provision of high-quality and safe patient-centred care. • Medical Expert is the central physician Role in the CanMEDS Framework and defines the physician's clinical scope of practice.

Excerpt from the CanMEDS 2015 Physician Competency Framework[a]

DEFINITION

As Medical Experts, physicians integrate all of the CanMEDS Roles, applying medical knowledge, clinical skills, and professional values in their provision of high-quality and safe patient-centred care. Medical Expert is the central physician Role in the CanMEDS Framework and defines the physician's clinical scope of practice.

DESCRIPTION

As Medical Experts who provide high-quality, safe, patient-centred care, physicians draw upon an evolving body of knowledge, their clinical skills, and their professional values. They collect and interpret information, make clinical decisions, and carry out diagnostic and therapeutic interventions. They do so within their scope of practice and with an understanding of the limits of their expertise. Their decision-making is informed by best practices and research evidence, and takes into account the patient's circumstances and preferences as well as the availability of resources. Their

clinical practice is up-to-date, ethical, and resource-efficient, and is conducted in collaboration with patients and their families,[b] other health care professionals, and the community. The Medical Expert Role is central to the function of physicians and draws on the competencies included in the Intrinsic Roles (Communicator, Collaborator, Leader, Health Advocate, Scholar, and Professional).

KEY COMPETENCIES

Physicians are able to:

1. Practise medicine within their defined scope of practice and expertise

2. Perform a patient-centred clinical assessment and establish a management plan

3. Plan and perform procedures and therapies for the purpose of assessment and/or management

4. Establish plans for ongoing care and, when appropriate, timely consultation

5. Actively contribute, as an individual and as a member of a team providing care, to the continuous improvement of health care quality and patient safety

a Bhanji F, Lawrence K, Goldszmidt M, Walton M, Harris K, Creery D, Sherbino J, Ste-Marie L-G, Stang A. Medical Expert. In: Frank JR, Snell L, Sherbino J, editors. *CanMEDS 2015 Physician Competency Framework*. Ottawa: Royal College of Physicians and Surgeons of Canada; 2015. Reproduced with permission.
b Throughout the CanMEDS 2015 Physician Competency Framework and Milestones Guide, references to the patient's family are intended to include all those who are personally significant to the patient and are concerned with his or her care, including, according to the patient's circumstances, family members, partners, caregivers, legal guardians, and substitute decision-makers.

KEY TERMS OF THE MEDICAL EXPERT ROLE

Expertise means the special skills or knowledge possessed by an individual.[3] The Dreyfus Model outlines five stages of expertise development: novice, advanced beginner, competent, proficient, expert.[4] There are a variety of domains of expertise:

- **Cognitive** means those skills pertaining to the mental processes of comprehension, judgment, memory, and reasoning, as contrasted with emotional and volitional processes.[5] Includes mental processes that are factual, conceptual and procedural.

- **Psychomotor skills** means those skills pertaining to the psychological processes associated with muscular movement and to the production of voluntary movements.

- **Visual perceptual processing**[6] is a group of discrete yet interrelated skills including visual discrimination, visual memory, visual sequential memory, visual form constancy, visual spatial relationships, and visual-motor integration.

- **Metacognitive**[7] means those skills pertaining to a knowledge about one's abilities, the demands of given tasks, and potentially effective learning strategies; it involves self-regulation via planning, predicting, monitoring, regulating, evaluating, and revising strategies.

- **Non-cognitive skills**[8] (or metacognitive learning skills) means those skills that have been related to successful performance persistence, self-control, curiosity, conscientiousness, grit and self-confidence.

Cognitive load refers to mental processing demands that a person can manage. When the mental processing demands exceed what the person can manage, performance is degraded or deteriorates resulting in errors and mistakes.[9]

Deliberate practice means repeated and purposeful effort to improve performance in a specific domain.[10] The amount of time someone spends in deliberate practice is what predicts expertise and continued learning in a given field. To develop expertise, learners need to invest considerable practice time and purposeful effort towards a reasonable yet appropriately challenging, goal (i.e. a goal that is neither too hard, nor too easy).[9]

Help-seeking is an active process between the learner, teacher and context. Help-seeking is self-regulating and a proactive learning strategy to help the learner achieve success and develop expertise.[11]

Scope of practice is a term that describes the clinical and non-clinical professional roles, responsibilities, activities, interests and competencies of a health-care practitioner. It is initially established by the successful completion of form education requirements and evolves in response to multiple personal and practice factors, including changing patient population needs. Scope of practice is foundational to the development and implementation of lifelong learning plans and contributes to processes and regulations related to licensure and privileging decisions.[12]

A *patient-centred* approach is one "providing care that is respectful of and responsive to individual patient preferences, needs, and values.[13] In day-to-day practice, physicians find common ground with their patients about the patient's problems, priorities and goals. Patient-centredness (i.e. the physician–patient relationship) is one of the four levels of relationships in a relationship-centred practice, which is described in more detail in the Collaborator Chapter of this Tools Guide.

An *encounter* is a purposeful patient-physician interaction.

Plain language is the use of common words that a patient can easily understand. This may mean avoiding technical or medical terms unless they are carefully defined or described.

Shared decision-making[14] is an important component of communication when patients and their health care professionals, including the physician, make decisions about the best course of action. These shared decisions are informed by the patient's preferences, needs, and values as well as by the available options and evidence, which are often conveyed by the health care professional. Shared decision-making involves patients to the degree that they wish; it allows patients to understand the decision-making process, and it increases patients' commitment to the plans.

© 2015 Royal College of Physicians and Surgeons of Canada

3. Preparing to teach the Medical Expert Role

In this section we help you prepare to teach Medical Expert by addressing some fundamental aspects of the Role.

3.1 Common misconceptions to address with learners

There are four misconceptions about the Medical Expert Role that you may want to address with your learners.

First, your learners may be inclined to define your specialty by the tools, therapeutics and technical acts associated with your specialty. Help reframe their thinking by reminding them that **patients care about what your specialty knows and how that knowledge contributes to addressing their needs**.

Another misconception associated with the Medical Expert Role is the idea that the physician's role is to "tell patients what to do". You may need to help your learners understand that the Medical Expert Role is deeply rooted in a patient-centred approach to care. **The type of patient-physician relationship should be defined by the patient's preferences and will always be respectful and responsive** to individual patient preferences, needs and values.

Some of your learners, and even some patients, may believe incorrectly that health care decisions are straightforward or dichotomous. It's important that we reframe their thinking to help them appreciate that it is much more complex. The truth is that most of the time the answer to many health care situations falls into a grey category of 'it depends'. **There are no simple answers to complex problems and becoming comfortable with uncertainty is an important part of the Medical Expert Role.**

Finally, one of the most common and divisive misconceptions is that the CanMEDS Intrinsic Roles are secondary to Medical Expert. It is important that your program's explicit and implicit curriculum help your learners understand that **a competent physician seamlessly integrates the competencies of all seven CanMEDS Roles.**

3.2 Patient-centred care – breaking it down for learners

Patient-centredness means being respectful to a patient – even when a patient or their family challenges the physician's skills. It means being responsive to individual patient preferences, needs and values even when those preferences, needs and values are different from those of the physician. It also means effectively sharing other perspectives with patients and their family.

Your learners should not equate the concept of patient-centredness with doing whatever the patient asks. Your learners will have patients whose expectations are inconsistent with care guidelines and/or with the learner's own beliefs. Your role is to help your learners work with their patients to build rapport, trust and common ground, so that the patient and care team can wisely plan the best action(s).

Help your residents understand that they will need to work with the patient to define the parameters of their patient-physician relationship. Table ME-3 below describes four different types of patient-physician relationships: informative, interpretive, deliberative and paternalistic.[15] It is important to underscore that the style of patient-physician relationship should be influenced by patient preferences and context as well as the physician's values.

You can help your learners by describing your own experiences with physician-patient relationships, in particular, times when you have taken on a deliberative relationship. You may also want to describe to them the types of relationships your patients typically prefer, which may or may not be related to your specialty. While informative and interpretive relationships are likely to be the most common physician-patient relationships, your learners will benefit from understanding what rare circumstances might warrant the physician to be more paternalistic as well as, what the variations in relationships are and when or where to move from informer, to counselor, to teacher roles.

3.3 Help others understand expertise and types of expertise in specialties

Health professions are 'tribal' in the sense that they have their own language, culture, ways of thinking about patient problems, and different skills and abilities. While each specialty group and subspecialty group has its own scope of practice, educational requirements and competencies, all physicians should still think of the whole patient.

Each specialty or subspecialty has a specific scope of practice including ways of thinking about patient problems, uniqueness via its minimal educational requirements, requisite specialist competencies and requirements for maintenance of specialist competence.

There are several key domains of expertise including; cognitive, psychomotor skills, visual perceptual processing, metacognitive and non-cognitive (or metacognitive learning skills).

TABLE ME-3. TYPES OF PATIENT-PHYSICIAN RELATIONSHIPS

Type[15]	Description	Physician approach	Patient approach	Example
Paternalistic	Patient wants the physician to provide significant direction, guidance or decisions on diagnostic and therapeutic interventions, risks and benefits in the clinical situation.	• Parent. • Authoritative and in control of information and situation.	Patient is passive and trusts physician to make decisions in their best interests and on their behalf.	Physician provides selected information and suggestions about treatment/care options. Physician presents information that encourages patient to consent to the intervention(s) that the physician views as best. *"I think you should…"*
Informative	Patient wants the information and medical expertise provided in a factual manner including possible diagnostic and therapeutic interventions, risks and benefits in the clinical situation.	• Informant. • Technical, rationale expert.	Patient consumes medical information making choices based on factual information provided.	Physician provides the facts about medical condition(s), options and plan. Patient asks questions about choices and then makes the decision(s). *"The options are…"*
Interpretative	Patient wants physician to help clarify values, needs and goals to inform the selection of diagnostic and therapeutic interventions, risk and benefits that meet those values, needs and goals in the clinical situation.	• Counselor. • Engaged, shared decision-making	Patient is knowledgeable about own wants and needs and communicates these expectations. Works with physician in selection of choices.	Physician explores patients' values, needs and goals to then offer diagnostic and therapeutic interventions that meet those values, needs and goals. *"How the options connect to your goals are…"*
Deliberative	Patient wants the physician to help clarify health-related values, clarify the issues arising from the various options for diagnostic and therapeutic interventions, risks and benefits in the clinical situation.	• Teacher or Coach	Patient engaged in dialogue and empowered to follow unexamined preferences or examined values.	Physician and patient explore values, needs and goals. Physician and patient dialogue about alternative health-related values including applicability and implications in the clinical situation. *"Have you considered that your goals might mean that…"*

The relative importance and attention of each of these areas of expertise varies, depending on clinical context, differing patient problems, and specialties:

- Examples of when problem solving cognitive skills are very important in practice are: selecting when, where and how to do a procedure; interpreting results or studies; treatment planning, triaging patient lists.

- Examples of when psychomotor skills are very important in practice are: physical maneuvers during assessments; completing procedures; processing laboratory samples.

- Examples of when visual perceptual processing skills are very important in practice are: interpreting radiologic studies; observing patient symptoms such as pallor, pain response, indrawing; diagnosing laboratory results;

monitoring patient progress during anesthesia; managing surgical field during procedure.

- Examples of when metacognitive skills are very important in practice are: mental rehearsal and planning for patient care; analysis of daily practice outcomes; considering options and priorities for action or improvement.

- Examples of when non-cognitive skills that are very important in practice are: awareness of limits, enthusiasm for improvement, tolerance of delays or frustrations, persistence through difficulty.

Help your learners understand which domains are emphasized in your specialty as well as, how the other less emphasized domains are also relevant to your specialty.

© 2015 Royal College of Physicians and Surgeons of Canada

3.4 Introduce learners to the value of deliberate practice

Doing more of the same does not improve practice or develop expertise. This is a well-researched area, and you may or may not be surprised that time on task alone does not develop expertise. For your learners this means they need to understand that to be present and engaged both physically and intellectually is key to becoming a Medical Expert.

The term 'deliberate practice' relates to the conditions necessary to reach high levels of performances.

Deliberate practice is more likely when individuals are:

1. given a specific task or activity with a well-defined goal that builds on pre-existing knowledge or skills,

2. motivated to improve,

3. provided with timely, specific feedback,

4. provided with ample opportunities for repetition, and

5. gradual refinements of their performance.[10]

Deliberate practice requires effort and determination and needs to be internally driven by each of your residents.

Help your learners develop habits associated with deliberate practice, which include:

- Using mental rehearsal to plan an encounter, procedure and clinical activity. Mental rehearsal includes working through both the 'usual' steps and sequence and also the mental rehearsal related to reviewing, preparing and anticipating the 'what if' related to alternate scenarios.

- Focused, specific practice of 'parts' of a challenging or personally troublesome aspect of practice. Perhaps your learner has a specifically troublesome aspect of an operation, procedure, activity to master to become efficient or effective. Learners need to be reminded that generally avoiding what we aren't good at catches up. They need to 'lean in' to the practice required to improve performance. Getting focused coaching and feedback from your faculty will be important to your residents' improvement. Acting on the coaching and feedback your residents get is equally important to their improvements.

- Reflection (with or without assistance) following an encounter. Compare what happened with the mental rehearsal. What are you pleased with? Were there any surprises? What is the follow up? What needs to be improved on 'next'?

- Watch others. Even when observing, notice "tricks" and techniques that others do.

For teachers, the concept of deliberate pracitce underscores the need to tailor instruction, feedback and coaching to individual learners' needs. Teachers need to remember to:

- Start with an accurate assessment of the learners' knowledge.

- Set specific goals for each session or learning activity.[9] Teachers can help by setting goals for performance at a reasonable and productive level of challenge.

- Help learners focus on what they need to learn rather than what they already know or may be more comfortable doing.

- Provide structure and support by using a variety of 'scaffolding' strategies. For example, teachers can use simulation, focused reading, group discussions, providing worked examples or cases, completing case reports. These strategies help learners practice specific skills at an appropriate level of challenge.

- Share the load of instruction, feedback and coaching by encouraging learners to seek assistance from another person or group (i.e. more senior learners, co-resident, other team members).

A caution about developing a culture of deliberative practice. For learners to take responsibilty for learning and to be comfortable identifying areas that need development requires that they feel supported in the process (i.e. that the teacher has their best interests at heart). Learners need to know and trust that in revealing 'deficiency' (either themselves or through direct observation by others) is viewed by all as an opportunity for coaching and improvement.

3.5 Bring learning to the "bedside"

There is an increasing emphasis on workplace-based education and practice and your new residents may need orientation to their dual role as both learners and workers.[16] Medical Expert competencies are typically developed in a work-based setting, which is sometimes simulated but mostly real. To avoid developing a culture and habit of being passive observers whose experiences are mostly taught or told, your learners need to avoid spending too much time in classrooms watching PowerPoints™. They need to understand that while learning happens in classrooms and labs, which they are accustomed to, now they must learn through and at work.

For your learners this means they need to assume ownership and responsibility for patients and for their learning. For some, this means accepting that part of work is just work.

© 2015 Royal College of Physicians and Surgeons of Canada

Work is not always new and exciting. Efficiency and routine are the realities of work and need to be understood and embraced. Help your learners to accept the routine aspects of clinical practice, but also to be inquisitive about the routine and watch for what can be learned or consolidated.

Remind your learners that as they learn in the workplace, they will also learn about the variety of workplaces. Your learners will encounter a variety of teacher styles and will also see that each of the practice contexts operate differently. Some of the practice context differences are concrete (e.g. drug formulary, electronic medical record system), while others are more subtle, such as the variety of styles of supervisors, culture of the team, approach to communication, and collaboration.

Your learners should not be 'surprised' when they move from one context to the next and notice differences. Anticipating variations and managing the difference is important to their functioning in the workplace.

Another part of learning in and from the workplace is to notice all of the work that is both related to patient care and supporting patient care. As such, it is important to alert your learners to both the reality of the considerable 'backstage' work that is done to prepare for a smoother clinical day (e.g. reviewing clinic lists and charts in advance, inventorying and hunting down test results to ensure efficient patient encounter, following up with the family physician or health professional collaborator to clarify issues and plans, mental rehearsal before procedures, and talking to patient family members).

As your learners progress towards completion of training, you should include all or most 'backstage' work to their role. This will build their metacognitive skills as they sort through the messiness of real practice. Remember to provide coaching for what is included on the 'to do' list of backstage work as well as, suggestions for improving their efficiency or effectiveness.

In day-to-day work, remind your learners to develop the habit of 'paying attention'. Again, reflection and review of how things might be done differently to improve satisfaction, efficiency or effectiveness are habits of paying attention and learning from work. With many different patients, patient problems, and team members concurrently interacting in the workplace to consider, if your residents are cued to what to pay attention to in the routine of daily practice, their observations can inform their mental rehearsal as well as improve their medical expertise. The key to learning from work is 'ownership' and attempts to learn from all patient cases, even the routine.

3.6 Encourage learners to attend to patient safety in daily practice

Establishing a safe working and learning environment is essential for your learners. Alert them to some of the safety issues that are likely to arise as well as who, where and how to get assistance to ensure patient safety and personal safety. Safety drills should be practices[d] for any high risk situation (e.g. radioactive or highly infectious agent is spilled) or potentially frequent situation (e.g. patient fall, aggressive patient).

It is equally important that your learners understand the implication of rushing through and/or resenting the routine parts of practice, which can negatively impact patients and patient care quality. For example, in the anticipation of doing a new procedure, the 'routine' lab results that are not carefully reviewed can have very real consequences to patients. Do not underestimate how much your residents will benefit from observing how you care for your patients.

Your residents need to learn to address concerns in a timely diplomatic and acceptable manner. Knowing who and how to report or manage patient safety issues is essential. (More detailed information about patient safety concepts, teaching and assessing patients is found in Leader Role.)

3.7 Introduce the concept of progression of competence

Within "expertise theory", time spent on task is an essential ingredient. In order to master a domain, time must be spent learning and in deliberate practice. The Royal College's approach to competency-based medical education (CBME) does not discount the valuable time spent in training (as would a pure, time-free, competency-based model). Instead, the Royal College will implement a hybrid competency-based system, called Competence by Design (CBD).

The new system will re-conceptualize time as a resource – not a limitation. Within the new model, residents will have the ability to achieve competencies (measured by milestones) at their own rate. Learners will have the same access as they do now to patient-level experiences. What will be improved is the structure. Milestones will be layered onto the experiences to provide learners with a clear path of learning goals. Learners will know what they need to learn and achieve at each stage, and the instructors will know what they need to observe and assess.

© 2015 Royal College of Physicians and Surgeons of Canada

Over the course of residency, learners gradually develop their medical expertise. During that time, they need to know the limits of their expertise and work within those limits. While acquiring medical expertise, your learners manage their work somewhat like a balancing act — they start by moving out into new practice areas with as much supervision and support as required, and as they become more competent over time, they will operate with greater autonomy.

It is important to help your learners practise within the limits of their expertise while they safely continue to expand their areas and depth of competence. Remember that a learner's cognitive load will be different than a teacher's, so set your expectations accordingly. Consider the factors which impact a persons' ability to manage the cognitive load[9]:

- type of task (e.g. simple vs. complex)
- number of concurrent tasks (e.g. distractions, multi-tasking)
- level of experience or previous practice with the task(s). When someone is more confident with a task the cognitive load is 'lighter'.

There are several approaches you can introduce that may help learners manage cognitive load as they learn to perform complex tasks. You can:

- encourage learners to focus on one skill at a time before asking them to integrate multiple skills,

- provide learners with worked examples and samples interspersed with problems to solve on their own,
- distinguish between the steps that are key and those that are secondary to skill development when teaching new skills,
- help learners set priorities including reasonable time for skill development, and
- remind learners to avoid distractions and interruptions when developing new skills.

Early in their training, learners are developing the Medical Expert knowledge, skills, and abilities that are required to be competent in the most common or frequent work scenarios with patients, teams, and systems. Over time, they develop their expertise and their competence becomes more sophisticated in a wider range of scenarios. As a teacher, you need to be aware of where your learners sit on this competence continuum, so that you can help them progress to the next levels (see Table ME-4). The new Royal College Competence by Design training model uses competency "milestones" and specialty specific tasks or Entrustable Professional Activities (EPAs) to help reduce some of the guess work involved for residents and faculty today.

Table ME-5 presents examples of the Medical Expert Role in day-to-day practice scenarios at two points in the Medical Expert competence continuum and illustrates the progression of Medical Expert from earlier to later in residency.

TABLE ME-4. FIVE STAGES OF THE LEARNER ON THE MEDICAL EXPERT COMPETENCE CONTINUUM

Requirements for residency	Transition to discipline	Foundations of discipline	Core of discipline	Transition to practice
Is oriented to residency and to the inventory of knowledge and skills	Has an awareness of and can act on key parts of high-volume routine cases, common situations, and straightforward problems	Handles high-volume routine cases, common situations, and straightforward problems on their own; has an awareness of complicated situations and problems. Recognizes co-morbidities that impact patient care	Handles with efficiency high-volume routine cases, common situations, and straightforward problems on their own; acts on complicated situations and problems with support. Manages co-morbidities that impact patient care. Prioritizes with increasing efficiency	Handles complex and complicated situations and problems on their own, and guides or supports others. Manages with various concurrent priorities. Develops judgment/wisdom to decide between various courses of action

TABLE ME-5. EXAMPLES OF MEDICAL EXPERT ACTIVITIES AT TWO POINTS IN THE MEDICAL EXPERT COMPETENCE CONTINUUM

Day-to-day practice scenario	Common situation and straightforward problem (i.e. earlier Medical Expert activity)	Complex or complicated problem (i.e. more developed Medical Expert activity)
Case report from learner to faculty	Learner gives a top-line summary of the patient history, inventory of problems, and planned treatment in a standard format to a faculty member who is a supportive teacher.	The blood work report that the learner requires to prepare an accurate treatment plan was delayed in being posted, and the learner, busy managing other patient priorities, did not discover this in sufficient time before case rounds to be able to hunt down the results with a phone call.
Rounds	Learner participates in teaching rounds with own team and on a topic with which the learner is quite familiar.	Learner presents a balanced overview of the literature and makes recommendations based on current best practice.
Phone consultation	Learner holds a conversation with the referring primary care physician about needed community follow-up.	Learner calls the referring specialist in another community to report that the requested intervention is not available for the patient (e.g. because of staff or equipment shortages resulting in backlogs). The learner then problem-solves with the referring specialist about alternatives to the requested intervention.
Goals of care	Learner meets with a patient and one family member before surgery to discuss elective surgical options.	Learner holds a post-operative meeting with a patient and three family members, all of whom have a limited comprehension of English and/or French, to review a serious pathology report and plan for identified further treatment with the assistance of a translator.

TABLE ME-6. HELP-SEEKING BARRIERS AND STRATEGIES[17, c]

Steps	Barriers	Strategies
1. Culture of Safety	• Asking for help is viewed as weakness • Help is not available	• Expectation that learners ask for help and that help is given without judgment • Supervision framed as teaching strategy • Faculty and senior residents model
2. Recognition of Need	• Lack of knowledge • Limitations of self-assessment	• Protocols for supervision • Direct observation as educational strategy • Interprofessional team encouraged to identify if help needed and share in problem solving
3. Willingness to Ask	• Independence valued instead of autonomy • Threats to credibility	• Teaching adaptive help seeking strategies • Learner assessment to include "asks for help appropriately"
4. Skills to asking for Help	• Does not recognize the need for help • Embarrassed to ask for help • No experience asking for help	• Practising "I don't' know" • Coaching to encourage improvement • Be clear, concise, deliberate in what you are asking for
5. Accessibility of Help	• Availability of teacher – physical proximity and timing of need • Approachability of teacher	• Establishing expectations for communication • Deliberate increase in number of interactions with learner • Teacher assessment

c Han Ra, Kim VH-D. *Setting a Climate for Help-Seeking in Postgraduate Medical Education: a Theoretical Framework for Understanding Barriers and Strategies for Successful Help-Seeking.* University of Toronto. 2015. Unpublished manuscript. Adapted with permission.

© 2015 Royal College of Physicians and Surgeons of Canada

3.8 Help learners see when CanMEDS Roles are being integrated

Experienced physicians appear to seamlessly weave together the different competencies embodied in the CanMEDS Framework. They make it look easy. In essence, it becomes second nature for them to use competencies from several CanMEDS Roles at the same time.

Your learners, however, will not have that same skill or skill level at the start. They will benefit from teachers who explicitly identify the competencies involved in various cases. By taking the time to deconstruct a common scenario and point out important competencies embedded within the scenario, you will help the learner more easily appreciate the complexity of the learning experience and take more away from it.

Many teachers become overwhelmed with the idea of needing to teach and assess all seven Roles. Remember that not all roles need to be taught all the time. **A rule of thumb is that when discussing Medical Expert related to a particular scenario, make connections with one or two Intrinsic Roles.** For example, in the course of a patient encounter or case study, besides Medical Expert, you could talk about one or two other roles such as:

- **Communicator Role**
  - help their patients translate and understand complex medical information and navigate the health care journey to achieve health and wellness goals.

- **Collaborator Role**
  - embrace the diversity of team members' views, and effectively engage their physician colleagues and other health care professionals in the care of their patients.

- **Health Advocate Role**
  - support patient health by incorporating relevant and appropriate health promotion, illness/injury prevention, and health surveillance into each encounter with a patient.

- **Leader Role**
  - act as resource stewards and engage in conversations with patients and colleagues to choose wisely[18] to avoid unnecessary tests, treatments, and procedures, and support effective operations, patient safety, and quality improvement of health care delivery.

- **Scholar Role**
  - take an active approach and develop a personal plan to keep up to date with current research, teach learner colleagues about a treatment plan and the reasons behind it, and enhance their knowledge and skills, both in areas that interest them and in areas where they know they are weak.

- **Professional Role**
  - manage the ethical issues arising in patient care, and prioritize professional duties and personal responsibilities when faced with multiple patients and problems.

With training and experience, your learners will be able to purposefully integrate multiple CanMEDS Roles concurrently.

3.9 Create a help-seeking/help-giving environment in your program

Learning in the workplace is best when the culture equates work with learning. Good teachers acknowledge that we are all learning every day; sometimes celebrating success and progress while at other times learning from our mistakes and from what did not go well.

Your learners undergo training in their specialty, which involves providing patient care under supervision of qualified teachers across a series of clinical placements. During this time, teachers and learners cope with a tension between adequate supervision and learner autonomy. Supervision is necessary to promote professional development and ensure quality care and patient safety. Over the course of their residency, learners are given graded responsibility and autonomy in patient care.

When should learners ask for help? You and your teachers need to create an environment where learners will ask for help when they need it.

Help-seeking[17] requires (See Table ME-6):

1. culture of safety for the learners

2. recognition of need for help by the learners

3. willingness to seek help by the learners

4. language for asking for help by the learners

5. the accessibility of help for the learners

© 2015 Royal College of Physicians and Surgeons of Canada

A crucial step in the process of help-seeking is the resident's willingness to ask for help once the need for help is recognized. This involves weighing the costs and benefits of help-seeking. However, asking for help can be difficult for the resident[19] given the high value on independence, concern about his or her credibility, effects on evaluation, and not wanting to be embarrassed in front of peers.[20] Factors such as stress, social difficulties, and depression may also affect the decision to ask for help[21] and underperformers have shown the biggest resistance to ask for help.[11]

Strategies to improve help-seeking behaviours include, addressing the medical culture and educating the resident. It is important to explicitly let the residents know that it is an accepted expectation to ask for help and that asking for help does not equate to being incompetent. Dr. Pencheon, a public health doctor, views "I don't know" as the three most important words in education[22]. You and your teachers can model this by demonstrating help-seeking behaviour. Senior residents should also be instructed about the benefits of accepting and expecting help-seeking behaviour from junior residents. It should be emphasized that the goal of training is not necessarily independent practice, but autonomous practice.

Independent practice threatens the development of competencies such as teamwork, help-seeking and collaboration[23]. You are preparing your learners for unsupervised practice, in which they interact with others rather than act independently. Autonomy and supervision can coexist. As your residents progress through training and demonstrate trustworthiness, the amount and style of supervision can be tailored, balancing patient needs. Entrustable professional activities can provide a framework for decisions about levels of supervision.[24]

4. Hints, tips and tools for *teaching* the Medical Expert Role

As a teacher your goal is to deliver the right content and in a way that helps your residents learn. A big part of your role as teacher is to support learners to take (and keep) control of their teaching and teaching plan. Sometimes you will teach directly. Other times you will facilitate and support the teaching of others. In all cases, you need to have a learning plan (e.g. why is this learner with you now? What are the key learning needs? What are the additional learner wants?).

There are parts of the Medical Expert Role that can be especially difficult for learners to relate to and understand in the context of their work. For this reason this section of the Tools Guide includes a short menu of tips and tricks that are highly effective for teaching the Medical Expert Role. You can treat the list as a buffet: pick and choose the tips that resonate most and that will work for you, your program and your learners.

Teaching Tip 1.
Integrate the Intrinsic Roles into your Medical Expert teaching

Medical expertise is at the core of specialist education and practice, and it often serves as the starting point for training individuals to become competent physicians. Given the primary and integrating position of the Medical Expert Role, there is a risk that attention to its competencies will crowd out work on skill development in the Intrinsic Roles. Sometimes others worry that there is too much to cover and that time spent on developing the competencies of the Intrinsic Roles diverts valuable time from teaching the Medical Expert Role.

As you work with your learners, don't think of your teaching time as being spent on either the Medical Expert Role or one of the Intrinsic Roles; rather, think about it being spent on the six Intrinsic Roles (i.e. Communicator, Collaborator, Leader, Health Advocate, Scholar, and Professional) through or with Medical Expert. For example, when you are faced with a challenging patient case that requires searching the literature, discuss your clinical reasoning (i.e. Medical Expert) with the learner; describe how and why you decided to do the search and whether you used primary research, systematic reviews, or another type of research (i.e. Scholar); and model how to incorporate that information into shared decision-making with the patient (i.e. Communicator). Explicit explanations of how the Intrinsic Roles influence your ability to function as a Medical Expert may help learners appreciate the importance of mastering all seven Roles.

Teaching Tip 2.
Establish a climate that supports help-seeking skills

There are a number of teaching strategies that can contribute to a culture of help-seeking behaviour including:

- Developing protocols that define the residents' scope of practice,

- Framing supervision as a learning strategy, and

- Including interdisciplinary team in feedback gathering.

© 2015 Royal College of Physicians and Surgeons of Canada

Protocols that define the learner's scope of practice can remove the reliance on judgment and uncertainty as to when the call for help should be made in specific contexts. For example, performing a neonatal resuscitation independently is beyond the expectations for an early-stage resident learner. A protocol could be developed that requires a senior resident or staff physician to be notified at the same time an early-level resident is called for a neonate in distress.

By framing supervision as a learning strategy, it is an opportunity for direct observation and specific feedback, rather than a loss of independence. For example, a resident with less experience might be permitted to start a neonatal resuscitation and perform to his/her abilities. The resident can request help if the need is identified, but as the supervising senior resident or staff has been called and is directly observing, they do not need to wait until the early-level resident recognizes the need before intervening as necessary.

Include interdisciplinary team in feedback gathering. Immediate patient care and future performance can be further refined through discussions with interdisciplinary team members who can provide additional points of view in assessing the need for help and feedback on performance. For example, the bedside nurse might recognize that the early level resident, who is normally quite competent in treating for a sick neonate, is overwhelmed in managing multiple sick patients. The culture of support could encourage the bedside nurse to communicate his/her concern to the entry level resident, and they could problem-solve solutions.

Teaching Tip 3.
Help your trainees learn during and from clinical care

Trainees learn during and from clinical care. Explore the key learning purposes, and your learners' interests and skills to identify opportunities for learners and supervisor to learn together. Set an agenda for what is on the 'watch', 'do', and 'don't' lists.

ONE-MINUTE PRECEPTOR[25, d]

The **one-minute preceptor** (OMP) model was developed to effectively and efficiently teach learners about teaching while simultaneously addressing patient needs. Teachers will need to practice, so this process can be done quickly and effectively in day to day practice.

STEPS to One Minute Preceptor.
1. Get a commitment
2. Probe for supporting evidence
3. Teach general rules
4. Reinforce what was done right
5. Correct mistakes and coach for improvement

This sequence fosters learner ownership of the clinical problem and allows you to identify gaps. Additionally, this approach encourages you and the learner to work together to plan for the patient.

More details
1. *Get a commitment*
   Ask an open ended question: "Tell me, what you think is going on"? "What are you considering for a treatment plan?" "What do you think our priorities are for this case?"

   - Here you are working with the learner to get them to commit to a diagnosis or treatment option

   - Avoid prompting or suggesting a diagnosis or treatment plan at this point

2. *Probe for supporting evidence*
   Ask specific questions that help clarify the thought processes and choices. "Why are you leaning to X and Y as your differentials? Did you think about alternative therapeutics? What sequence of diagnostic tests would you consider optimal?

   - Avoid asking 'text book questions'. Stay grounded in the case.

3. *Teach general rules*
   - Try to teach a 'rule of thumb' or key principle that guide and inform you in this/similar cases.

   - Point out how the principle can be applied in other cases.

4. *Reinforce what was done right*
   - Identify two or three things that were done well. Clarify what was on track.

   - Positive feedback is motivating to learners.

5. *Correct mistakes and coach for improvement*
   - Identify two or three things that need to be done differently.

   - Focus on the 'next' part of improving performance that is within their reach.

   - Offer specific concrete advice on how to improve.

---

d Adapted from Neher JO, Stevens NG. The one-minute preceptor: shaping the teaching conversation. *Fam Med.* 2003;35(6):391-3. Reproduced with permission.

Help your learners become skilled at observing themselves and others during clinical care, so they can be attentive to learning opportunities, understand when they are consolidating skills, and use clinical care experiences to develop new skills in themselves or in others. Help your learners appreciate what the workplace can offer them in learning new competencies, consolidating competencies that are already developed, and developing the comfort to use competencies independently. If a learner tends to focus only on new or novel cases, encourage him or her to embrace opportunities to actively learn from moments in their day-to-day practice and to recognize that each patient is unique and presents a new learning opportunity. The One Minute Preceptor is a teaching strategy that can be built into day-to-day teaching.

Although it may be necessary to teach your learners about medical expertise away from the clinical setting at times, consider the clinical setting to be the primary venue for instruction about this Role.

Teaching Tip 4.
Help your learners navigate from the common to the complex as they learn about your specialty

There are general principles of education even with advanced or "adult learners." Remember that your learners may need help to understand and apply the mountain of new, detailed medical information and clinical skills related to their specialty, the competencies, and the activities of day-to-day practice in their specialty, as well as when, how, where, and why to employ that information.

Use general principles of good learning and teaching as you help your learners move along the competence continuum as Medical Experts (see Table ME-5). The use of feedback and assessment for learning is key to developing medical expertise. (For more information on feedback and assessment, see the Leader Role.) Over the course of a rotation, a year, or a residency, learners acquire increasing responsibility with incremental expertise.

Teaching Tip 5.
Identify how ambiguity and uncertainty may influence practice and the value of patient input

Show your learners that they practise medicine in complex systems where decisions must be made and actions carried out in the face of uncertainty. Among many factors, they will need to weigh risks, patient preferences, resource availability, priorities, and their own capacity to care for patients.

Teach them to avoid the trap of thinking that information and evidence are by themselves solutions or that there is just one solution to a complex challenge. Instead, information and evidence need to be situated in the context and applied thoughtfully when making clinical decisions: "The practice of evidence-based medicine means integrating individual clinical expertise with the best available external clinical evidence from systematic research. By individual clinical expertise we mean the proficiency and judgment that individual clinicians acquire through clinical experience and clinical practice."[26] Information and evidence must also be applied in the context of patient's preferences, so that you respect their autonomy.

Prepare your learners to accept ambiguity and uncertainty as part of everyday work and to be aware if uncertainty is negatively impacting patient care. For example, discomfort with ambiguity can lead to tests or referrals that reduce your discomfort but have little impact on decision-making and may produce harm or waste resources or be overly burdensome to the patient. Show your learners how to attend to the patient's voice, how to empower patients in decision-making and the impact of the choices they face.

Sample teaching tools

You can use the sample *Teaching Tools for Medical Expert* at the end of this section as is, or you can modify or use them in various combinations to suit your objectives, the time allocated, the sequence within your residency program, and so on.

Easy-to-customize electronic versions of the *Teaching for Medical Expert* (in .doc, .ppt and .pdf formats) are found at: canmeds.royalcollege.ca

The tools provided are:

- T1 Lecture or Large Group Session: Foundations of the Medical Expert Role

- T2 Presentation: Teaching the Medical Expert Role

- T3 Guided Reflection: Medical Expert Role competence continuum in day-to-day practice

- T4 Simulation: Patient-centeredness in patient-physician relationships

- T5 Ward Rounds: Oral case presentations via SNAPPS

- T6 Coaching: One minute preceptor template for coaching the Medical Expert Role

- T7 Coaching: I don't know activity to develop help-seeking behaviours

- T8 Tools and Strategies: Summary sheet for the Medical Expert Role

© 2015 Royal College of Physicians and Surgeons of Canada

5. Hints, tips and tools for *assessing* the Medical Expert Role

Assessment for learning is a major theme in this CanMEDS Tools Guide and a growing emphasis in medical education. You can and should use assessment as a strategy to inform a resident's learning plan (e.g. to alert or signpost to learners what is important to learn as well as what and how they will be assessed). This section of the Tools Guide offers a number of hints to help you develop a program of assessment that will ensure that both teachers and learners have a clear understanding of their performance and what needs improvement.

Assessment Tip 1.
Incorporate the Intrinsic Roles when assessing the Medical Expert Role

Although evaluation of Medical Expert competencies might be the central or primary purpose of a given assessment, do not miss the opportunity to include competencies of one or two additional CanMEDS Roles in the assessment. This means assessing the Intrinsic Roles with and through the day-to-day practice of the Medical Expert Role.

Assessment Tip 2.
Work within (or build) an assessment plan or map using the Specialty Training Requirements (or Competency Training Requirements if you are working in the Competence by Design system)

Start with your specialty's expectations for learners and residency education. Organize the regular assessments (e.g. per block or quarter) that will be conducted over the course of training to ensure a good balance of:

- regular purposeful direct observations of key tasks to ensure development and progress of expertise (e.g. informally, encounter form assessment, mini clinical evaluation exercises [mini-CEx], observed/assessed encounters);

- assessments that involve scanning large amounts of knowledge and knowledge application (e.g. annual or semi-annual in-training written exams, oral exams); and

- regular assessments of demonstrations in simulated settings/situations (e.g. simulation lab assessments, case reports, teaching sessions, objective structured clinical exams [OSCEs]).

Build a culture of feedback and coaching by providing a small dose of on-the-spot feedback in the course of each day of clinical practice.

Your assessment plan or map also needs to consider general assessment tips:

- Learners pay attention to what is assessed. Remember that assessments signal to your learners that something is important. When time is tight (and it almost always is), most learners set their learning and studying priorities on the basis of assessments that 'count.'

- When you start working with learners, clarify your expectations and explain whether the learners will be assessed (if at all). If there will be an assessment, will it be formative and for feedback purposes? Or will it be summative, with a score submitted to the residency program? What elements are of most interest to you in this location, at this time, with these learners? What do you expect of learners, and what can they expect of you?

- Define the role of the learner in the different aspects of the assessment plan — in other words, which parts they are responsible for on their own through self-study, what they are expected to track (e.g. case logs, portfolios), what you will need them to report on (e.g. research reports, semi-annual meetings with the program director).

- Assessments also help cue faculty to what aspects of care are of most interest in this location, at this time, with these learners.

- Identify how learners can provide input and feedback (e.g. placing resident reps on committees, creating a process for providing feedback to teachers, organizing an annual retreat).

- Include as wide a variety of different assessment tools as is feasible for the assessors and learners.

- Share the responsibility for conducting individual assessments across faculty and the health care team. Short assessments done frequently are better than long assessments done infrequently.

- Share the responsibility for interpreting learners' assessment results and progress (or lack of) with a group of faculty (e.g. residency program committee, evaluation committee). Look for episodes and trends of progress to identify who is on, behind, or ahead of the usual trajectory of expertise development.

- Create and demonstrate a safe learning environment.

Medical Expert

Sample assessment tools

You can use the sample *Assessment Tools for Medical Expert* found at the end of this section as is, or you can modify or use them in various combinations to suit your objectives, the time allocated, the sequence within your residency program, and so on.

Easy-to-customize electronic versions of the *Assessment Tools for Medical Expert* (in .doc, .ppt and .pdf formats) are found at: canmeds.royalcollege.ca

The tools provided are:

- A1 Multisource Feedback: Types of expertise

- A2 O-SCORE: The Ottawa surgical competency operating room evaluation (O-SCORE)

6. Suggested resources

- **Ericsson KA. Deliberate practice and acquisition of expert performance: a general overview. *Acad Emerg Med* 2008; 15(11):988-994.** A straightforward and important resource on the definition, description and approach to deliberative practice to develop medical expertise.

- **Ferenchick G, Simpson D, Blackman J, DaRosa D, Dunnington G. Strategies for efficient and effective teaching in the ambulatory care setting. *Acad Med.* 1997; 72(4): 277-80.** Five strategies for teaching in the ambulatory care setting are described. They discuss the practical realities of how to ensure educational effectiveness while simultaneously providing high-quality, cost-effective patient care.

- **Kennedy TJ, Regehr G, Baker GR, Lingard L. Preserving professional credibility: grounded theory study of medical trainees' requests for clinical support. *BMJ* 2009;338:b128.** A systematic review of the effect of clinical supervision on patient and education outcomes. Medical trainees acknowledge that they may lack the expertise required to recognize how or when to call for help

- **For specialty-specific training requirements, see the Royal College website (last retrieved July 11, 2015):** English: http://www.royalcollege.ca/portal/page/portal/rc/credentials/specialty_information French: http://www.collegeroyal.ca/portal/page/portal/rc/credentials/specialty_information

7. Other resources

- Greenhalgh T. Narrative based medicine: narrative based medicine in an evidence-based world. *BMJ.* 1999;318(7179):323.

- Hodges B. A tea-steeping or i-Doc model for medical education? *Acad Med.* 2010;85(9 Suppl):S34-44.

- Schmidt HG, Boshuizen HPA. On acquiring expertise in medicine. *Educ Psychol Rev* 1993; 5(3): 205-221.

- Goldszmidt M. Faden L, Dornan T, van Merrienboer J, Bordage G, Lingard L. Attending Physician Variability: A model of four supervisory styles. *Acad Med.* 2015 Apr 17 EPub ahead of print.

© 2015 Royal College of Physicians and Surgeons of Canada

8. MEDICAL EXPERT ROLE DIRECTORY OF TEACHING AND ASSESSMENT TOOLS

You can use the sample *teaching and assessment tools for the Medical Expert Role* found in this section as is, or you can modify or use them in various combinations to suit your objectives, the time allocated, the sequence within your residency program, and so on. Tools are listed by number (e.g. T1), type (e.g. Lecture), and title (e.g. Foundations of the Medical Expert Role).

Easy-to-customize electronic versions of the sample *teaching and assessment tools for the Medical Expert Role* in .doc, .ppt and .pdf formats are found at: canmeds.royalcollege.ca

TEACHING TOOLS

ASSESSMENT TOOLS

T1. FOUNDATIONS OF THE MEDICAL EXPERT ROLE

Created for the *CanMEDS Teaching and Assessment Tools Guide* by S Glover Takahashi. Reproduced with permission of the Royal College.

This learning activity includes:

1. Presentation: Teaching and Assessing Medical Expert (T2)

2. Worksheet: Medical Expert Competence Continuum in day-to-day practice (T3)

Instructions for Teacher:

Sample learning objectives

- Recognize common words related to the process and content of the Medical Expert Role

- Describe the Role of Medical Expert within the *CanMEDS 2015 Framework*

- Apply the Medical Expert competence continuum to your own program or specialty

- Identify opportunities to integrate other CanMEDS Roles into the teaching and assessment of Medical Expert

Audience: All learners

How to adapt:

- Consider whether your session's needs and goals match the sample ones provided in this slide deck. Select from, modify, or add to the sample content as required.

- The sample PowerPoint presentation and worksheets are generic and foundational. Consider whether you'll need additional slides to meet your objectives. Modify, add or delete questions as you view appropriate, to include specific information related to your discipline and context.

Logistics:

- Allocate about 20 minutes for each worksheet/group activity: this time will be used for you to explain the activity and for your learners to complete the worksheet individually, share their answers with their small group, discuss, prepare to report back to the whole group, and then deliver their small group's report to the whole group.

- Depending on the group and time available, you may wish to assign one or more worksheets as homework to be completed before the session or as a follow-up assignment.

- Depending on the group and time available, you may also wish to explore the Specialty Training Requirements (STRs) or work through applying the teaching tips and/or the assessment tips to the specialty or program. See the Royal College website for STRs: English: http://www.royalcollege.ca/portal/page/portal/rc/credentials/specialty_information French: http://www.collegeroyal.ca/portal/page/portal/rc/credentials/specialty_information

Setting:

- This teaching session is best done in a small-group format (i.e. less than 30 learners) if possible. It can also be effectively done with a larger group if the room allows for learners to be at tables in groups of five or six. With larger groups, it is helpful to have additional teachers or facilitators available to answer questions arising from the worksheet activities.

Medical Expert

© 2015 Royal College of Physicians and Surgeons of Canada

T2. TEACHING THE MEDICAL EXPERT ROLE

Created for the *CanMEDS Teaching and Assessment Tools Guide* by S Glover Takahashi. Reproduced with permission of the Royal College.

Instructions for Teacher:

- Setting and Audience: Faculty and all learners
- How to use: Use as an orientation to the Role.
- How to adapt: Slides can be modified to match the specialty or the learners' practice context
- Logistics: Equipment – laptop, projector, screen

Slide	Words on slide	Notes to teachers
1.	Foundations of Teaching and Assessing Medical Expert	• Add information about presenters and modify title
2.	**Objectives and agenda** 1. Recognize common words related to the process and content of the Medical Expert Role 2. Describe the role of Medical Expert within the CanMEDS 2015 Framework 3. Apply the Medical Expert competence continuum to your own program or specialty 4. Identify opportunities to integrate other CanMEDS Roles into the teaching and assessment of Medical Expert	• SAMPLE goals and objectives of the session – revise as required. • CONSIDER doing a 'warm up activity' • Review/revise goals and objectives. • Insert agenda slide if desired
3.	**Why the Medical Expert Role matters** • Medical Expert is central to a physician's competence and identity. • Medical Expert competencies by themselves are not sufficient to practice medicine. • Medical Expertise must be integrated with the Intrinsic Roles to optimize patient care.	• Reasons why this Role is important
4.	**The details: What is the Medical Expert Role?**[a] As Medical Experts, physicians integrate all of the CanMEDS Roles, applying medical knowledge, clinical skills, and professional values in their provision of high-quality and safe patient-centred care. Medical Expert is the central physician Role in the CanMEDS Framework and defines the physician's clinical scope of practice.	• Definition from the *CanMEDS 2015 Physician Competency Framework* • Avoid including competencies for learners • If you are giving this presentation to teachers or planners, you may want to add the key and enabling competencies
5.	**ABOUT MEDICAL EXPERT** 1. Patients care about what your specialty knows and how that knowledge contributes to addressing their needs. 2. The type of patient-physician relationship should be defined by the patient's preferences and will always be respectful and responsive. 3. There are no simple answers to complex problems and becoming comfortable with uncertainty is an important part of the Medical Expert Role. 4. A competent physician seamlessly integrates the competencies of all seven CanMEDS Roles.	• Truth behind misconceptions
6.	**Key definitions** • Cognitive load • Deliberate practice • Expertise • Help seeking • Patient-centred • Shared decision-making	• Definitions in Tools Guide text • Provide examples of these terms in your specialty

a Bhanji F, Lawrence K, Goldszmidt M, Walton M, Harris K, Creery D, Sherbino J, Ste-Marie L-G, Stang A. *Medical Expert.* In: Frank JR, Snell L, Sherbino J, editors. CanMEDS 2015 *Physician Competency Framework*. Ottawa: Royal College of Physicians and Surgeons of Canada; 2015. Reproduced with permission.

Medical Expert

T2. TEACHING THE MEDICAL EXPERT ROLE (continued)

Slide	Words on slide	Notes to teachers
7.	**Recognizing Medical Expert PROCESS** • Assess • Clinical decision-making • Diagnose • Plan • Treat	• Trigger words for process
8.	**Recognizing Medical Expert CONTENT** • Best practices • Clinical practice • Clinical skills • Diagnostic interventions • High-quality care • Intervention • Management plan • Medical knowledge • Patient-centred • Patient Safety • Professional values • Scope of practice • Therapy	• Trigger words for content
9.	**Four Types of patient-centred relationships** 1. Paternalistic 2. Informative 3. Interpretive 4. Deliberative	• Review examples or experiences about how the four types of patient-centred relationships applies to your specialty. • SEE T4 activity
10.	**Preparing to teach the Medical Expert Role** Five Stages of Competence by Design Entry to residency Transition to discipline Foundations of discipline Core of discipline Transition to practice	• Table ME-4. Five stages of the learner on the Medical Expert competence continuum
11.	T3 – Medical Expert competence continuum in day-to-day practice	• Can do on own or in groups • Groups are appropriate when everyone is in the same specialty as examples will vary with each specialty • Explore answers in small groups or with the whole group
12.	Samples of the Medical Expert competence continuum in day-to-day practice	• Table ME-5. Examples of Medical Expert activities at two points in the Medical Expert competence continuum • Explore how generic samples do/do not apply to their specialty
13.	**HELP-SEEKING:** *Steps*[b] Culture of safety Recognition of need Willingness to ask Skills to asking for help Accessibility of Help	• Table ME-6. Review Barriers and Supports to Help Seeking. • Review how this applies to your specialty. If your specialty is working within the Competence by Design system change STR to Competency Training Requirements
14.	Recap, revisiting objectives, and next steps	• Revisit session goals and objectives

b Karabenick, Stuart A., and John R. Knapp. Relationship of academic help seeking to the use of learning strategies and other instrumental achievement behavior in college students. *J Educ Psychol.* 1991;83(2):221.

© 2015 Royal College of Physicians and Surgeons of Canada

T2. TEACHING THE MEDICAL EXPERT ROLE (continued)

Slide	Words on slide	Notes to teachers
OTHER SLIDES		
15.	**Medical Expert Key Competencies**[a] ***Physicians are able to:*** 1. Practise medicine within their defined scope of practice and expertise 2. Perform a patient-centred clinical assessment and establish a management plan 3. Plan and perform procedures and therapies for the purpose of assessment and/or management 4. Establish plans for ongoing care and, when appropriate, timely consultation 5. Actively contribute, as an individual and as a member of a team providing care, to the continuous improvement of health care quality and patient safety	• Key Competencies from the *CanMEDS 2015 Physician Competency Framework* • Avoid including competencies for learners • You may wish to use this slide if you are giving the presentation to teachers or planners
16.	**Medical Expert Key Competency 1**[a] ***Physicians are able to:*** 1. Practise medicine within their defined scope of practice and expertise 1.1 Demonstrate a commitment to high-quality care of their patients 1.2 Integrate the CanMEDS Intrinsic Roles into their practice of medicine 1.3 Apply knowledge of the clinical and biomedical sciences relevant to their discipline 1.4 Perform appropriately timed clinical assessments with recommendations that are presented in an organized manner 1.5 Carry out professional duties in the face of multiple, competing demands 1.6 Recognize and respond to the complexity, uncertainty, and ambiguity inherent in medical practice	• From the *CanMEDS Framework* • Use one slide for each key competency and associated enabling competencies
17.	**Medical Expert Key Competency 2**[a] ***Physicians are able to:*** 2. Perform a patient-centred clinical assessment and establish a management plan 2.1 Prioritize issues to be addressed in a patient encounter 2.2 Elicit a history, perform a physical exam, select appropriate investigations, and interpret their results for the purpose of diagnosis and management, disease prevention, and health promotion 2.3 Establish goals of care in collaboration with patients and their families, which may include slowing disease progression, treating symptoms, achieving cure, improving function, and palliation 2.4 Establish a patient-centred management plan	• From the *CanMEDS Framework*

© 2015 Royal College of Physicians and Surgeons of Canada

T2. TEACHING THE MEDICAL EXPERT ROLE (continued)

Slide	Words on slide	Notes to teachers

18.	**Medical Expert Key Competency 3**[a]
	Physicians are able to:
	3. Plan and perform procedures and therapies for the purpose of assessment and/or management
	   3.1 Determine the most appropriate procedures or therapies
	   3.2 Obtain and document informed consent, explaining the risks and benefits of, and the rationale for, a proposed procedure or therapy
	   3.3 Prioritize a procedure or therapy, taking into account clinical urgency and available resources
	   3.4 Perform a procedure in a skilful and safe manner, adapting to unanticipated findings or changing clinical circumstances
		• From the *CanMEDS Framework*

19.	**Medical Expert Key Competency 4**[a] ***Physicians are able to:*** 4. Establish plans for ongoing care and, when appropriate, timely consultation 4.1 Implement a patient-centred care plan that supports ongoing care, follow-up on investigations, response to treatment, and further consultation	• From the *CanMEDS Framework*

20.	**Medical Expert Key Competency 5**[a]
	Physicians are able to:
	5. Actively contribute, as an individual and as a member of a team providing care, to the continuous improvement of health care quality and patient safety
	   5.1 Recognize and respond to harm from health care delivery, including patient safety incidents
	   5.2 Adopt strategies that promote patient safety and address human and system factors
		• From the *CanMEDS Framework*

21.	**Medical Expert resources** Specialty Training Requirements http://www.royalcollege.ca/portal/page/portal/rc/credentials/specialty_information	• Insert resources, including Royal College Specialty Training Requirement http://www.royalcollege.ca/portal/page/portal/rc/credentials/specialty_information

© 2015 Royal College of Physicians and Surgeons of Canada

T3. MEDICAL EXPERT ROLE COMPETENCE CONTINUUM IN DAY-TO-DAY PRACTICE

Created for the *CanMEDS Teaching and Assessment Tools Guide* by S Glover Takahashi. Reproduced with permission of the Royal College.

See Medical Expert Role teacher tips appendix for this teaching tool

Completed by:_____

Learner Instructions:

• Use the Medical Expert Competence Continuum and examples as a reference tool (SEE Tables ME-1 and ME-2).

1. Complete the table below, providing specific details from your specialty.

Day-to-day practice scenario	Common situation and straightforward problem (i.e. earlier Medical Expert activity)	Complex or complicated problem (i.e. more developed Medical Expert activity)
SCENARIO #1		
SCENARIO #2		

Comments:

T3. MEDICAL EXPERT ROLE COMPETENCE CONTINUUM IN DAY-TO-DAY PRACTICE (continued)

2. For each of the scenarios you chose in question 1, identify the one or two additional CanMEDS Roles you could most easily highlight when teaching or assessing Medical Expert.

Day-to-day practice scenario	Common situation and straightforward problem (i.e. earlier Medical Expert activity)		Complex or complicated problem (i.e. more developed Medical Expert activity)	
SCENARIO #1 from above	Additional CanMEDS Roles most easily highlighted when teaching or assessing the Medical Expert		Additional CanMEDS Roles most easily highlighted when teaching or assessing the Medical Expert	
SCENARIO #2 from above	Additional CanMEDS Roles most easily highlighted when teaching or assessing the Medical Expert		Additional CanMEDS Roles most easily highlighted when teaching or assessing the Medical Expert	

Comments:

© 2015 Royal College of Physicians and Surgeons of Canada

T3. MEDICAL EXPERT ROLE COMPETENCE CONTINUUM IN DAY-TO-DAY PRACTICE (continued)

LEARNER RESOURCES

TABLE 1: FIVE STAGES OF THE LEARNER ON THE MEDICAL EXPERT COMPETENCE CONTINUUM

1. Entry to residency	2. Transition to discipline	3. Foundations of discipline	4. Core of discipline	5. Transition to practice
Is oriented to residency and to the inventory of knowledge and skills	Has an awareness of and can act on key parts of high-volume routine cases, common situations, and straightforward problems	Handles high-volume routine cases, common situations, and straightforward problems on their own; has an awareness of complicated situations and problems	Handles with efficiency high-volume routine cases, common situations, and straightforward problems on their own; acts on complicated situations and problems with support. Prioritizes with increasing efficiency	Handles complex and complicated situations and problems on their own, and guides or supports others. Manages with various concurrent priorities. Develops judgment/ wisdom to decide between various courses of action

EARLIER ← ――――――――――――――――――――――――― → END
in Residency   of Residency

TABLE 2: EXAMPLES OF MEDICAL EXPERT ACTIVITIES AT TWO POINTS ON THE COMPETENCE CONTINUUM

SAMPLE day-to-day scenario	Common situation and straightforward problem (i.e. earlier Medical Expert activity)	Complex or complicated problem (i.e. more developed Medical Expert activity)
Case report from learner to faculty	Learner gives a top-line summary of the patient history, inventory of problems, and planned treatment in a standard format to a faculty member who is a supportive teacher.	The blood work report that the learner requires to prepare an accurate treatment plan was delayed in being posted, and the learner, busy managing other patient priorities, did not discover this in sufficient time before case rounds to be able to hunt down the results with a phone call.
Rounds	Learner participates in teaching rounds with own team and on a topic with which the learner is quite familiar.	Learner presents a balanced overview of the literature and makes recommendations based on current best practice.
Phone consultation	Learner holds a conversation with the referring primary care physician about needed community follow-up.	Learner calls the referring specialist in another community to report that the requested intervention is not available for the patient (e.g. because patients from that region are not eligible owing to limited resources/funding). The learner then problem-solves with the referring specialist about alternatives to the requested intervention.
Goals of care	Learner meets with a patient and one family member before surgery to discuss elective surgical options.	Learner holds a post-operative meeting with a patient and three family members, all of whom have a limited comprehension of English and French, to review a serious pathology report and plan for identified further treatment with the assistance of a translator.

EARLIER ← ――――――――――――――――――――――――― → END
in Residency   of Residency

Medical Expert

T4. PATIENT-CENTEREDNESS IN PATIENT-PHYSICIAN RELATIONSHIPS

Created for the *CanMEDS Teaching and Assessment Tools Guide* by S Glover Takahashi. Reproduced with permission of the Royal College.

See Medical Expert Role teacher tips appendix for this teaching tool

Instructions for Learner:

- This activity will give you an opportunity to 'try out' a variety of patient-physician relationships.

- See back of worksheet for description of different terms.

- Remember to stay 'patient-centred'.

- You will be assigned a scenario. Choose one or two of the physician relationships that you would like to role play.

- Take a moment to complete the table and prepare for your role play.

- Role-play with one or more peers and then reflect on the experience. What did you learn from the experience? Would it change your practice in any way?

Type of patient-physician relationship[a]	Questions or statements the physician might say
Paternalistic (PARENTAL)	
Informative patient-physician relationship (INFORMANT)	
Interpretive patient-physician relationship (COUNSELLOR)	
Deliberative patient-physician relationship (TEACHER OR COACH)	

a   Emanuel EJ, Emanuel LL. Four Models of the Physician-Patient Relationship. *JAMA.* 1992;267(16):2221-6.

© 2015 Royal College of Physicians and Surgeons of Canada

T4. PATIENT-CENTEREDNESS IN PATIENT-PHYSICIAN RELATIONSHIPS (continued)

LEARNER INFORMATION

Types of patient-physician relationships

Type	Description	Physician approach	Patient approach	Example
Paternalistic[a]	Patient wants the physician to provide significant direction, guidance or decisions on diagnostic and therapeutic interventions, risks and benefits in the clinical situation.	• Parent. • Authoritative and in control of information and situation.	Patient is passive and trusts physician to make decisions in their best interests and on their behalf.	Physician provides selected information and suggestions about treatment/care options. Physician presents information that encourages patient to consent to the intervention(s) that the physician views as best. *"I think you should..."*
Informative	Patient wants information and medical expertise provided in a factual manner including possible diagnostic and therapeutic interventions, risks and benefits in the clinical situation.	• Informant. • Technical, rationale expert.	Patient consumes medical information making choices based on factual information provided.	Physician provides the facts about medical condition(s), options and plan. Patient asks questions about choices and then makes the decision(s). *"The options are..."*
Interpretative	Patient wants physician to help clarify values, needs and goals to inform the selection of diagnostic and therapeutic interventions, risk and benefits that meet those values, needs and goals in the clinical situation.	• Counsellor. • Engaged, shared decision-making	Patient is knowledgeable about own wants and needs and communicates these expectations. Works with physician in selection of choices.	Physician explores patients' values, needs and goals to then offer diagnostic and therapeutic interventions that meet those values, needs and goals. *"How the options connect to your goals are..."*
Deliberative	Patient wants the physician to help clarify health-related values, clarify the issues arising from the various options for diagnostic and therapeutic interventions, risks and benefits in the clinical situation.	• Teacher or Coach	Patient engaged in dialogue and empowered to follow unexamined preferences or examined values.	Physician and patient explore values, needs and goals. Physician and patient dialogue about alternative health-related values including applicability and implications in the clinical situation. *"Have you considered that your goals might mean that..."*

Medical Expert

T5. ORAL CASE PRESENTATION VIA SNAPPS[a]

See Medical Expert Role teacher tips appendix for this teaching tool

Instructions for Learner:

- Refer to the SNAPPS reference sheet provided with this tool.
- Observe and take (non-identifying) notes on your case.
- Remember to be cautious about privacy when taking notes.
- Review with faculty as arranged or initiate a review of your ward round presentation to get feedback.

S – summarize the case

_____

_____

N – narrow the differential

_____

_____

A – analyze the differential

_____

_____

P – probe the preceptor

_____

_____

P – plan management

_____

_____

S – select an issue for self-directed learning

_____

_____

a Wolpaw DR, Papp KK. SNAPPS: a learner-centered model for outpatient education. *Acad Med.* 2003. 78(9):893-8.

© 2015 Royal College of Physicians and Surgeons of Canada

T5. ORAL CASE PRESENTATION VIA SNAPPS (continued)

LEARNER INFORMATION

Ward rounds or verbal case presentation via **SNAPPS**[a]

S – summarize the case

N – narrow the differential

A – analyze the differential

P – probe the preceptor

P – plan management

S – select an issue for self-directed learning

Summarize the case

- The learner obtains a history, performs an appropriate examination of a patient, and presents a concise summary to the preceptor.

- Though the length may vary, depending on the complexity of the case, the summary should not occupy more than 50% of the learning encounter and, generally, should be no longer than three minutes.

- The summary should be condensed to relevant information because the preceptor can readily elicit further details from the learner.

- In this step, the learner should be encouraged to present the case at a higher level of abstraction (e.g. to use semantic qualifiers: yesterday becomes acute, third time becomes recurrent) because successful diagnosticians use these qualifiers early in their presentations.

Narrow the Differential

- Limit your differential to two to three relevant possibilities.

- The learner verbalizes what he or she thinks is going on in the case, focusing on the most likely possibilities rather than on "zebras."

- For a new patient encounter, the learner may present two or three reasonable diagnostic possibilities.

- For follow-up or sick visits, the differential may focus on why the patient's disease is active, what therapeutic interventions might be considered, or relevant preventive health strategies.

- This step requires a commitment on the part of the learner by presenting an initial differential to the preceptor before engaging the preceptor to expand or revise the differential.

Analyze the Differential

- Compare and contrast the relevant diagnostic possibilities and discriminating findings.

- A learner's discussion of the cause of a patient's chest pain might proceed as follows: "I think that angina is a concern because the pain is in his anterior chest. At the same time I think that a pulmonary cause is more likely because the pain is worse with inspiration, and I heard crackles when I examined the lungs."

- Often the learner may combine this step with the previous step of identifying the diagnostic possibilities, comparing and contrasting each in turn.

- This discussion allows the learner to verbalize his or her thinking process and can stimulate an interactive discussion with the preceptor.

- Learners will vary in their fund of knowledge and level of diagnostic sophistication, but all are expected to utilize the strategy of comparing and contrasting to discuss the differential.

Probe the Preceptor

- Ask questions about uncertainties, difficulties, or alternative approaches.

- During this step, the learner is expected to reveal areas of confusion and knowledge deficits and is rewarded for doing so.

- This step is the most unique aspect of the learner-driven model because the learner initiates an educational discussion by probing the preceptor with questions rather than waiting for the preceptor to initiate the probing of the learner.

- The learner is taught to utilize the preceptor as a knowledge resource that can readily be accessed. The learner may access the preceptor's knowledge base with questions or statements ranging from general to specific. Examples include, "What else should I include in the differential?," or "I'm not sure."

- How to examine for a knee effusion," or "We could taper his corticosteroids since his Crohn's flare is nearly resolved, but what protocols can be used to avoid problems with steroid withdrawal?"

- The preceptor can learn a great deal about the learner's thought process and knowledge base by such interactions.

Medical Expert

T5. ORAL CASE PRESENTATION VIA SNAPPS (continued)

Plan Management

- The learner initiates a discussion of patient management with the preceptor and must attempt either a brief management plan or suggest specific interventions.

- This step asks for a commitment from the learner, but encourages him or her to access the preceptor readily as a rich resource of knowledge and experience.

Select a Case-related Issue for Self-directed Learning

- Self-directed learning can occur at any point in the SNAPPS process and does not have to wait till the end.

- This final step encourages the learner to read about focused, patient-based questions.

- The learner may identify a learning issue at the end of the patient presentation or after seeing the patient with the preceptor.

- The learner should check with the preceptor to focus the reading and frame relevant questions.

- The learner should devote time to reading as soon after the office encounter as possible.

- For example, a learner would be encouraged to read to answer a question such as, "What is the rationale for the use of ace inhibitors in congestive heart failure?" rather than reading an entire chapter in a review text on heart failure.

- Learners should be expected to have an index card or personal digital assistant with them in the office to note learning issues.

- At the next meeting with the preceptor, the learner can utilize the preceptor as a resource as he or she refers to the list and further probes the preceptor with questions based on the readings.

© 2015 Royal College of Physicians and Surgeons of Canada

T6. ONE MINUTE PRECEPTOR[a] TEMPLATE FOR COACHING THE MEDICAL EXPERT ROLE

Created for the *CanMEDS Teaching and Assessment Tools Guide* by S Glover Takahashi. Reproduced with permission of the Royal College.

Instructions for Learner:

- This approach encourages you to 'own' the clinical problem, sort out your thinking and ensure you and the teacher work together to plan for the patient.

- Fill out the template or use it to mentally prepare for the teacher to ask a series of questions as part of a case presentation dialogue.

- This tool encourages feedback.

1. Learner provides specific answers/commitment about a SPECIFIC case (e.g. differential, diagnostic or therapeutic intervention, procedures).

_____

_____

2. Learner answers teacher probes for supporting evidence about answers to question one above. These questions will be SPECIFIC to the case.

_____

_____

3. Teacher provides general rules for this and similar case(s) (e.g. rules of thumb)

_____

_____

4. Teacher comments on what the learner did right for the SPECIFIC case

_____

_____

5. Teacher comments on errors or mistakes and coaching advice on how to improve for this/similar case(s) in the future

_____

_____

LEARNER take away notes:

---

a Adapted from Neher JO, Stevens NG. The one-minute preceptor: shaping the teaching conversation. *Fam Med.* 2003;35(6):391-3.

Medical Expert

T7. I DON'T KNOW ACTIVITY TO DEVELOP HELP-SEEKING BEHAVIOURS[a]

Instructions for Teacher:

- Ask a learner questions of increasing difficulty.

- Stay neutral as the questions become increasingly less accurate. Just accept the answers.

- Eventually — and it may take a while — a learner will say: "I don't know."

- When the learner says, "I don't know" reward them (e.g. applause, box of Smarties)

- Then discuss the importance of those three words

- Discuss how to become comfortable with not knowing, asking for help, where/how to get help.

- You may adapt this approach by making it a subtheme for rounds on a given day and done in groups.

Comments:

_____

_____

_____

_____

_____

_____

_____

_____

_____

---

a   Adapted from Smith R. Thoughts for new medical students at a new medical school. *BMJ*. 2003; 327.7429: 1430.

© 2015 Royal College of Physicians and Surgeons of Canada

Medical Expert

T8. SUMMARY SHEET FOR THE MEDICAL EXPERT ROLE

Created for the *CanMEDS Teaching and Assessment Tools Guide* by S Glover Takahashi. Reproduced with permission of the Royal College.

See Medical Expert Role teacher tips appendix for this teaching tool

MEDICAL EXPERT

1. Patients care about what your specialty knows and how that knowledge contributes to addressing their needs.

2. The type of patient-physician relationship should be defined by the patient's preferences and will always be respectful and responsive.

3. There are no simple answers to complex problems and becoming comfortable with uncertainty is an important part of the Medical Expert Role.

4. A competent physician seamlessly integrates the competencies of all seven CanMEDS Roles.

Trigger words relating to the PROCESS of Medical Expert:

- Assess
- Diagnose
- Treat
- Clinical decision-making
- Plan
- Quality Improvement

Trigger words relating to the CONTENT of Medical Expert:

- Best practices
- Clinical skills
- High-quality care
- Management plan
- Patient-centred
- Professional values
- Therapy
- Clinical practice
- Diagnostic interventions
- Intervention
- Medical knowledge
- Patient Safety
- Scope of practice

Expertise means the special skills or knowledge possessed by an individual, including:

- ***Cognitive skills*[b]** (i.e. factual, conceptual and procedural processes for comprehension, judgment, memory.

- ***Psychomotor skills*** (i.e. voluntary muscular movements) Visual perceptual processing (i.e. visual discrimination, visual memory, visual sequential memory, visual spatial relationships, visual-motor integration)

- ***Metacognitive*[c]** (i.e. planning, predicting, monitoring, regulating, evaluating, revising strategies).

- ***Non-cognitive skills*[d]** (or metacognitive learning skills) (i.e. persistence, self-control, curiosity, conscientiousness, grit, self-confidence.)

Deliberate practice, necessary for Expert performance, requires:

1. investment of considerable practice time,

2. purposeful effort, and

3. working towards a reasonable yet appropriately challenging goal.

Help-seeking is an active learning strategy to help the learner achieve success and develop expertise.[c]

Cognitive load is the mental processing demands that a person can manage. When overloaded, performance is degraded or deteriorates resulting in errors and mistakes.[f]

a Online Dictionary. Cognitive Last retrieved August 4, 2015 http://dictionary.reference.com/browse/cognitive.
b Miller-Keane Encyclopedia and Dictionary of Medicine, Nursing, and Allied Health. Seventh Edition. © 2003 by Saunders, an imprint of Elsevier, Inc.
c Tough P. *How Children Succeed: Grit, Curiosity, and the Hidden Power of Character.* Houghton, Minton and Harcourt; 2012.
d Karabenick, Stuart A., and John R. Knapp. Relationship of academic help seeking to the use of learning strategies and other instrumental achievement behavior in college students. *J Educ Psychol* 83.2 (1991): 221.
e Ambrose SA, Bridges MW, DiPietro M, Lovett MC, Norman MK, editors. 2010, How learning works: seven research-based principles for smart teaching, John Wiley & Sons, Inc,, Jossey-Bass, San Francisco, CA. pp 104.

T8. SUMMARY SHEET FOR THE MEDICAL EXPERT ROLE (continued)

Types of patient-centred relationships. Patient-centred means respectfully and responsively finding common ground and sharing decision-making with their patients about their values, needs, problems, priorities and goals.

Type[f]	Description	Physician approach	Patient approach	Example
Paternalistic	Patient wants the physician to provide significant direction, guidance or decisions on diagnostic and therapeutic interventions, risks and benefits.	• Parent • Authoritative and in control of information and situation	Patient is passive and trusts physician to make decisions in their best interests and on their behalf.	Physician provides selected information and suggestions about how care is best treated. Presents information that encourages patient to consent to intervention the physician views as best. ***"I think you should..."***
Informative	Patient wants information and medical expertise provided in a factual manner including possible diagnostic and therapeutic interventions, risks and benefits.	• Informant • Technical, rationale expert	Patient as consumer of medical information making choices based on factual information provided.	Physician provides the facts about medical condition, options and plan. Patient asking questions and deciding on own about choices. ***"The options are..."***
Interpretative	Patient wants physician to help clarify values, needs and goals to inform the selection of diagnostic and therapeutic interventions, risk and benefits that meet those values, needs and goals.	• Counsellor • Engaged, shared decision-making	Patient knowledgeable about wants and needs and communications same. Works with physician in selection of choices.	Physician explores patients' values, needs and goals to then offer diagnostic and therapeutic interventions, that meet those values, needs and goals. ***"How the options connect to your goals are...***
Deliberative	Patient wants the physician to help clarify health-related values, clarify the issues arising from the various options for diagnostic and therapeutic interventions, risks and benefits	• Teacher or Coach	Patient engaged in dialogue and empowered to follow unexamined preferences or examined values.	Physician and patient explore values, needs and goals. Physician and patient dialogue about alternative health-related values including applicability and implications in the clinical situation. ***"Have you considered that your goals might mean that..."***

HELP-SEEKING: Steps[g]	Barriers	Strategies
Culture of safety	• Asking for help is viewed as a weakness • Help is not available	• Expectation that learners ask for help and that help is given without judgment • Supervision framed as teaching strategy • Faculty and senior residents model
Recognition of need	• Lack of knowledge • Limitations of self-assessment	• Protocols for supervision • Direct observation as educational strategy • Interprofessional team encouraged to identify if help needed and share in problem solving
Willingness to ask	• Independence valued instead of autonomy • Threats to credibility	• Teaching adaptive help seeking strategies • Learner assessment to include "asks for help appropriately"
Skills to asking for help	• Do not recognize need for help • Embarrassed to ask for help • No experience asking for help	• Practising "I don't' know" • Coaching to encourage improvement
Accessibility of Help	• Availability of teacher – physical proximity and timing of need • Approachability of teacher	• Establishing expectations for communication • Deliberate increase in number of interactions with learner • Teacher assessment

f   Emanuel EJ, Emanuel LL. Four Models of the Physician-Patient Relationship. *JAMA.* 1992;267(16):2221-6.
g   Adapted from Han, Ra and Kim, Vy Hong-Diep. May 2015. Setting a Climate for Help-Seeking in Postgraduate Medical Education: a Theoretical Framework for Understanding Barriers and Strategies for Successful Help-Seeking. University of Toronto. Unpublished manuscript. Adapted with permission.

   © 2015 Royal College of Physicians and Surgeons of Canada

Medical Expert

A1. TYPES OF EXPERTISE

Created for the *CanMEDS Teaching and Assessment Tools Guide* by S Glover Takahashi. Reproduced with permission of the Royal College.

See Medical Expert Role teacher tips appendix for this assessment tool.

Instructions for Teacher:

- The FOCUS of this activity is an opportunity for formative assessment and coaching to guide learners about what aspects of expertise need attention.

- Could also be adapted to a summative tool with addition of more description on expectation for learner level and program

Instructions for Assessor:

- Using the form below, please help this resident physician gain insight into his/her skills by providing valuable confidential feedback.

- This information will be shared with the learner in aggregate form and for the purposes of helping him/her improve.

- Please return this form in a confidential sealed envelope to the attention of:

_____

RESIDENT Name: _____

Postgraduate year (PGY): _____

Indicate ☑ all that apply. I am a:
- ☐ Health professional team member
- ☐ Resident
- ☐ Medical student (including clerk)
- ☐ Faculty member
- ☐ Other, please specify_____

Degree of interaction
- ☐ Considerable interaction from this resident
- ☐ Occasional or one interaction with this resident
- ☐ Other, please specify_____

AREA OF EXPERTISE	Examples of what is done well	Examples of what needs improvement	Plans for improvement
Cognitive			
Psychomotor skills			
Visual perceptual processing			
Metacognitive			
Non cognitive skills			
Other:			

© 2015 Royal College of Physicians and Surgeons of Canada

A2. THE OTTAWA SURGICAL COMPETENCY OPERATING ROOM EVALUATION (O-SCORE)[a]

Trainee#:	Level: 1 2 3 4 5	Staff:
Procedure:		Date:

Relative complexity of this procedure to average of same procedure   Low   Medium   High

The purpose of this scale is to evaluate the trainee's ability to perform this procedure safely and independently. With that in mind please use the scale below to evaluate each item, irrespective of the resident's level of training in regards to **this** case.

Scale

1 – "I had to do" – i.e. Requires complete hands on guidance, did not do, or was not given the opportunity to do

2 – "I had to talk them through" – i.e. Able to perform tasks but requires constant direction

3 – "I had to prompt them from time to time" – i.e. Demonstrates some independence, but requires intermittent direction

4 – "I needed to be in the room just in case" – i.e. Independence but unaware of risks and still requires supervision for safe practice

5 – "I did not need to be there" – i.e. Complete independence, understands risks and performs safely, practice ready

1. Pre-procedure plan   1   2   3   4   5
Gathers/assesses required information to reach diagnosis and determine correct procedure required

2. Case preparation   1   2   3   4   5
Patient correctly prepared and positioned, understands approach and required instruments, prepared to deal with probable complications

3. Knowledge of specific procedural steps   1   2   3   4   5
Understands steps of procedure, potential risks and means to avoid/overcome them

4. Technical performance   1   2   3   4   5
Efficiently performs steps avoiding pitfalls and respecting soft tissues

5. Visuospatial skills   1   2   3   4   5
3D spatial orientation is accurate and is able to position instruments/hardware where intended

6. Post-procedure plan   1   2   3   4   5
Appropriate complete post-procedure plan

7. Efficiency and flow   1   2   3   4   5
Obvious planned course of procedure with economy of movement and flow

8. Communication   1   2   3   4   5
Professional and effective communication/utilization of staff

9. Resident is able to safely perform *this* procedure *independently* (circle)   Y   N

10. Give at least one *specific* aspect of procedure done well _____

11. Give at least one *specific* suggestion for improvement _____

Signatures: Staff_____

Trainee _____

a   Gofton WT, Dudek NL, Wood TJ, Balaa F, Hamstra SJ. The Ottawa surgical competency operating room evaluation: a tool to assess surgical competence. *Acad Med.* 2012;87(10):1401-7. Reproduced with permission.

© 2015 Royal College of Physicians and Surgeons of Canada

Medical Expert

MEDICAL EXPERT ROLE TEACHER TIPS APPENDIX

T3 GUIDED REFLECTION: COMPETENCE CONTINUUM

Instructions for Teacher:

- Setting and Audience: All learners.

- How to use: Plan for about 20 minutes for the worksheet.

  - Allow individuals to read the worksheet and spend about five minutes working on the answers.

  - Compare and discuss answers in small groups.

  - Reporting back by group.

  - Summary of key points by faculty.

- How to adapt:

  - You may wish to assign the worksheet as homework to be completed before the session or as a follow-up assignment.

  - Select only those questions that apply to your teaching. Modify questions as appropriate to match the specialty or the learners' practice context.

- Logistics:

  - Copies of worksheets, flip chart paper.

  - Extra pens for learners.

T4 SIMULATION: PATIENT-CENTEREDNESS

Instructions for Teacher:

- FOCUS of this activity is an opportunity to 'try out' a variety of patient-physician relationships while staying patient-centred.

- Assign learners a scenario and one or two of the physician relationships.

- You can use the sample scenarios as part of small group activity to explore the style and type of patient-physician relationship. Please add appropriate details to scenarios (e.g. script development for standardized patient) to maximize the learning.

- This approach and cases can also be used to develop online simulations or simulated examinations such as OSCEs.

- Another adaptation is to use this framing to debrief patient-centredness in the workplace.

SAMPLE SCENARIOS (add detail to maximize learning)

- Patient with end stage dementia has stopped eating, drinking and has a urinary tract infection.

- Patient with breast cancer trying to decide what treatment to have.

- Patient with new diagnosis of young onset Parkinson's disease.

- Patient who is frail with diabetes, kidney disease and cataracts.

- Patient who abuses prescription medication is hospitalized for a fractured arm from a fall down a flight of stairs in the community.

T5 WARD ROUNDS: ORAL CASE PRESENTATION

Instructions for Teacher:

- Teaching your learners to present cases in the SNAPPS[a] format encourages them to reflect on the problem and possible solutions before quizzing you. SNAPPS is a good way to promote higher level clinical reasoning skills. While similar to the One-minute Preceptor, SNAPPS is much more learner-driven. This approach is particularly effective when used in longitudinal clinics, horizontal curriculums or where the learner-teacher have a series of opportunities to work together.

- This tool can be assigned to prepare for ward rounds.

- This tool could also be used as a portfolio submission.

- Indicate the number of case presentations via SNAPPS to be completed and when they are to be presented.

- After the ward rounds are completed, it is important to review and debrief, reinforce learning, focus areas for clarification or improvement.

T8 SUMMARY SHEET FOR THE MEDICAL EXPERT ROLE

Instructions for Teacher:

- The summary sheet is intended to be a cheat sheet for the teacher as well as the learner. It is a one page resource on key concepts, frameworks and approaches.

- You may wish to review and customize the summary sheet based on local information important to your learners.

---

a Wolpaw TM, Wolpaw DR, Papp KK. SNAPPS: a learner-centered model for outpatient education. *Acad Med.* 2003; 78(9):893-8.

© 2015 Royal College of Physicians and Surgeons of Canada

Medical Expert

Medical Expert

MEDICAL EXPERT ROLE TEACHER TIPS APPENDIX (continued)

A1 MULTISOURCE FEEDBACK: TYPES OF EXPERTISE

Instructions for Teacher:

- The FOCUS of this activity is an opportunity for formative assessment and coaching to guide learners about what aspects of expertise need attention.

- Could also be adapted to a summative tool with addition of more description on expectation for learner level and program

- Modify the form by adding or removing criteria that do/ not apply.

- To optimize learning and to protect the identity of those who provide feedback, be mindful of the size and composition of your data sample.

- Be sure to provide your 'assessors' with clear instructions and provide guidance on your rating scale. You may plan faculty development to support assessors and improve consistency in completion.

- It is a good idea to notify your learners of your intention and rationale for collecting feedback on their teaching skills. Be clear about the timeframe when you will collect the data, how you will maintain confidentiality and how and when you will present the data back to the learner.

- Plan to share the summary of feedback with your learner in written format and in a face to face meeting. A face to face meeting will allow valuable coaching around areas of strength and areas for improvement.

© 2015 Royal College of Physicians and Surgeons of Canada

REFERENCES

1. Canadian Association of Occupational Therapy(CAOT), The Profile of Occupational Therapy in Canada. Ottawa; 2007. Last retrieved July 11, 2015 from: https://www.caot.ca/pdfs/otprofile.pdf

2. National Physiotherapy Advisory Group. *Physician Competeny Profile for Physiotherapists in Canada.* 2009. Available from: http://www.physiotherapyeducation.ca/Resources/Essential%20Comp%20PT%20Profile%20 2009.pdf

3. Learner's Dictionary. *Expertise.* Last retrieved July 11, 2015 from www.learnersdictionary.com/definition/expertise

4. Dreyfus H, Dreyfus S. *Mind over machine: the power of human intuitive expertise in the era of the computer.* New York: Free Press; 1986.

5. Online Dictionary. *Cognitive.* Last retrieved August 4, 2015 http://dictionary.reference.com/browse/cognitive

6. Uttal WR. *A taxonomy of visual processes.* Psychology Press, 2014.

7. *Miller-Keane Encyclopedia and Dictionary of Medicine, Nursing, and Allied Health.* Seventh Edition. © by Saunders, an imprint of Elsevier, Inc. 2003.

8. Tough P. *How Children Succeed: Grit, Curiosity, and the Hidden Power of Character.* Houghton, Mifflin and Harcourt; 2012.

9. Ambrose SA, Bridges MW, DiPietro M, Lovett MC, Norman MK, editors. *How learning works: seven research-based principles for smart teaching.* San Francisco, p 104.

10. Ericsson, KA. Deliberate practice and acquisition of expert performance: a general overview. *Acad Emerg Med* 2008; 15(11):98894.

11. Karabenick SA, Knapp JR. Relationship of academic help seeking to the use of learning strategies and other instrumental achievement behavior in college students. *Educ Psychol* 1991;83(2):221.

12. Scope of practice definition. Scope of practice working group. Royal College of Physician and Surgeons of Canada. 2015.

13. Committee on Quality of Health Care in America, Institute of Medicine. 2001. *Crossing the quality chasm: a new health system for the 21st century.* Washington, D.C.: National Academy Press. Last retrieved July 11, 2015, from http://iom.edu/Reports/2001/Crossing-the-Quality-Chasm-A-New-Health-System-for-the-21st-Century.aspx

14. This definition has been developed on the basis of information found on Wikipedia: *Shared decision-making.* Last retrieved July 11, 2015, from http://en.wikipedia.org/wiki/Shared_decision-making

15. Emanuel EJ, Emanuel LL. Four Models of the Physician-Patient Relationship. *JAMA.* 1992;267(16):2221-6.

16. Houston P, Conn R, Rajan, M, Sinha R. *Issues Related to Residents as Workers and Learners.* Members of the FMEC PG consortium; 2011. Last retrieved July 11, 2015 from: https://www.afmc.ca/pdf/fmec/09_Houston_Worker%20and%20 Learners.pdf

17. Han R, Kim VH-D. Setting a Climate for Help-Seeking in Postgraduate Medical Education: a Theoretical Framework for Understanding Barriers and Strategies for Successful Help-Seeking. University of Toronto. 2015. Unpublished manuscript.

18. Choosing Wisely Canada. *What is CWC?* Last retrieved July 3, 2015, from http://www.choosingwiselycanada.org/about/what-is-cwc/

19. Christakis DA, Feudtner C. Ethics in a short white coat: The ethical dilemmas that medical students confront. *Acad Med.* 1993; 68(4): 249-54.

20. Kennedy TJT, Regehr G, Baker FR, Lingard L. Preserving professional credibility: Grounded theory study of medical trainees' requests for clinical support. *BMJ.* 2009;338,b128.

21. Payakachat N, Gubbins PO, Ragland D, Norman SE, Flowers SK, Stowe CD, Dettart RM, Pace A, Hastings JK. Academic help-seeking behavior among student pharmacists. *Am Pharm Ed.* 2013; 77(1): 7.

22. Smith R. Thoughts for new medical students at a new medical school. *BMJ.* 2003;327(7429):1430-3.

23. Schumacher DJ, Bria C, Frohna G. The quest toward unsupervised practice – promoting autonomy, not independence. *JAMA.* 2013;310(24):2613-4.

24. Ten Cate O. Viewpoint: Competence-based postgraduate training: Can we bridge the gap between theory and clinical practice? *Acad Med.* 2007;82(6):542-7.

25. Adapted from Neher JO, Stevens NG. The one-minute preceptor: shaping the teaching conversation. *Fam Med.* 2003;35(6):391-3.

26. Sackett DL, Rosenberg WMC, Muir Gray JA, Haynes RB, Richardson WS. Evidence-based medicine: what it is and what it isn't. *BMJ.* 1996;312(7023):71-2.

© 2015 Royal College of Physicians and Surgeons of Canada

BOUNDARIES
Building rapport
Conveying THERAPEUTIC
RELATIONSHIP
INFORMED CONSENT
History EMPATHIZING
taking
ACTIVE LISTENING Common ground
COMMUNICATOR
Difficult discussion **DISCHARGE PLANNING**
PATIENT-CENTRED
Shared decision-making
Documentation NON-VERBAL
COMMUNICATION SKILLS
Categorization
SIGNPOSTING

Sue Dojeiji

Dawn Martin

Susan Glover Takahashi

1. Why the Communicator Role matters

Communicating effectively with patients is an essential element of the practice of medicine. Evidence shows that patients have better outcomes and are more satisfied when they have helpful conversations about their health care with their doctors. Similarly, the ability to communicate well in writing is vitally important to patient care in many specialties where core activities regularly include preparing patient documents such as consultation letters, reports on test results, and various procedural reports.

There are numerous studies[1] of the impact of effective and ineffective physician-patient communication.

The evidence says that effective communication skills are an essential element for creating a "culture of safety" that supports the safe delivery of patient care. Furthermore, effective communication results in:[2, 3]

- increased accuracy, which improves patient understanding, recall, and compliance, and increases efficiency for patients and physicians;

- improved outcomes of care (physiological and psychological);

- heightened perceptions by patients that they are being supported by their physicians, resulting in improved relationships between patients and caregivers and higher satisfaction for patients and physicians;

- reduced rates of adverse events and medical errors, and

- better protection against complaints and malpractice claims.

Evolving technology, health care systems, and societal expectations can challenge the ability of patients and physicians to establish strong therapeutic relationships. For this reason, learners need to acknowledge the value of their relationships with their patients and be encouraged to leverage opportunities to reinforce positive relationships. They must also build on the basic communication skills acquired at the undergraduate level, so they can explore with patients their needs, values, and preferences, while also developing and then honing new specialty skills.

2. What the Communicator Role looks like in daily practice

The CanMEDS Framework is an educational construct that organizes complex competencies into seven major themes or roles; as much as possible, these Roles are meant to be distinct and intuitive with regard to the competencies. Experience tells us, however, that learners sometimes struggle to distinguish between different Roles in their daily practice. This is understandable, given that experienced physicians often switch between Roles seamlessly. It is important that teachers highlight the competencies to help learners identify the different Roles.

In day-to-day practice, the Communicator Role is often intertwined with the Medical Expert Role because of the centrality of communication in the clinical encounter. Two examples of where and how the Communicator Role can be intertwined with other CanMEDS Roles include:

- **Professional Role:** When completing a social history (e.g. medications and drug history, sexual history, family history) with a patient, the physician uses an empathetic, patient-centred approach to the encounter to be sensitive to the patient's discomfort (i.e. Communicator) while ensuring professional boundaries are respected (i.e. Professional).

- **Health Advocate Role:** When talking with the patient to identify barriers to a healthy diet caused by a low income (i.e. Health Advocate), the physician focuses on using an empathetic approach to elicit the patient's perspective on the issue so that solutions can be found together (i.e. Communicator). Compassion is empathy in action.

© 2015 Royal College of Physicians and Surgeons of Canada

Key features of good communication in daily practice

1. **Good communication is an interaction** rather than a monologue, speech, or other one-way transmission. Aim for communication that is like a boomerang, which comes back to you.

2. **Good communication is dynamic** and responsive to several factors (e.g. one size does not fit all):

   - the nature of the problem: acute versus chronic, severe versus mild, major versus minor

   - the setting: outpatient community clinic, emergency department, inpatient hospital unit, operating room, laboratory

   - the patient: age, education level, values, beliefs, preferences, physical and cognitive impairments, health literacy, culture

   - the physician: values, beliefs, biases, experience, expertise

3. **Good communication reduces uncertainty.** Uncertainty leads to anxiety, which in turn can block effective communication. Imagine a patient who is entering an electrodiagnostic clinic for the first time and doesn't know what to expect. A quick orientation to the testing process may help reduce the patient's apprehension and facilitate communication for the rest of the interaction.

4. **Good communication is preceded by planning and thinking about purposes and outcomes.** It's important to think about your intentions and goals before communicating with a patient. If, after the interaction, the outcome is not what you had intended, you can consider how to modify your approach the next time.

5. **Good communication evolves with practice, feedback, and reiteration.** As with other skills in clinical practice, communication skills are not static. The communication skills learned in medical school (which are mostly related to data gathering) are not sufficient in residency. In residency, learners will be expected, for example, to accurately explain diagnoses and options for treatment in plain language as well as to negotiate treatment plans with their patients. Once learners can competently explain information to a patient in a clear and organized manner using minimal medical jargon, they can progress to explaining a plan in a more challenging clinical scenario, such as breaking bad news to a patient with a different cultural background from their own (i.e. situations that are more complex and may be emotionally charged).

6. **Patient-centred does not mean 'patient controlled'.** The communication approach should reflect the needs of the patient (i.e. more physician directed in highly acute medical situations).

If your learners are struggling to distinguish the Communicator Role among the various CanMEDS Roles, encourage them to listen for some of the following trigger words and phrases, (see Table COM-1) which can be associated with communication skills. When they hear or use these words and phrases, they can be relatively confident that they are functioning within the Communicator Role of the CanMEDS Framework.

Communicator

TABLE COM-1. TRIGGER WORDS RELATING TO THE COMMUNICATOR ROLE

• Acknowledging feelings/ideas	• Bad news
• Active listening	• Biomedical and social history
• Building rapport	• Boundaries
• Conveying	• Common ground
• Developing a therapeutic relationship	• Discharge planning
• Empathizing	• Disclosure of harmful patient safety incidents
• Facilitating conversations	• Documentation
• Incorporating perspectives	• Electronic medical information
• Providing structure to the interview	• Family meeting
• Setting an agenda	• Informed consent
• Sharing information	• Patient-centred
	• Sexual history taking

© 2015 Royal College of Physicians and Surgeons of Canada

Communicator

Excerpt from the CanMEDS 2015 Physician Competency Framework[a]

DEFINITION

As Communicators, physicians form relationships with patients and their families[b] that facilitate the gathering and sharing of essential information for effective health care.[c]

DESCRIPTION

Physicians enable patient-centred therapeutic communication by exploring the patient's symptoms, which may be suggestive of disease, and by actively listening to the patient's experience of his or her illness. Physicians explore the patient's perspective, including his or her fears, ideas about the illness, feelings about the impact of the illness, and expectations of health care and health care professionals. The physician integrates this knowledge with an understanding of the patient's context, including socio-economic status, medical history, family history, stage of life, living situation, work or school setting, and other relevant psychological and social issues. Central to a patient-centred approach is shared decision-making: finding common ground with the patient in developing a plan to address his or her medical problems and health goals in a manner that reflects the patient's needs, values, and preferences. This plan should be informed by evidence and guidelines.

Because illness affects not only patients but also their families, physicians must be able to communicate effectively with everyone involved in the patient's care.

KEY COMPETENCIES

Physicians are able to:

1. Establish professional therapeutic relationships with patients and their families

2. Elicit and synthesize accurate and relevant information, incorporating the perspectives of patients and their families

3. Share health care information and plans with patients and their families

4. Engage patients and their families in developing plans that reflect the patient's health care needs and goals

5. Document and share written and electronic information about the medical encounter to optimize clinical decision-making, patient safety, confidentiality, and privacy

---

a Neville A, Weston W, Martin D, Samson L, Feldman P, Wallace G, Jamoulle O, François J, Lussier M-T, Dojeiji S. Communicator. In: Frank JR, Snell L, Sherbino J, editors. CanMEDS 2015 Physician Competency Framework. Ottawa: Royal College of Physicians and Surgeons of Canada; 2015. Reproduced with permission.
b Throughout the CanMEDS 2015 Physician Competency Framework and Milestones Guide, references to the patient's family are intended to include all those who are personally significant to the patient and are concerned with his or her care, including, according to the patient's circumstances, family members, partners, caregivers, legal guardian, and substitute decision-makers.
c Note that the Communicator Role describes the abilities related to a physician–patient encounter. Other communication skills are found elsewhere in the framework, including health care team communication (Collaborator) and academic presentations (Scholar).

© 2015 Royal College of Physicians and Surgeons of Canada

KEY TERMS OF THE COMMUNICATOR ROLE[4]

To help your learners familiarize themselves with the Communicator Role, have them review key words that are central to the Communicator Role:

Three types of communication skills[4]

1. *Content communication skills* are what doctors communicate. The skills revolve around the substance of the physician's responses to the patient's questions, the information the physician gathers and gives, and the treatment the physician discusses with the patient.

2. *Process communication skills* are how doctors communicate. These skills include the ways doctors go about obtaining the history or providing information, the verbal and non-verbal skills the physician uses, how the physician develops therapeutic relationships with patients, and the way the physician organizes and structures communication in a clinical encounter.

3. *Perceptual communication skills* are often referred to as intra-personal communication (communication within self) or personal capacities. Perceptual skills are the core of communication skills — they are what you feel and think. They include authenticity, commitment, integrity, trust, and trustworthiness. These capacities impact on our communication skills. Personal capacities apply across all CanMEDS Roles; they are particularly relevant in the Professional Role, yet they are highlighted in Communicator owing to their significant interrelationship with communication skills. For example, irritation with a patient (perceptual) can interfere with active listening and lead us to miss important patient cues (process).

Empathy[4] is a key skill in developing the physician-patient relationship. It has two parts: the understanding and sensitive appreciation of another's predicament or feeling; and the communication of that understanding back to the patient in a supportive way. It does not necessarily equate to agreeing with the patient's feelings. An example is "I can see that your husband's memory loss has been very difficult for you to cope with." Empathy is often confused with sympathy, which is feeling pity or concern from outside of the patient's perspective.

The *therapeutic relationship* is the working alliance between the physician and patient. Respect (i.e. unconditional positive regard), genuineness, and empathy have been correlated with good therapeutic outcomes.[5]

A *patient-centred approach* is one "providing care that is respectful of and responsive to individual patient preferences, needs, and values, and ensuring that patient values inform all clinical decisions."[6,d]

An *encounter* is a purposeful patient–physician interaction.

Common ground forms the basis for trust and relationship-building; it involves using an encounter(s) to help the physician and patient identify with one another. It doesn't mean the doctor and the patient necessarily agree with each other, but they understand and acknowledge the other perspective.[1] Common ground provides a basis for mutual interest or agreement.[7]

Shared decision-making[8] is an important component of communication when patients and their health care professionals, including the physician, make decisions about the best course of action.[1] These shared decisions are informed by the patient's preferences, needs, and values as well as by the available options and evidence, which are often conveyed by the health care professional. Shared decision-making involves patients to the degree that they wish; it allows patients to understand the decision-making process, and it increases patients' commitment to the plans.

Plain language is the use of common words that a patient can easily understand. This may mean avoiding technical or medical terms unless they are carefully defined or described.

---

d Patient-centredness (e.g. the physician–patient relationship) is one of the four levels of relationships in a relationship-centred practice, which is described in more detail in the Collaborator Role of this Tools Guide.

© 2015 Royal College of Physicians and Surgeons of Canada

A *difficult discussion* is a patient-physician interaction related to the patient's health care preferences, needs, and values that can be challenging because of the high level or intensity of the emotion involved. The topics considered challenging or difficult vary on the basis of the patient's characteristics or personality, preferences, needs, and values; the physician's characteristics or personality, preferences, needs, values, and comfort level; and the environmental, cultural, and health care contexts.

Non-verbal communication skills[4] are the skills involved in transmitting information without the use of words. They include body language (e.g. facial expressions, eye contact, gestures), paraverbal skills (e.g. pace, tone, pitch, rhythm, volume, articulation, use of pauses), touch, smell, space, and clothing. Non-verbal communication is responsible for conveying most of our attitudes, emotions, and affect. If there is disconnect between verbal and non-verbal communication, non-verbal communication can override the words we speak.

Signposting is a process skill used throughout the clinical encounter and especially in the explanation and planning portion. Signposting involves the use of bridging statements to alert patients that you are changing topics or direction in the encounter. Signposts help the patient understand where the interview is going and why. They also help provide structure to the interview and act as guide markers to keep you organized and the patient focused. An example is "I've just finished getting a history of your stomach pain; now I would like to do a physical exam. Is that okay?"[4]

Categorization is a process skill used in the explanation and planning portion of the clinical encounter. Categorization helps orient the patient to specific details about how information is going to be discussed. It also aids in patient recall. For example, "There are three important things I want to explain about your nerve injury: (1) how it happened, (2) how it will heal, and (3) how we will treat it." This skill can be used effectively with signposting: "We have talked about how it happened; now let's talk about how the nerve is going to heal…"[4]

Chunking and checking is a process skill used in the explanation and planning portion of the clinical encounter. The physician provides one piece of information and then pauses to verify that the patient understands before giving another piece. It is a technique used to gauge how much information to give to a patient. This approach aids in achieving a shared understanding with the patient, and in improving patient recall of information.[4]

A *safety net* is a component of closing the clinical encounter whereby a set of contingency plans is discussed at the end of the clinical encounter. Providing a safety net for the patient involves explaining what the patient should do if things do not go according to plan, telling them how they should contact you, and discussing what developments might require back-up.[4]

© 2015 Royal College of Physicians and Surgeons of Canada

3. Preparing to teach the Communicator Role

The Communicator Role includes verbal and written or electronic competencies. Communication with patients is how your learners will develop an understanding of their patients' health care preferences, needs, and values. Communication is also about gathering and sharing of patient-related information through written and electronic documentation in support of the patient's health care preferences, needs, and values. In this section we review some key concepts that will help you prepare to teach the Communicator Role by addressing some common misconceptions about the Role and exploring how to integrate the content and process of the Communicator Role into practice.

3.1 Common misconceptions to address with learners

One of the first misconceptions that you may address with your learners is the idea that you can not teach or assess communication skills. Many people think that communication skills are subjective or related to personal style and that they are fundamentally linked to one's personality and being nice. Many people feel that good communicators are just "born that way" — in other words, you either have it or you don't. The research shows otherwise. Some people might be more natural communicators, but **communication skills are skills that can be readily defined, taught, and assessed in an objective and systematic manner.**

The second misconception is that communication skills "naturally" improve over time. During day-to-day practice, learners are often focused on developing their clinical knowledge and skills and few pay much attention to how they communicate what they know. Learners' **communication skills need to be intentionally developed and refined over time in the same way as all essential clinical skills in medicine.**

Not only do communication skills deteriorate over time, less than optimal communication approaches left uncorrected become bad habits. For example, learners may begin patient encounters using a closed approach because they believe it is more effective and efficient than an open-ended approach, not recognizing that the latter approach not only gives patients the opportunity to be heard and acknowledged but also often elicits more accurate and time-efficient histories. As with other areas of expertise, there is no ceiling to communication skills.

The third misconception is that communication skills improve through passive observation. In the same way that they learn other skills (e.g. physical examination), your learners benefit from first learning a framework for good communication, watching and analyzing the use of the framework, and then engaging in iterative loops of practice with specific, focused feedback. Your learners **need to actively engage in the development of their communication skills through deliberate practice** that is observed and assessed both informally and formally.

3.2 Help learners understand patient communication challenges

Communication with anyone in a noisy, action-filled clinical setting can be problematic, so learners should be prepared to invest effort and attention to communicate effectively with a patient who is unwell, is injured, or has other stressors. Many patients do not have the necessary knowledge or skills to manage their health care needs adequately (i.e. to understand medication-taking instructions). For learners, this means they may need to work on developing specialized communication skills for patients who:

- are children or youth,
- have socio-cultural and/or ethnic backgrounds that require the participation of family members or the use of an interpreter,
- have difficulty hearing,
- have cognitive impairments (e.g. from a stroke, head trauma, medication) or have mental health conditions.

Furthermore, the demands of seeing many patients in the course of a day who have different needs and preferences can be challenging. It is easy to become complacent, take shortcuts, and become less attentive as the day unfolds. Help learners look for opportunities to minimize the possibility that their patients will misinterpret their intentions. Remind them that making assumptions about a patient's understanding, level of agreement, needs, and preferences is a common pitfall leading to misunderstanding. Learners need to ask clear questions, clarify information, and provide their rationale. They also must not be afraid to apologize if an assumption has led to a misunderstanding.

Communicator

3.3 Use a communication skills framework to teach learners verbal communication skills

Clinician teachers generally focus on teaching content skills, otherwise known as the "what" of communication (e.g. features of the traditional medical history, such as the history of the presenting illness). They often overlook the "how" or process of communication (e.g. strategies to improve patient understanding and recall). Integrating content and process skills improves the efficiency of the task under way and better meets the needs of both patients and physicians. But the task is made difficult by curricula that teach the "what" and "how" elements separately (i.e. the medical history-taking course is taught separately from communication skills courses).

There are many communication skills frameworks. Choosing a structured framework is essential to guide teaching, facilitate assessment, and create a common lexicon of communication "jargon" for teachers and learners. Kurtz et al suggest that a framework will serve as a "life raft" for learners struggling with their communication and provide validation for those who are doing well.[1] As well, a framework is helpful to teachers unfamiliar with communication skills and training.

If you don't already have a preferred framework for your own teaching, you can begin teaching communication skills with the Calgary-Cambridge Observation Guide[9], which outlines six communication tasks in a framework that is widely used to teach learners. (Figure COM-1).

Portions of the framework can be used at the bedside to observe discrete aspects of the patient-learner interaction (i.e. how well did the learner explain the impression and plan to the patient?), or the entire framework can provide the basis for an academic half-day formal session on communication skills related to explanation and planning.

Tables COM-2 and COM-3 illustrate how content and process can be taught together by integrating the usual steps of the clinical encounter with the tasks of the Calgary–Cambridge Observation Guide.

FIGURE COM-1 CALGARY-CAMBRIDGE OBSERVATION GUIDE[e,f,1,9]

PROVIDING STRUCTURE
- Making organization overt
- Attending to flow

INITIATING THE SESSION
- Preparation
- Establishing initial rapport
- Identifying the reason(s) for the consultation

GATHERING INFORMATION
- Exploration of the patient's problem to discover:
  - Biomedical perspective
  - The patient's perspective
  - Background information-context

PHYSICAL EXAMINATION

EXPLANATION AND PLANNING
- Providing the correct amount and type of information
- Aiding accurate recall and understanding
- Achieving a shared understanding: incorporating the patient's illness framework
- Planning: shared decision-making

CLOSING THE SESSION
- Ensuring appropriate point of closure
- Forward planning

BUILDING THE RELATIONSHIP
- Using appropriate nonverbal behaviour
- Developing rapport
- Involving the patient

---

e Silverman J, Kurtz S, Draper J. *Skills for communicating with patients.* 3rd ed. London: Radcliffe Publishing. Copyright © 2013. Reproduced by permission of Taylor & Francis Books UK.
f Kurtz S, Silverman J, Draper J. *Teaching and learning communication skills in medicine.* 2nd ed. London: Radcliffe Publishing. Copyright © 2005. Reproduced by permission of Taylor & Francis Books UK.

© 2015 Royal College of Physicians and Surgeons of Canada

TABLE COM-2. COMMUNICATION SKILLS CONTENT AND PROCESS

#	Communication skills task	When used in encounter
1.	Initiating the session	Beginning
2.	Gathering information and physical exam	Middle
3.	Explanation and planning	End
4.	Closing the session	End
5.	Providing structure	Ongoing
6.	Building the relationship	Ongoing

TABLE COM-3. CONTENT AND PROCESS COMMUNICATION SKILLS IN A CLINICAL ENCOUNTER USING THE CALGARY-CAMBRIDGE OBSERVATION GUIDE[1]

#	COMMUNICATION TASK	PURPOSES	"WHAT" SAMPLE Content to Discover	"HOW" SAMPLE Process Skills to Use
1.	INITIATING THE SESSION	• Establishing initial rapport • Identifying the reason for the visit	• Clear understanding of the patient's reason for initiating or being invited to the visit (reduces uncertainty) • Clarify information about the presenting problem	• Greets the patient • Listens attentively to the patient's opening statement without interrupting
2.	GATHERING INFO AND PHYSICAL EXAM	• Exploration of the patient problem to discover: • Biomedical perspective (disease) • Patient perspective (illness) • Background information – context	• Sequence of events; symptom analysis; medical management to date • Past history; family history • Patient's concerns, ideas (beliefs about cause)	• Uses open and closed questioning techniques, appropriately moving from one to the other • Actively explores patient's ideas, feelings, expectations, and concerns of the presenting issue(s) and the impact of the issue(s) on the patient's life
3.	EXPLANATION AND PLANNING	• Providing the correct type and level of information • Aiding accurate recall and understanding • Achieving a shared understanding – incorporating the patient's perspective • Planning – shared decision-making	• Differential diagnosis, or hypothesis; Investigations; Treatment plan; lifestyle changes • What the patient has understood of what he/she's been told • Patient's perspective on the information provided and proposed treatment plan	• Gives information in manageable chunks, then checks for understanding • Uses explicit categorization (e.g. "There are three important things that I would like to discuss: first,..." • Picks up and responds to verbal and non-verbal cues • Explores management options
4.	CLOSING THE SESSION	• Ensuring appropriate point of closure • Forward planning	• Clear plan of action • What to do if Plan "A" does not work	• Summarizes session briefly and clarifies plan of care • Establishes a safety net on what to do if plan is not working
5.	BUILDING THE RELATIONSHIP	• Developing a therapeutic alliance • Involving the patient	• Patient feels empowered to be active participants in their own health care	• Shares thinking with patient to encourage patient's involvement (e.g. "What I am thinking now is....")
6.	PROVIDING STRUCTURE	• Making organization overt • Attending to flow	• Patient has the opportunity to tell his or her story within a structured framework that attends to the patient's and physician's needs	• Progresses from one section to another using signposting and transitional statements • Structures interview in logical sequence

© 2015 Royal College of Physicians and Surgeons of Canada

Communicator

3.4 Help learners manage pitfalls and problems with verbal communication

In addition to teaching and supporting good communication, it is important to know when and where there may be problems and how to fix them. Table COM-4 shows common communication pitfalls, their negative impact on the patient or on the encounter, and how you can get the learner back on track. You might also want to share with your learners the following that may assist in reducing the chances for miscommunication.

3.5 Teach learners written communication skills by integrating content and style

Physicians are required to document and share written and electronic information about the medical encounter in a way that optimizes clinical decision-making, patient safety, confidentiality, and privacy. Documentation is a medico-legal requirement as well.

A common example of written communication is the consultation letter, where the specialist sends a letter to a referring physician about their patient's presenting problem. Other forms of written communication include the inpatient discharge summary, inpatient progress notes, operative notes, diagnostic imaging interpretation reports, and laboratory interpretation reports.

HINTS FOR PATIENT-CENTREDNESS

1. **Orient yourself to the patient**

   Before you start a conversation with a patient, it is important to be situationally aware and oriented to the relationship with this patient — in other words, make sure you are patient-centred. Situational factors that need to be considered each time include:

   - Is there a prior patient-physician relationship? (Is this the first time you have had a conversation, or is this a follow-up visit? Or is this a long-standing patient-physician relationship? How have any past encounters proceeded?)

   - What type of problem does the patient have? (minor or serious)

   - What is the nature of the patient's problem? (acute, urgent or chronic)

   - What are the particular needs of this patient? (e.g. health literacy, personality, age, gender)

   - Where will the communication take place? (e.g. office, clinic, emergency department, health facility)

   - What orienting information is available? (e.g. charts, health care professional debriefing or handover information)

2. **Watch for signals and cues**

   During a patient-physician encounter, it is important to pay attention to signals and cues that provide feedback about understanding, misunderstanding, or disagreement, such as:

   - signals of shared understanding (e.g. smiles, nods, relaxed or open body language) and

   - cues to misunderstanding or disagreement (e.g. looking away, shaking head, arms crossed, tensed muscles, silence, closed body language).

   Be cautious about interpreting signals and cues, since they vary by person and are influenced by the patient's experience and background. For example, silence is not necessarily a sign of understanding and agreement. Seek confirmation frequently, provide opportunities for questions, and encourage patients' concerns.

3. **Be careful about labels**

   - Be careful about using labels such as 'minor' and 'mild'.

   - Sometimes what a physician views as 'minor' and 'mild' will be perceived very differently by the patient, who has different views and needs. For example, a 'minor' sprained ankle or 'mild' stroke may not be viewed as 'minor' or 'mild' by the patient.

© 2015 Royal College of Physicians and Surgeons of Canada

TABLE COM-4. SAMPLE VERBAL COMMUNICATION PITFALLS AND THEIR IMPACTS AND FIXES

Communication skills pitfall[1,9]	Impact on the patient or on the encounter	Suggested fix
1. INTRODUCTION Learner forgets to introduce self, role or responsibility	• Missed opportunity to build a trusting relationship with the patient • In some cases, the patient doesn't realize the physician was in to visit • Confusion and uncertainty	While it may seem fairly intuitive, the majority of the time when communication breaks down, it has to do with the very beginning — physicians do not explain clearly who they are and what their role is in the patient's care before jumping into the medical encounter. Encourage learners to take the time to introduce themselves and to explain their role on the health care team
2. GATHERING INFORMATION Physician-centred approach	The physician-centred questions (e.g. where is the pain, when did it start, where does it go, what makes it better or worse) are critical. However, to better understand the patient problem, learners need to better understand the patient's context. Critical information to guide the management plan will be missed. This may impact on patient adherence	Remind the learner that asking patients about their perceptions of their presenting problem at the beginning of the encounter will often elicit useful information
3. EXPLANATION AND PLANNING The soliloquy – i.e. learners often share information in long run-on sentences, moving from topic to topic without pausing in-between	Patient is overwhelmed and does not know what information to attend to	Work with the learner to break up the content into manageable chunks. Encourage the learner to pause after each chunk to check for patient understanding and for the patient to ask questions
4. CLOSING THE SESSION Learner assumes Plan A is going to unfold as planned	Unless a safety net is stated explicitly, patients may improvise or stop a plan when common side effects occur or unexpected problems arise; patients may go to the emergency room or to their family physician unless they are told explicitly who to contact if a treatment plan is not proceeding as expected	When reviewing cases with the learner, take a moment to discuss the plan "B" in the event plan "A" does not work — this is the safety net for the patient. Patient uncertainly and anxiety will lessen when there is an explicit discussion of what to do in the event of treatment failure. Tell the learner to provide patients with clear direction on what to do, if more questions or issues arise
5. BUILDING THE RELATIONSHIP Learner does not pay attention to their own non-verbal communication	*How* words are said has far more impact on patients than *what* is said. Learners need to be mindful of their own non-verbal communication skills as these can impact on the patient interaction (e.g. closed posture with arms and legs crossed, eye contact focused on the paper/computer, speaking quickly)	Regularly get learners to reflect on what they were thinking and feeling during an encounter (i.e. perceptual skills) Some options to consider when training non-verbal communication: • directly observe learner's non-verbal communication • videotape simulated encounter and discuss NVC seen in interaction
6. PROVIDING STRUCTURE Learner mistakes a patient-controlled approach with being patient-centred	Often learners will come away from a complex patient interaction completely overwhelmed by details of the history, particularly if the patient was in complete control of the encounter. Learners confuse allowing the patient to tell their story with allowing the patient to control the encounter	Tell the learner that there is a fine line between allowing the patient to provide their story and ensuring the needs of the patient and physician are met by obtaining the essential details from the patient. Remind the learner that the patient may be driving the bus, but physicians have a say on the route taken

Communicator

As with verbal communication skills, there are content considerations (i.e. what essential information needs to be included?) and process considerations (i.e. how should the letter or note be organized so that it is easy for the reader to scan?) for written communication skills. Often, process considerations in written communication are referred to as the style of the letter (e.g. length of sentences and paragraphs, and whether to use tables and graphics).

Written communication skills require your specific attention during residency training. Skills acquisition is most successful when specific skills are delineated (i.e. what makes a consultation letter or discharge summary effective?), when learners are given the opportunity to practise and reiterate the skills, and when clinical teachers provide regular, specific, timely, and intentional feedback on how learners can improve their written communications.

A framework can be helpful in teaching residents written communication skills. Table COM-5 outlines a sample structure for written communications that focuses on content and style and their respective purposes:

- The purpose of content is to convey what is considered essential, important, or relevant based on the specific patient, population, and context.
- The purpose of style is to make the documentation easier to read.

Table COM-6 illustrates a framework for incorporating content and style for specific communication tasks such as a consultation letter. What goes into the written communication (content) will be influenced by the purpose of the document, but the general principles of style (such as simplified language, use of white space) will likely be the same no matter what is being written.

3.6 Help learners manage pitfalls and problems with written communication

Table COM-7 shows areas where learners commonly struggle with their written communication skills, along with the negative impact of these pitfalls on the patient or the referral source.

TABLE COM-5. SAMPLE CONSULTATION LETTER COMMUNICATION FRAMEWORK

CONTENT		Sample details
1.	History	• Chief problem/reason for referral • Chief complaint • Relevant past history • Current medications, as appropriate • Other history appropriate to presenting problem: psychosocial history, functional history, family history, review of systems, etc.
2.	Physical Exam	• Details and facts on what has been done: for example, describe physical examination findings relevant to presenting problem
3.	Impression and Management	• Diagnosis and/or differential diagnosis • Management plan • Rationale for the management plan (education) • Report on whether the management plan was discussed with patient • Notes on who will be responsible for elements of the management plan and follow-up • Answer the referring physicians question (if present)
STYLE		**Sample details**
4.	Clarity and Brevity	• Words used: - short (less than three syllables) - active voice - minimal medical jargon; minimal filler words/phrases - no word or phrase repetition • Length of sentences: - one idea per sentence - each sentence less than three lines long • Length of paragraphs: - one topic per paragraph - each paragraph less than four to five sentences long
5.	Organization of Letter	• Use of headings • Layout visually appealing with lots of white space • Use of bulleted or numbered lists, tables, or graphics as appropriate • Information easy to scan

© 2015 Royal College of Physicians and Surgeons of Canada

TABLE COM-6. EXAMPLES OF WRITTEN COMMUNICATION SKILLS FRAMEWORK

COMMUNICATION TASK	PURPOSE	CONTENT	STYLE
CONSULTATION LETTER	Communicates findings and opinions to the referring physician effectively and efficiently Acts as the record for the consultant	**Referring physicians want:** • The consultant's impressions (dx and answer to the referring question) • Management plan (who will do what and when) • Medication changes • Rationale for recommendations • Who is providing ongoing care • Guidance and education (e.g. articles, advice, guidelines) **Consultants want:** • Record of the history and physical exam • Context that enables the interpretation of investigations • Proof the consultation took place	**Simplify Language:** • Few or no abbreviations and acronyms (i.e. use only institution approved acronyms) • Short words (less than three syllables) • Active instead of. passive voice ("I saw Ms. X …" vs "Ms. X was seen …") **Increase visual impact (i.e. more white space):** • Headings to organize material • Bullet points for some sections • Short sentences (one idea per sentence) • Short paragraphs (four or five sentences) • Graphics: lists, tables • Margins: left justify, ragged right • Appropriate font style and size
DISCHARGE SUMMARY	Post-discharge management	• Admission diagnosis • Pertinent physical exam • Pertinent lab results • Procedures completed • Complications in hospital • Discharge diagnosis • Discharge medications • Active medical problems • Follow-up plans — who will do what • Highlighted expectations of the referring or primary care physician	**Simplify Language:** • Few or no abbreviations and acronyms (i.e. use only institution approved acronyms) • Short words (less than three syllables) • Active instead of. passive voice ("I saw Ms. X …" vs "Ms. X was seen …") **Increase visual impact (i.e. more white space):** • Headings to organize material • Bullet points for some sections • Short sentences (one idea per sentence) • Short paragraphs (four or five sentences) • Graphics: lists, tables • Margins: left justify, ragged right • Appropriate font style and size

INPATIENT RECORD	Record of patient	• Individual hospital, province, and specialty will vary on record-keeping policies
		
		Key elements:
		• Admission history and physical (e.g. HPI, PMH, medications, allergies, physical exam, treatment plan)
		• Progress notes (e.g. care directions, procedures, new chief complaints, description and duration of symptoms, symptoms present, positive and negative physical exam findings, imaging, lab, consultant requests, diagnosis, treatment plan, advice provided to patient, doses/duration of medications
		• Consistency between written orders and progress notes
		• All notes must be signed with legible name, signature, and credentials
		
		Provide explicit information that:
		• Abnormal tests have been reviewed and are being followed
		• Periodic assessments are being done
		• Issues are being addressed and by whom
			• Style elements are similar to consultation letters (SEE above)
			• Also:
			  - Minimize use of abbreviations and acronyms
			  - Use SOAP format to organize progress notes (Subjective, Objective, Assessment Plan)
			  - Ensure the text is legible

© 2015 Royal College of Physicians and Surgeons of Canada

Communicator

TABLE COM-7. WRITTEN COMMUNICATION SKILLS PITFALLS AND THEIR IMPACTS

Type of written communication	Pitfall	Impact on patient or on referral source
CONSULTATION LETTER	• No attention to what information should be included in the letter: what is essential, important, or relevant is not considered (e.g. a lot of detail on the assessment, with little detail on the impression and treatment plan). The letter did not answer the referring physician's question. • The letter is not written and sent in a timely fashion. • Content is disorganized; there is a lack of content planning; wordiness (i.e. letter is filled with medical jargon and filler words that don't add to the meaning of the letter); no attention to visual layout with no white space, making the letter difficult to scan by a busy clinician.	• The length of the letter is irrelevant as long as the content is organized discretely and clearly. However, learners need to reflect on what content is deemed essential, important, or relevant to the patient population they are managing • Without a working knowledge of what is important, essential information may be hidden in the letter, rendering it unhelpful to the referring source and the treating physician; as well, learners have wasted time producing an ineffective letter • Delay in patient care if information not provided in a timely manner • Referring physician frustration as referring question not answered; this may generate another referral
DIAGNOSTIC IMAGING CONSULTATION REPORT	• Description of findings is poor, vague, variable, or inconclusive, with a lack of detail	• Frustration on referring physician's part • Potential for misunderstanding regarding diagnosis and next steps, leading to inappropriate use of resources (e.g. unnecessary additional tests) • Patient safety may be compromised if there is a delay in treatment because it was not clear that additional tests were needed
LABORATORY CONSULTATION REPORT	• Poor or vague impressions of the case with an unclear statement of reasons for the uncertainty • Incomplete report (missing parameters) • Incorrect use of language • Use of non-conventional terminology	• Report reader may make incorrect assumptions, potentially impacting treatment recommendations • Delays in treatment • Requests for second opinion via clinician • Improper grammar and ambiguities may lead to reader misunderstanding of the severity of findings
SURGICAL OPERATIVE REPORT	• Abbreviations used without citing specifics (e.g. AVSS) • Missing pertinent information (e.g. intraoperative findings, blood loss, placement of drains, pathology pending, intraoperative complications experienced, etc.) • Incorrect or incomplete procedure recorded	• Using abbreviations that are not known can result in misunderstanding of patients needs and/or delaying further intervention or alterations in management due to confusion • Missing information that can direct and alter post-operative care, investigations, or monitoring • Incorrect drains, etc., may be removed (especially in cases of multiple drains) • Perception of patient having undergone incorrect procedure leads to miscommunication with the patient, family, and consultants, and creates potential for confusion and loss of faith in the system and team
SURGICAL CONSULTATION REPORT	• A diagnosis but no recommendations	• Further investigations • Improper follow-up • Inaccurate expectations around recovery process • Missed opportunity to educate the physician
DISCHARGE SUMMARIES	• Lack of a discharge plan, with far too much focus on the details of what transpired and little information on the next steps and who is responsible for following up on the issues identified • Delay in discharge note	• Patient safety is jeopardized or compromised • Confusion and frustration for the primary care physician and community services providing follow-up • Delay in needed services

© 2015 Royal College of Physicians and Surgeons of Canada

Communicator

4. Hints, tips and tools for *teaching* the Communicator Role

As a teacher your goal is to deliver the right content and in a way that helps your learners learn. Sometimes you will teach directly. Other times you will facilitate and support the teaching of others or self-directed activities by learners. There are parts of the Communicator Role that can be especially difficult for learners to relate to and understand in the context of their work. For this reason this section of the Tools Guide includes a short menu of tips and tricks that are highly effective for teaching the Communicator Role. You can treat the list as a buffet: pick and choose the tips that resonate most and that will work for you, your program and your learners.

Teaching Tip 1.
Focus your learners equally on the "how" and the "what" of communication during a medical encounter

Patient-physician communication comprises a series of learned process and content skills, and both need to be taught to learners using a structured communication skills framework.

You may be tempted or find it more comfortable to focus your learners on the content part of the medical encounter, but it is the process skills that patients (and complaints and lawsuits) repeatedly indicate are problematic. Physicians are more easily forgiven for what they say than for how they say it. In teaching verbal communication skills, it is important to delineate both the process and the content.

Teaching Tip 2.
Take every opportunity to observe your learners communicating with patients and families; do not rely just on the learner's report of what was or was not said or done

Listening to a learner as he or she provides the details of a patient's history does not allow you to determine how the learner got the information from the patient. Nor does it give you the opportunity to give feedback on the actual encounter. The only way you can really know how learners communicate with patients is to observe them directly, have others observe them, or ask patients to provide their perspective.

After watching how your learners communicate with patients, it is important to provide specific, focused coaching on those process and content skills that need further improvement. Use a structured communication skills framework (e.g. the Calgary-Cambridge Observation Guide[1]) to make your feedback more explicit.

You can also help learners build their skills by having them participate in academic half-day workshops where they can practise and get feedback, or watch videos of themselves or others. These sessions will help learners become more aware of their communication process skills and give them the opportunity to explore what worked (or not) and what might work better next time with the same patient or in a similar situation. Such sessions are an excellent way to practise highly challenging or emotionally charged medical encounters (e.g. breaking bad news, disclosing a medical error).

Teaching Tip 3.
Demonstrate your content and process skills for your learners

Your learners will benefit from watching you conduct your patient interactions. Prime your learner on what to observe during the interaction. For example, if you are about to give a patient some bad news, ask the learner to focus on the process skills that you use. Once the interaction is over, debrief with the learner on what they observed you doing and how they felt the interaction went. You can give them a copy of the communication skills framework you are using as a guide for their observations.

Teaching perceptual communication skills is often overlooked but can provide some of the most helpful learning to learners.. Whenever opportunity permits, unpack your own thoughts and feelings about patient encounters. Share why you made the decisions you did. For example, discuss why you paused when you did, why you took the conversation in one direction and not another, and why you did or did not focus on certain information. Help your learners know when and why you may find the encounter challenging. Discuss how you attend to the patient's preferences, needs, and values when there are time constraints, limited options, or insufficient evidence, or when you are having genuine difficulty connecting with the patient. Knowing how faculty work through these everyday challenges (regardless of success) will help learners know that what looks easy on the outside involves knowledge and skill. As well, in working through these everyday challenges with patient interactions, you role model the back-and-forth reflection skills critical to providing optimal patient care.

Teaching Tip 4.

Provide or help your learners develop communication scripts for challenging topics and common activities in your specialty

Inventory the topics that are particularly challenging to communicate with patients in your specialty, and help your learners draft scripts for those issues — or provide the scripts yourself. For example, discussing driving ability with a patient who has had a stroke or has progressive dementia can be stressful for both patient and physician. Explain to learners the content and process skills you use for managing this encounter.

Consider, as well, activities that recur frequently in your specialty, program, or location. If consent is frequently required for certain procedures in your specialty, help your learners by providing them with a communication script that includes the necessary content and process skills. Videotape staff members holding conversations with simulated patients on challenging subjects that come up frequently in your specialty so that learners can review them as many times as they want. Video review is a great way to learn key phrases and to observe non-verbal styles.

Also, when your learner is going to use a script in a day-to-day case review with a specific patient, identify the top one or two learning points that might be relevant for that patient and work with the learner on how to talk to their patient about those topics.

Teaching Tip 5.

Provide samples and examples of documentation and information-sharing that meet the needs of the patients and physicians in a particular context

Develop samples of key documents (e.g. electronic records, consultation letter) used in a specific location and review them with your learners when you orient them to your rotation. Teach the basics of the three to five most frequent issues or challenges for documentation and the expectations for information sharing in that location. The list of frequent issues and challenges and the samples can be made readily available to your learners on a website or as handouts.

Sample teaching tools

- You can use the sample *Teaching Tools for Communicator* in this chapter as is, or you can modify or use them in various combinations to suit your objectives, time allocated, sequence within your residency program, and so on.

- Easy-to-customize electronic versions of the *Teaching Tools for Communicator* (in .doc, .ppt and .pdf formats) are found at: canmeds.royalcollege.ca

- The tools provided are:

  - T1 Lecture or Large Group Session: Foundations of the Communicator Role

  - T2 Presentation: Teaching the Communicator Role

  - T3 Small Group Activity: Communication scripts for day-to day communication

  - T4 Guided Reflection and Coaching: Exploring verbal and written communication tasks and skills in day-to-day practice

  - T5 Curriculum Planning Tool: Guidelines for developing communication skills curricula

  - T6 Coaching: Verbal communication skills – exploring common pitfalls

  - T7 Coaching: Resident coaching on common written communications

  - T8 Tools and Strategies: Summary sheet for the Communicator Role

5. Hints, tips and tools for *assessing* the Communicator Role

Assessment for learning is a major theme in this CanMEDS Tools Guide and a growing emphasis in medical education. You can and should use assessment as a strategy to inform a learner's learning plan (i.e. to alert or signpost to learners what is important to learn as well as, what and how they will be assessed). This section of the Tools Guide offers a number of hints to help you develop a program of assessment that will ensure that both teachers and learners have a clear understanding of their performance and what needs improvement.

© 2015 Royal College of Physicians and Surgeons of Canada

Assessment Tip 1.

Observe your learners directly as much as you can with a communication skills tool

Directly observing your learners remains the best method of assessing your learners' communication abilities in practice. When doing so, be sure that you and the learner use the same structured communication skills framework or guide as the basis for the interaction and assessment. Direct observation is not always possible under all circumstances; therefore, other tips are described below.

When giving feedback on the patient-learner encounter, you can use the language and process skills in the framework to select your questions. For example, begin by asking what the learner's intent was going into the encounter, and then ask what they perceived was the outcome. If the intent and the outcome are not in alignment, ask what could be done differently the next time.

Assessment Tip 2.

Assess in the clinical setting with the help of other health care professionals and/or patients

Communication between the learner and patient can, at times, be observed by other health care team members. Get feedback on learner communication skills from team members or patients using multisource feedback (MSF) forms or session encounter forms or by asking for input for the interim or end-of-rotation in-training evaluation (ITER) form.

When you are soliciting feedback from other sources, it is best to prime the patient or team member in advance with the specific areas or aspects of communication you would like addressed. Many patients will say they "liked" the learner but struggle with being specific. Without more nuanced feedback, learners will not know what to continue doing or what to change. Tools are available to assist patients and team members in formulating their feedback.

Assessment Tip 3.

Use formal assessment methods to supplement those used at the bedside and the feedback from patients, caregivers, and other health care professionals

Many methods are available to strengthen your assessment of the communication skills of your learners. Examples include Objective Structured Clinical Exams (OSCEs), with or without video, and portfolios to demonstrate growth in practice.

Assessment Tip 4.

Include communication process and content questions in case presentations, case reports, and rounds

In day-to-day cases, ask questions about a specific patient-physician encounter such as:

- What do you think the patient's agenda was today?
- What, if any, challenges or issues did you encounter when being patient-centred?
- What, if any, challenges or issues did you encounter with the shared decision-making process?
- What did you discuss with the patient regarding healthy behaviours?
- What choices in your treatment and management plan did you make based on the patient's perspectives and preferences?
- What did you do to involve the patient in the management plan?

Take advantage of focused coaching opportunities to improve your learners' communication process and content when they answer about what worked (or not) with that patient.

Assessment Tip 5.

Assess documentation quality and efficiency

When assessing learners' documentation, ask whether it matches the exemplars or criteria.

Documentation has very specific content and process for each specialty and each context, including location, patient population, and problem type. You need to help learners develop documentation skills that meet quality requirements in a time-efficient manner. Monitor and assess both the quality of documentation and the time and effort it took to complete. Sometimes you may need to coach your learners on quality related issues and/or efficiency related issues. Set expectations early on in the learner's rotation about when progress notes, operative notes, consultation notes, or discharge summaries should be completed.

In the same way that verbal communication benefits from direct observation, written communication can be assessed by analyzing copies of dictated consultation letters, discharge summaries, and other handwritten or typed health records or medical letters. Dictated consultation letters may be formally assessed using a validated, reliable rating scale.[10] As well, learners can be taught to assess their own letters and to provide feedback on peer and faculty consultation letters using this tool.

Communicator

Sample assessment tools

You can use the sample *Assessment Tools for Communicator* found at the end of this section as is, or you can modify or use them in various combinations to suit your objectives, the time allocated, the sequence within your residency program, and so on.

Easy-to-customize electronic versions of the *Assessment Tools for Communicator* (in .doc, .ppt and .pdf formats) are found at: canmeds.royalcollege.ca

The tools provided are:

- A1 Encounter Form: Communication assessment tool

- A2 Coaching: Consultation letter rating scale

- A3 Written Questions and Answers: for the Communicator Role

- A4 Objective Structured Clinical Exam (OSCE): for the Communicator Role

6. Suggested resources

- **Silverman J, Kurtz S, Draper J. Skills for communicating with patients. 3rd ed. London: Radcliffe Publishing. 2013.**

- **Kurtz S, Silverman J, Draper J. Teaching and learning communication skills in medicine. 2nd ed. London: Radcliffe Publishing. 2005.** This compendium set is an excellent, evidence-informed resource for clinical teachers and educators interested in communication skills training in undergraduate and postgraduate medicine. The books provide the evidence for why we teach communication skills and why we teach the specific communication skills outlined. The Calgary-Cambridge Observation Guide lists all of the communication skills, which can be used as a whole or in segments (i.e. one specific communication task or process skill) depending on the needs of the learner and teacher.

- **Keely E, Dojeiji S, Myers K. Writing effective consultation letters: 12 tips for teachers.** *Med Teach.* **2002;24(6):585–9.** This and subsequent articles by the authors provide an approach to teaching and assessing consultation letters. This article describes the creation and validation of a consultation letter rating scale that can be used for formative and summative assessments of consultation letter quality.

- **Canadian Patient Safety Institute. Tools and resources. Last retrieved July 11, 2015 from: http://www.patientsafetyinstitute.ca/English/toolsResources/Pages/default.aspx**

- **Teamwork and Communication Working Group. 2011. Improving patient safety with effective teamwork and communication: literature review needs assessment, evaluation of training tools and expert consultations. Edmonton, AB: Canadian Patient Safety Institute. Last retrieved July 11, 2015, from http://www.patientsafetyinstitute.ca/english/toolsresources/teamworkcommunication/documents/canadian%20framework%20for%20teamwork%20and%20communications.pdf.** This document provides a framework for patient safety and outlines objectives within each Role, including the Communicator Role.

7. Other resources

- Kurtz S, Silverman J, Benson J, Draper J. Marrying content and process in clinical method teaching: enhancing the Calgary-Cambridge guides. *Acad Med.* 2003;78(8):802–9.

- Kurtz SM, Silverman JD. The Calgary-Cambridge Referenced Observation Guides: an aid to defining the curriculum and organizing the teaching in communication training programmes. *Med Educ.* 1996;30(2):83–9.

- Platt FW, Gordon GH. *Field Guide to the Difficult Patient Interview* 2 ed. Wolters Kluwer; 2004.

- Martin D. Martin's map: a conceptual framework for teaching and learning the medical interview using a patient-centred approach. *Med Educ.* 2003;37(12):1145–53.

- Canadian Medical Protective Association website. Last retrieved July 11, 2015, from www.cmpa-acpm.ca.

- Makoul G, Krupat E, Chang CH. Measuring patient views of physician communication skills: development and testing of the Communication Assessment Tool. *Patient Educ Couns.* 2007;67(3):333–42.

© 2015 Royal College of Physicians and Surgeons of Canada

8. COMMUNICATOR ROLE DIRECTORY OF TEACHING AND ASSESSMENT TOOLS

You can use the sample *teaching and assessment tools for the Communicator Role* found in this section as is, or you can modify or use them in various combinations to suit your objectives, the time allocated, the sequence within your residency program, and so on. Tools are listed by number (e.g. T1), type (e.g. Lecture), and title (e.g. Foundations of the Communicator Role).

Easy-to-customize electronic versions of the sample *teaching and assessment tools for the Communicator Role* in .doc, .ppt and .pdf formats are found at: canmeds.royalcollege.ca

Communicator

T1. FOUNDATIONS OF THE COMMUNICATOR ROLE

Created for the *CanMEDS Teaching and Assessment Tools Guide* by S Glover Takahashi. Reproduced with permission of the Royal College.

This learning activity includes:

- Presentation: Foundations of Communicator (T2)

- Small group activity: Communication scripts for day-to-day communication (T3)

- Guided reflection and coaching: Exploring verbal and written communication tasks and skills in day-to-day practice (T4)

Instructions for Teacher:

Sample learning objectives

1. Recognize common words related to the Communicator Role

2. Apply key Communicator steps to examples from day-to-day practice

3. Develop a personal Communicator resource for common patient needs

Audience: All learners

How to adapt:

- Consider whether your session's objectives match the sample ones. Select from, modify, or add to the sample objectives as required.

- The sample PowerPoint presentation and worksheets are generic and foundational and tied to simple objectives. Consider whether you'll need additional slides to meet your objectives. Modify, add or delete content as required. You may want to include specific information related to your discipline and context.

- Depending on whether you are using these materials in one session (e.g. Communicator Basics Workshop) or a series of two to four academic half days will determine which activities you select and in what sequence.

- You may wish to review and customize the Communicator Role Summary Sheet with your learners as an additional activity.

Logistics:

- Select one or two activities for each teaching session.

- Plan for about 20 minutes for each group activity: this time will be used for you to explain the activity and for your learners to complete the worksheet individually, share their answers with their small group, discuss, prepare to report back to the whole group, and then deliver their small group's report to the whole group.

- Allow individuals to read the worksheet and spend about five minutes working on the answers on their own before starting to work in groups. This format allows each person to develop his or her own understanding of the topic.

- Depending on the group and time available, you may wish to assign one or more worksheets as homework to be completed before the session or as a follow-up assignment.

Setting:

- This information is best taught in a small-group format (i.e. less than 30 learners) if possible. It can also be effectively done with a larger group if the room allows for learners to be at tables in groups of five or six. With larger groups, it is helpful to have additional teachers or facilitators available to answer questions arising from the activities.

© 2015 Royal College of Physicians and Surgeons of Canada

T2. TEACHING THE COMMUNICATOR ROLE

Created for the *CanMEDS Teaching and Assessment Tools Guide* by S Glover Takahashi. Reproduced with permission of the Royal College.

Instructions for Teacher:

* Setting and Audience: Faculty and all learners

* How to use: Use as an orientation to the Role: refer to Notes to Teachers below.

* How to adapt: Slides can be modified to match the specialty or the learners' practice context

* Logistics: Equipment – laptop, projector, and screen

Slide #	Words on slide	Notes to teachers
1.	Communicator	• Add information about presenters and modify title
2.	Objectives and agenda	• SAMPLE goals and objectives of the session – revise as required. • CONSIDER doing a 'warm up activity' • Review/revise goals and objectives
3.	**Why the Communicator Role matters** • increased accuracy: • improved outcomes of care (physiological and psychological); • heightened perceptions by patients that they are being supported by their physicians • reduced rates of adverse events and medical errors, and • better protection against complaints and malpractice claims.	• Link evidence to practice/ experience
4.	**Communication skills** • are skills that can be readily defined, taught, and assessed • communication skills need to be intentionally developed and refined as all essential clinical skills • need to actively engage in the development of their communication skills via deliberate practice	
5.	**The details: What is the Communicator Role**[a] As Communicators, physicians form relationships with patients and their families[b] that facilitate the gathering and sharing of essential information for effective health care.[c]	• Avoid including competencies for learners • If you are giving this presentation to teachers or planners, you may want to add the key and enabling competencies
6.	**Key terms** • therapeutic relationship • patient-centred approach • empathy	• Provide examples
7.	• Common ground • Shared decision-making • Signposting • Categorization • Chunking and checking • Safety net	• Provide examples

a Neville A, Weston W, Martin D, Samson L, Feldman P, Wallace G, Jamoulle O, François J, Lussier M-T, Dojeiji S. Communicator. In: Frank JR, Snell L, Sherbino J, editors. CanMEDS 2015 Physician Competency Framework. Ottawa: Royal College of Physicians and Surgeons of Canada; 2015. Reproduced with permission.

b Throughout the CanMEDS 2015 Physician Competency Framework and Milestones Guide, references to the patient's family are intended to include all those who are personally significant to the patient and are concerned with his or her care, including, according to the patient's circumstances, family members, partners, caregivers, legal guardian, and substitute decision-makers.

c Note that the Communicator Role describes the abilities related to a physician–patient encounter. Other communication skills are found elsewhere in the Framework, including health care team communication (Collaborator) and academic presentations (Scholar).

Communicator

T2. TEACHING THE COMMINICATOR ROLE (continued)

Slide #	Words on slide	Notes to teachers
8.	**Key features of good communicator**[d] • Interactive • Dynamic and responsive • Reduces uncertainty • Planned, purposeful • Welcomes practice and feedback	• Provide examples
9.	**Verbal communication skills framework** 1. PROVIDING STRUCTURE (ONGOING) 2. BUILDING THE RELATIONSHIP (ONGOING) 3. INITIATING THE SESSION 4. GATHERING INFO AND PHYSICAL EXAM 5. EXPLANATION AND PLANNING 6. CLOSING THE SESSION	• Provide specialty examples • Review purpose of each step • Explore how to prepare for, act on, and evaluate each step in your specialty, based on experience — you can draw on either learners' or teachers' experience
10.	**HINTS on patient-centredness** 1. Orient yourself to this patient and needs. aka patient-centred 2. Watch for signals and cues. Seek confirmation. Silence may not be agreement 3. Be careful about labels to patients or their problems	• Explore each of the steps with the whole group • Explore how to prepare for, act on, and evaluate each step in your specialty, based on experience — you can draw on either learners' or teachers' experience
11.	T3 Activity	• Communication scripts for day-to-day communication
12.	Written communication skills framework • CONTENT (what is considered essential to include) • STYLE (visual layout)	
13.	T4 Activity	• Assessing verbal and written communication tasks and skills in day-to-day practice • T4 activity can be used for guided self-reflection, to assess videotaped samples, or to assess role plays
14.	Sample written communication	**Consult letters** • Consider focusing each session on one or two of the topics • Consider focusing each session on one or a small number of patient issues • Orient learners to these issues and explore them with the whole group
15.	Recap, revisiting objectives, and next steps	• Revisit session goals and objectives

---

d Kurtz S, Silverman J, Draper J. *Teaching and learning communication skills in medicine.* 2nd ed. London: Radcliffe Publishing. Copyright © 2005. Reproduced by permission of Taylor & Francis Books UK.

© 2015 Royal College of Physicians and Surgeons of Canada

T2. TEACHING THE COMMINICATOR ROLE (continued)

Slide #	Words on slide	Notes to teachers
OTHER SLIDES		
16.	**Communicator key competencies**[a] ***Physicians are able to:*** 1. Establish professional therapeutic relationships with patients and their families 2. Elicit and synthesize accurate and relevant information, incorporating the perspectives of patients and their families 3. Share health care information and plans with patients and their families 4. Engage patients and their families in developing plans that reflect the patient's health care needs and goals 5. Document and share written and electronic information about the medical encounter to optimize clinical decision-making, patient safety, confidentiality, and privacy	• Avoid including competencies for learners • You may wish to use this slide if you are giving the presentation to teachers or planners
17.	Communicator enabling competencies	• Avoid including competencies for learners • Use one slide for each key competency and associated enabling competencies
18.	Consultation letters	• Provide blinded sample letters. • Use T7
19.	Diagnostic radiology documentation hints	• Use as time allows and for appropriate learner group
20.	Pathology documentation hints	• Use as time allows and for appropriate learner group
21.	Surgical documentation hints	• Use as time allows and for appropriate learner group
22.	CAT tool	• Use as time allows and for appropriate learner group

Communicator

T3. COMMUNICATION SCRIPTS FOR DAY-TO-DAY COMMUNICATION

Created for the *CanMEDS Teaching and Assessment Tools Guide* by S Glover Takahashi.
Reproduced with permission of the Royal College.

See Communicator Role teacher tips appendix for this teaching tool

Completed by:_____

1. Complete the table below, providing details from your clinical practice over the past month.

Clinical location(s) (include details about when, where, how long, type of service)	Common or repeated communication topics or subjects	Challenging communication topics or subjects

2. Select one of the two examples of common or repeated communication topics or subjects, and then write a patient scenario of no more than three sentences for that topic or subject.

_____

_____

_____

_____

_____

_____

_____

_____

Communicator

© 2015 Royal College of Physicians and Surgeons of Canada

T3. COMMUNICATION SCRIPTS FOR DAY-TO-DAY COMMUNICATION
(continued)

Communicator

3. You will be drafting a communication script for part of the scenario you just wrote. First, choose one or two communication skills tasks from the six listed below. Then, fill out the corresponding row(s) in the table for your scenario.

Outline the core content used to discuss common or challenging communication scenarios; for verbal communication, you may wish to include some key phrases that you find particularly helpful.

☐ 1. Initiating the session
☐ 2. Gathering information
☐ 3. Explanation and planning
☐ 4. Closing the session
☐ 5. Providing structure
☐ 6. Building the relationship

Communication skills task[a]	Potential script wording	Content skills to highlight
1. Initiating the session		
2. Gathering information		
3. Explanation and planning		
4. Closing the session		
5. Building the relationship		
6. Providing structure		

a Kurtz S, Silverman J, Draper J. *Teaching and learning communication skills in medicine.* 2nd ed. London: Radcliffe Publishing. Copyright © 2005. Reproduced by permission of Taylor & Francis Books UK.

T3. SAMPLE SCRIPT #1: BREAKING BAD NEWS – "THE DRIVING TALK"

(continued)

Created for the *CanMEDS Teaching and Assessment Tools Guide* by S Dojeiji. Reproduced with permission of the Royal College.

SCENARIO

- You've just examined a young woman with a sensory motor peripheral polyneuropathy with significant arm and leg weakness and poor proprioception in the lower legs.

- You're concerned about her ability to drive, and you need to discuss this.

- She was referred to you for the leg and arm weakness, so she's not expecting to discuss her driving ability.

SKILLS FOCUS of this script:

- Explanation and planning (Communication skills task #3)

- Closing the session (Communication skills task #4)

- Building the relationship (Communication skills task #5)

Communication skills task	Potential script wording and other tips	CONTENT skills to highlight	PROCESS skills to highlight
3. Explanation and planning	• Begin by asking how the patient perceives her driving ability • Provide an assessment of the patient's function in plain language using the content above in the scenario • Ask if the patient feels her driving is safe, and depending on the situation, ask "what do you think I'm going to say about your driving?" • Pause regularly to gauge reaction to the information • Check for body language throughout the interaction (the patient may say little verbally but express a lot of emotion through eye contact, posture, etc.) • Allow time for questions	• Highlight what is needed for safe driving: good eyes, brain, and strong arms and legs • Summarize the weakness and sensory loss so the patient has a good understanding of deficits • Explain that it is the Ministry of Transportation that makes the final decision about ability to drive; however, physicians are mandated (in some provinces) to report concerns about driving safety if the patient has a condition that may affect their ability to drive	• Assess patient's starting point • Organize information into discrete chunks • Regular chunks and checks • Pick up and respond to verbal and non-verbal cues • Check with patient to determine if she accepts the information and if her concerns are being addressed
4. Closing the session	• Provide support by offering to explore other transportation options • Finish by asking if the patient has further questions about what was said or the next steps • Offer to discuss again once the patient has had time to reflect on the information further (some will be stunned enough by the interaction that they say very little, but then a few days later, there will be a call). Provide permission for a follow-up call to happen with an agreement to discuss again (this is an example of forward planning)		• Contract with the patient for next steps • Do a final check that the patient agrees with the plan and ask if there are any other questions
5. Building the relationship	• Provide the content in an empathic and sensitive manner • Respond with empathy at the reaction (sometimes can be quite forceful and negative; allow the patient to express her emotion). For example, I know the driving was not a topic that you were expecting to discuss with me today. I can see that the information that I have given you is unexpected. This builds on picking up on verbal and non-verbal cues from above and shows the learner is acknowledging the emotion and is reflecting back understanding to the patient		• Uses empathy to communicate understanding and appreciation of the patient's predicament (overtly acknowledges patient's views and feelings)

© 2015 Royal College of Physicians and Surgeons of Canada

Communicator

T3. SAMPLE SCRIPT #2: SHARING INFORMATION – "TEST RESULTS AND CONSENT" (continued)

Created for the *CanMEDS Teaching and Assessment Tools Guide* by S Dojeiji. Reproduced with permission of the Royal College.

SCENARIO

* You are seeing Mrs. X for a follow-up appointment to discuss the results of a biopsy, which are positive to cancer, and to plan next steps.

SKILLS FOCUS of this script:

* Initiating the session (Communication skills task #1)
* Gathering information (Communication skills task #2)
* Explanation and planning (Communication skills task #3)
* Closing the session (Communication skills task #4)

Communication skills task	Potential script wording and other tips	CONTENT skills to highlight	PROCESS skills to highlight
1. Initiating the session	"Good to see you back, Mrs. X, I can imagine it's been a long two weeks." "As you know, the purpose of today's appointment is to discuss the results of your biopsy. I'm going to start there, discuss what they mean, answer any questions you may have about the results, then move to discussing next steps. Does that sound reasonable?" "Unfortunately the biopsy showed … which means …" "What are your thoughts at this point?"	Will vary by specialty	• Have results ready • Provide privacy • Sit down • Make eye contact • Greet patient with empathy for the wait • Set the agenda • Provide the result in plain language immediately. Pay attention to reaction • Pause after presenting the result and meaning • Empathetically acknowledge reaction
2. Gathering information	"I need to get some further history and to ask about your preferences so we can come up with next steps that work for you."	Will vary by specialty	• Signpost – provide rationale for needing to ask further questions
3. Explanation and planning	"Based on the results and your history, we have two surgical treatment choices: a lumpectomy or a mastectomy. I am going to describe each procedure, and discuss the risks and benefits. I'll start with the lumpectomy and then move to the mastectomy." "A lumpectomy is a surgical procedure where they go in and remove the cancerous tissue. On the day of surgery ..[details]…." "Do you have any more questions before I move on to talk about the risks and benefits of this choice?"	Will vary by specialty	• Categorize • Draw pictures • Chunk and check • Use plain language • Pause frequently for questions.
4. Closing the session	"Okay, let's summarize the plan to ensure we are both on the same page. Can you repeat in your own words the next steps?" "Let's talk about what to do if you have not heard back about a surgical date in two weeks or feel you are experiencing changes that are important for me to know."	Will vary by specialty	• Repetition • (Repeat OR ask the patient to repeat the plan) • Safety net

© 2015 Royal College of Physicians and Surgeons of Canada

Communicator

T4. EXPLORING VERBAL AND WRITTEN COMMUNICATION TASKS AND SKILLS IN DAY-TO-DAY PRACTICE[a]

Created for the *CanMEDS Teaching and Assessment Tools Guide* by S Glover Takahashi and S Dojeiji. Reproduced with permission of the Royal College.

Instructions for Learners:

- Critically analyze your strengths and weaknesses in verbal and written communication.

- In completing the tables, you can draw on patient encounters in clinical setting, videotapes of simulated encounters, or practice scenarios.

- This can be "homework" for discussion with faculty at an educational session or it could be inserted in your portfolio.

- Report on the verbal communication tasks provided in the table below.

Verbal communication tasks	Rating from 1–5			Example(s) of when you did this well over the past few months	Example(s) of when you could have been more effective
	1 Could be better	3 Good, competent	5 Strong		
1. INITIATING THE SESSION • Establishing initial rapport • Identifying the reason for the visit					
2. GATHERING INFORMATION AND PHYSICAL EXAM • Exploration of the patient problem • Biomedical perspective (disease) • Patient perspective (illness) • Background information – context					
3. EXPLANATION AND PLANNING • Providing the correct type and level of information • Aiding accurate recall and understanding • Achieving a shared understanding — incorporating the patient's perspective • Planning — shared decision-making					
4. CLOSING THE SESSION • Ensuring appropriate point of closure • Forward planning					

a Kurtz S, Silverman J, Draper J. *Teaching and learning communication skills in medicine.* 2nd ed. London: Radcliffe Publishing. Copyright © 2005. Reproduced by permission of Taylor & Francis Books UK.

© 2015 Royal College of Physicians and Surgeons of Canada

Communicator

T4. EXPLORING VERBAL AND WRITTEN COMMUNICATION TASKS AND SKILLS IN DAY-TO-DAY PRACTICE (continued)

Verbal communication tasks	Rating from 1–5			Example(s) of when you did this well over the past few months	Example(s) of when you could have been more effective
	1 Could be better	3 Good, competent	5 Strong		
5. PROVIDING STRUCTURE • Making organization overt • Attending to flow					
6. BUILDING THE RELATIONSHIP • Developing a therapeutic alliance • Involving the patient					
Other communication SKILLS					
Analyse the features of YOUR communication • Interactive • Dynamic and responsive • Reduces uncertainty • Planned, purposeful					
Analyse the features of YOUR Non-verbal communication skills • body posture • facial expressions • eye contact • gestures • touch • space • smell and clothing					
Analyse the features of YOUR Paraverbal skills • tone • pitch • pace • volume of speech • articulation • use of pauses					
Summary of OVERALL VERBAL COMMUNICATION SKILLS					

Communicator

Communicator

T4. EXPLORING VERBAL AND WRITTEN COMMUNICATION TASKS AND SKILLS IN DAY-TO-DAY PRACTICE (continued)

2. In what verbal communication task are you most skilled? Please illustrate with an example.

_____

_____

_____

_____

3. With what verbal communication task are you most comfortable? Please illustrate with an example.

_____

_____

_____

_____

4. Report on the written communication tasks provided in the table below (i.e. gather input and feedback).

Written communication tasks	Generally, how well do you do this?			Example(s) of when you did this well over the past few months	Example(s) of when you could have been more effective
	1 Can do better	3 Good, competent	5 Strong		
1. CONTENT					
2. STYLE **Language:** • Plain language • No abbreviations or acronyms • Short words (less than three syllables) • Active vs. passive voice ("I saw Ms. X ..." vs. "Ms. X was seen ...") **Visual display:** • Organized • Bullet points • Short sentences (one idea per sentence) • Short paragraphs (four or five sentences) • Section headings • Graphics • Right amount of information • Edited					

© 2015 Royal College of Physicians and Surgeons of Canada

T4. EXPLORING VERBAL AND WRITTEN COMMUNICATION TASKS AND SKILLS IN DAY-TO-DAY PRACTICE (continued)

3. Opening statement • Reason for referral					
4. Presentation of findings and physical exam					
5. Opinion, rationale, recommendations, and planning					
6. Closing statement					
OVERALL WRITTEN COMMUNICATION SKILLS					

5. In what consultation letter task do you require improvement? Please illustrate with an example and how it might be improved.

_____

_____

_____

_____

6. In what written communication processes do you require improvement? Please illustrate with an example and describe how it might be improved.

_____

_____

_____

_____

© 2015 Royal College of Physicians and Surgeons of Canada

Communicator

T5. GUIDELINES FOR DEVELOPING COMMUNICATION SKILLS CURRICULA

Created for the *CanMEDS Teaching and Assessment Tools Guide* by S Dojeiji. Reproduced with permission of the Royal College.

This resource is designed as a primer / refresher for teachers. It is a quick and easy summary of what you can and should do when developing communication skills curricula. You can also use this resource as a teaching aid for some of your more advanced learners if they will be involved in designing curricula.

1. Consider the following factors when developing your curricula:

   - **the level of expertise of your learners**

   - **the priority topics for your specialty**

   - **the sequence of topics**

   - **the time** that you can devote to communication skills teaching

   - **the processes** for teaching and assessing communication skills. Your specialty committee can provide guidance based on established objectives and standards of training documents.

2. **Integrate communication training into both formal teaching and clinical setting teaching** — both are needed. For example, if you have an academic session on breaking bad news, ensure that you then observe the communication skills of learners when they break bad news to a patient in the clinical setting. Be sure to provide the learners with feedback on what you observe.

3. Your curriculum needs to be **discipline specific and relevant to your specialty**. Have your learners review a selection of challenging cases from their own experience as part of an academic half-day. Encouraging them to draw from their own professional experience allows them to reflect on and practise in a safe environment. This will help create learner buy-in.

4. Your curriculum needs to **include evidence for the utility of good communication skills** (i.e. the "why bother" information) to encourage buy-in with your learners. Learners, in particular, are interested to learn about the risk of malpractice suits as a result of poor communication.

5. Your curriculum needs to **use a communication skills framework** to teach and assess communication skills. This framework is the "anatomy and physiology" of communication, and you need to know it and be able to use it every day.

6. Your curriculum needs to delineate the difference between **content skills (what to ask the patient) and process skills (how to ask the patient)**. Both are essential to effective communication. Often learners struggle with communication process skills because they have a weak knowledge base. Ensure they know what to ask, before focusing on how they ask.

7. Your curriculum needs to **teach process skills before it addresses special topics skills**. This means you should help your residents develop the process skills for building relationships and for explanation and planning before you attempt to teach breaking bad news, which is a special type of explanation and planning.

8. Your curriculum needs to **teach the various components of communication skills more than once**. Communication skills need to be rehearsed, reiterated, repeated, and refined, with feedback along the way.

9. Your curriculum needs to emphasize **direct observation of learners with a communication skills framework**, as it remains the best method for teaching and assessing communication skills. Consider using videotaped recordings of clinical interactions so that learners can review nuances of non-verbal communication skills.

   Your curriculum can also include:

   - OSCE with or without video

   - Multisource feedback with feedback providers primed before the encounter

   - Portfolios to demonstrate growth in practice

© 2015 Royal College of Physicians and Surgeons of Canada

Communicator

T5. GUIDELINES FOR DEVELOPING COMMUNICATION SKILLS CURRICULA

(continued)

10. **Observe your learners communicating with patients and families** at every opportunity and provide feedback using a communication skills framework as a guide. You can choose to focus on one aspect of communication just as you would when assessing a learner's knee examination (i.e. did the learner use plain language or medical jargon when giving information to the patient). You may not always have time to give feedback on the entire knee examination, but you can give feedback on hand placement for the Lachman test for anterior cruciate ligament laxity. When providing feedback, focus on the learner's intent and outcome – what did the learner intend to do and what actually happened. If the outcome was unexpected, what could the learner do differently next time.

11. **Identify one or more leads (i.e. champions)** for the teaching and assessment of the Communicator Role in your program. The lead(s) can support your program.

12. **Share the load.** Consider liaising with other similar specialties to share some of the communication skills teaching within your formal curriculum (e.g. subspecialties in your department).

© 2015 Royal College of Physicians and Surgeons of Canada

Communicator

Communicator

T6. VERBAL COMMUNICATION SKILLS – EXPLORING COMMON PITFALLS

Created for the *CanMEDS Teaching and Assessment Tools Guide* by S Dojeiji, D Martin and S Glover Takahashi. Reproduced with permission of the Royal College.

Instructions for Teachers:

- Observe part(s) or all of a clinical encounter.
- Provide feedback and coaching using a communication skills framework such as the one below.
- Discuss any noted gaps, areas of strength or areas for improvement.

Communication skills pitfall[a,b]	Impact on the patient or on the encounter	Suggested fix
1. INTRODUCTION • Learner forgets to introduce self, role or responsibility	• Missed opportunity to build a trusting relationship with the patient • In some cases, the patient does not realize the physician was in to visit • Confusion and uncertainty	• While it may seem fairly intuitive, the majority of the time when communication breaks down, it has to do with the very beginning — physicians don't explain clearly who they are and what their role is in the patient's care before jumping into the medical encounter • Encourage the learner to take the time to introduce themselves and to explain their role on the health care team
• Learner and patient can't agree on why the patient is there	• Patient is confused if they have been referred or if they communicated the reason for the visit to another party • Missed opportunity to build rapport and trust • Patient safety may be compromised • Interferes with time management as additional time is needed to clarify the reason for the visit • Expectation of care is not set up	• For specialists, summarizing the referral note from the family physician on patient arrival at the clinic ensures both patient and physician are on the same page about the purpose for the visit. Expectations can be clarified. • For family physicians and specialists, encouraging patients to elaborate on their reasons for the visit ensures that patients have the opportunity to express their ideas, expectations, and concerns. The majority of patients can do this within 60–90 seconds, but most physicians interrupt within the first 18 seconds.
2. GATHERING INFORMATION • Physician-centred approach	• The physician-centred questions (e.g. where is the pain, when did it start, where does it go, what makes it better or worse?) are critical. However, to better understand the patient problem, learners need to better understand the patient's context Critical information to guide the management plan will be missed. This may impact on patient adherence.	• Remind the learner that asking patients about their perceptions of their presenting problem at the beginning of the encounter will often elicit useful information: - Identifies patient fears, which may act as a barrier to accepting the diagnosis or to engaging in treatment - Provides a beginning understanding of how the condition is impacting the patient's ability to function at home and work, which enables the physician to tailor further questions and history - Provides a benchmark to better understand the patient's level of health literacy, perspective, and knowledge of their problem • Encourage the learner to begin encounters with an opportunity for the patient to talk • Establish the gap between medical reality and patient's knowledge about their condition by incorporating some of the strategies here

a Silverman J, Kurtz S, Draper J. *Skills for communicating with patients.* 3rd ed. London: Radcliffe Publishing. Copyright © 2013. Reproduced by permission of Taylor & Francis Books UK.

b Kurtz S, Silverman J, Draper J. *Teaching and learning communication skills in medicine.* 2nd ed. London: Radcliffe Publishing. Copyright © 2005. Reproduced by permission of Taylor & Francis Books UK.

© 2015 Royal College of Physicians and Surgeons of Canada

T6. VERBAL COMMUNICATION SKILLS – EXPLORING COMMON PITFALLS

(continued)

Communication skills pitfall[1,9]	Impact on the patient or on the encounter	Suggested fix

• Patient non-verbal communication skills not noted by the learner	• Learners need to be mindful of patients' non-verbal communication (e.g. body language, eye contact, tone of voice) as it can tell a lot about how a patient may be feeling (e.g. anxious) Patients may not divulge sensitive information if their non-verbal communication is not acknowledged and addressed.
	• Learners need to be mindful of their own non-verbal communication skills as these can impact the patient interaction (e.g. closed posture with arms and legs crossed and eye contact focused on the paper/computer and not on the patient gives the impression that there is no invitation to speak; the patient may not feel comfortable to disclose essential content relevant to the presenting problem)
		• Consider these options when teaching non-verbal communication skills:
		  - Observe the learner directly with a patient and comment on non-verbal communication skills and their impact on the patient interaction
		  - Videotape a simulated interaction and comment specifically on non-verbal communication skills
		  - Videotape a live patient interaction and review it at the end of clinic with the learner

3. EXPLANATION AND PLANNING • The soliloquy – i.e. learners often share information in long run-on sentences, moving from topic to topic without pausing in-between	• Patient is overwhelmed and does not know what information to attend to	• Work with the learner to break up the content into manageable chunks • Encourage the learner to pause after each chunk to check for patient understanding and for the patient to ask questions
• Learner uses medical jargon that the patient does not understand	• Risk that the patient will not understand, recall ,or comply with recommendations made by the learner	• Listen closely to the words used by the learner to explain information to the patient. Medical jargon is ubiquitous — we take many words for granted • Ask the patient for their understanding of the information provided after the learner completes their explanation. This technique is a nice way to verify learners' abilities to explain, and it also, by having the patient repeat the information heard, increases the likelihood of the patient remembering
• Learner "tells" rather than sharing and asking	• Because there is a power differential, patients may not raise concerns or questions as there is no apparent invitation to do so. Many learners mistake silence for approval • Patient safety can be compromised as the patient does not have the information they need or the motivation to comply with the treatment plan	• Encourage the learner to invite questions from their patients by asking if there are questions and also what patients think of the plan — fears, concerns, barriers to success, reasonableness, and so on • Remind the learner that it's best to get concerns and barriers on the table early on so that they may be addressed as a partnership. This is the true hallmark of shared decision-making

T6. VERBAL COMMUNICATION SKILLS – EXPLORING COMMON PITFALLS

(continued)

Communicator

Communication skills pitfall	Impact on the patient or on the encounter	Suggested fix
4. CLOSING THE SESSION • Learner assumes Plan A is going to unfold as planned	• Unless a safety net is stated explicitly, patients may improvise or stop a plan when common side effects occur or unexpected problems arise • Patients may go to the emergency room or to their family physician unless they are told explicitly who to contact if a treatment plan isn't proceeding as expected	• When reviewing cases with the learner, take a moment to discuss the plan B in the event plan A doesn't work — this is the safety net for the patient. Patient uncertainly and anxiety will lessen when there is an explicit discussion of what to do in the event of treatment failure • Tell the learner to provide patients with clear direction on what to do if more questions or issues arise
• The hand-on-the-door-handle question, or the "hidden agenda" emerges	• Research shows that if physicians don't elicit patient concerns or provide opportunities for the patient to contribute their ideas and understanding during the encounter, patients will share this information at the end of the encounter • Patients are often blamed for having hidden agendas, but more often than not it is the physician who has not asked the right question(s)	• Encourage the learner to obtain patient goals and expectations right at the beginning of the interaction (i.e. as soon as introductions are made and the reason for referral has been established) • Remind the learner that expectation mismatch can be addressed right at the beginning so the patient feels they've been heard and have a solid understanding of the goals of the interaction • Encourage the learner to empathetically acknowledge patients' concerns and frustration with healing time. Surgeons who acknowledge emotional cues during a post-surgical visit (i.e. responding to "I'm concerned about the swelling in my foot after the bunion surgery") are more likely to finish the patient interaction in less time than a surgeon who doesn't address the emotional cue provided[a]
5. BUILDING THE RELATIONSHIP • Learner does not pay attention to their own non-verbal communication	• How words are said have far more impact on patients than what is said • Learners need to be mindful of their own non-verbal communication skills as these can impact on the patient interaction e.g. closed posture with arms and legs crossed, eye contact focused on the paper/computer, speaking quickly) Any of the examples will give the patient the impression that they don't have an invitation to speak. The may result in an incomplete or inaccurate history.	• Regularly get learners to reflect on what they were thinking and feeling during an encounter (i.e. perceptual skills)
• Learner fails to build trust with their patient	• Establishing trust is essential to successful therapeutic relationships with patients. Without trust, patients are likely to discredit information provided, risking non-compliance with the management plan	• Ensure the learner adopts an open and non-judgmental approach and tone in their patient interactions • Teach an empathic response — learners can be intentional in acknowledging the emotion they are witnessing and linking it to a potential cause. The empathic response tells the patient that their physician is listening and trying to understand the their perspective. Remind the learner that empathy is a powerful tool for building therapeutic relationships and trust

a Levinson W, Gorawara-Bhat R, Lamb J. A study of patient clues and physician responses in primary care and surgical settings. *JAMA.* 2000;284(8):1021-7.

© 2015 Royal College of Physicians and Surgeons of Canada

T6. VERBAL COMMUNICATION SKILLS – EXPLORING COMMON PITFALLS

(continued)

Communication skills pitfall	Impact on the patient or on the encounter	Suggested fix
6. PROVIDING STRUCTURE • Learner mistakes a patient-controlled approach with being patient-centred	• Often learners will come away from a complex patient interaction completely overwhelmed by details of the history, particularly if the patient was in complete control of the encounter • Learners confuse allowing the patient to tell their story with allowing the patient to control the encounter	• Tell the learner that there is a fine line between allowing the patient to provide their story and ensuring the needs of the patient and physician are met by obtaining the essential details from the patient • Remind the learner that the patient may be driving the bus, but physicians have a say on the route taken • For junior learners new to a particular area of medicine, it is helpful to have a conversation in advance of the patient interaction about the critical elements to be obtained and covered during the interaction. Patients may veer in multiple directions, but the template you provide to your learners will be their anchor and help them cover critical ground in an efficient manner • Teach junior learners how to set agendas at the beginning of the encounter so they have a roadmap of what they are to achieve • Give the learner permission to redirect a patient who may be going off course and tips on how to do this. This can be done in a neutral, professional, and compassionate manner, using signposting as a communication skill
• Awkward history-taking	• Learners often ask sensitive questions without providing a rationale for why they are asking (e.g. sexual health, high-risk behaviours) • Often patients will experience confusion and anger when questions seem inappropriate	• Work with the learner to create a series of orienting phrases providing a rationale for why certain questions are being asked. For example, for a patient presenting with back pain: "The nerves going to the legs also go to the bladder, bowel, and sexual organs. I need to ask how those things are working…" • Or for a patient presenting with a polyneuropathy and the rationale for asking about illicit drug use: "I ask the next series of questions of everyone as these things can affect the health of our nerves…" • Ensure learners' knowledge about what to ask (i.e. clear that this is not a Medical Expert issue).
• Disjointed history-taking	• Learners with no framework often miss important questions and get lost in the interview. Disjointed history-taking sometimes represents poor knowledge of the topic area, other times no framework. It is also disorienting for patients, who are trying to follow the learner's logic and answer questions accurately	• Provide an organizational framework for history-taking • Help the learner recognize the different "pockets" of information they need to retrieve • Help the learner develop a logical sequence for retrieving information without jumping back and forth • Ensure basic knowledge of what to ask is present.

Communicator

T7. RESIDENT COACHING ON COMMON WRITTEN COMMUNICATIONS

Created for the *CanMEDS Teaching and Assessment Tools Guide* by S Dojeiji, D Martin and S Glover Takahashi. Reproduced with permission of the Royal College.

As residents or learners develop their verbal and written communication skills they tend to experience many of the same pitfalls. If you have one or more learners that tend to experience any of these common pitfalls, consider using this tool as the basis for a one-on-one coaching session. Your learners will benefit from actively engaging in the development of their communication skills through deliberate practice that is observed and assessed both informally and formally.

Start your coaching session by asking the learner if he/she can identify his/her own strengths and weaknesses. Explore any relevant pitfall(s) identified by either you or the learner. Ask the learner to articulate the potential impact on the patient. Talk through suggested fixes and make a commitment to observe the learner on his/her approach. Commit to providing timely feedback and coaching.

Instructions for Teachers:

- Have the learner select a written communication for review.

- Review it together discuss any areas of strength or areas for improvement

- If you identify any of the common pitfalls below discuss the impact and explore possible fixes

Type of written communication	Pitfall	Impact on patient or on referral source	Suggested fix
CONSULTATION LETTER	CONTENT • No attention to what information should be included in the letter: what is essential, important, or relevant is not considered • A lot of detail on the assessment, with little detail on the impression and treatment plan • Letter not written and sent in a timely fashion • Did not answer the referring physician's question	• The length of the letter is irrelevant as long as the content is organized discretely and clearly. However, learners need to reflect on what content is deemed essential, important, or relevant to the patient population they are managing • Without a working knowledge of what is important, essential information may be hidden in the letter, rendering it unhelpful to the referring source and the treating physician; as well, learners have wasted time producing an ineffective letter • Delay in patient care if information not provided in a timely manner • Referring physician frustration as referring question not answered; this may generate another referral	• Create templates for specific patient populations seen • Tell the learner to focus on the impression and plan as this is the area most physicians will review first • Provide samples of what a good consultation letter looks like in your specialty for your learner to review and compare and contrast with their own • Explicitly set expectations with the learner for when the letter needs to be done • Tell the learner to always answer the referring physician's question posed in the referral letter
	STYLE • Disorganized content and lack of content planning • Wordy • No attention to visual layout with no white space	• Lack of content planning, organization, and white space, making the letter difficult to scan by a busy clinician • Wordy letter filled with medical jargon and filler words that do not add to the meaning of the letter	• Encourage the learner to use templates for conditions commonly seen • Tell the learner to review all dictations before sending so they can pay attention to the visuals of the letter (white space) and check for errors • Encourage the learner to use bullet points in the body of dictation (e.g. history of presenting illness, physical examination) • Encourage the learner to use numbered lists (e.g. past medical history, medications, plan) • Encourage the learner to use tables to reflect a lot of information in a visually effective manner (e.g. table for muscle grading numbers)

© 2015 Royal College of Physicians and Surgeons of Canada

T7. RESIDENT COACHING ON COMMON WRITTEN COMMUNICATIONS

(continued)

Type of written communication	Pitfall	Impact on patient or on referral source	Suggested fix
DIAGNOSTIC IMAGING CONSULTATION REPORT	• Description of findings is poor, vague, variable, or inconclusive, with a lack of detail	• Frustration on referring physician's part • Potential for misunderstanding regarding diagnosis and next steps, leading to inappropriate use of resources (i.e. unnecessary additional tests) • Patient safety may be compromised if there is a delay in treatment because it was not clear additional tests were needed	• Variable approaches in diagnostic imaging are a common problem. Ensure the learner chooses one approach that they are able to articulate and routinely use • Create a template of acceptable phrases for common findings and opinions • Teach the learner to synthesize and consolidate clear findings, opinions, and management plans
LABORATORY REPORT, CONSULTATION REPORT	• Poor or vague impressions of the case with an unclear statement of reasons for the uncertainty	• Report reader may make incorrect assumptions, potentially impacting treatment recommendations • Delays in treatment • Requests for second opinion via clinician	• Provide templates for common diagnoses • Teach the learner to outline the key concepts to be transmitted before writing the draft report
	• Incomplete report (missing parameters)	• Delayed treatment • Requests for review of case (duplication of work)	• Rather than rely on electronic synoptic reporting systems, the learner may write a draft report, including all necessary parameters • Encourage reference to College of American Pathologists' cancer reporting protocols for draft writing
	• Incorrect use of language • Use of non-conventional terminology	• Improper grammar and ambiguities may lead to reader misunderstanding of the severity of findings • Delays in treatment • Requests for review of case (duplication of work)	• Provide a list of standardized (conventional) terminology • Teach the learner to outline the key concepts to be transmitted before writing a draft
SURGICAL – OPERATIVE REPORT	• Abbreviations used without citing specifics (e.g. AVSS) • Missing pertinent information (e.g. intraoperative findings, blood loss, placement of drains, pathology pending, intraoperative complications experienced, etc.) • Incorrect or incomplete procedure recorded	• Using abbreviations that are not known can result in misunderstanding of patients needs and / or delaying further intervention or alterations in management due to confusion • Missing information that can direct and alter post-operative care, investigations, or monitoring • Incorrect drains, etc., may be removed (especially in cases of multiple drains) • Perception of patient having undergone incorrect procedure leads to miscommunication with the patient, family, and consultants, and creates potential for confusion and loss of faith in the system and team	• Teach the learner to look up and record the appropriate specific pertinent vitals (HR, BP, SaO2, Temp, urine output) • Teach the learner to ask for and record the various important surgical aspects • Teach the learner to clearly label and record positions of drains (use diagram if necessary) • Teach the learner to discuss procedure performed with MRP so that it can be adequately reported in the chart

Communicator

T7. RESIDENT COACHING ON COMMON WRITTEN COMMUNICATIONS

(continued)

Type of written communication	Pitfall	Impact on patient or on referral source	Suggested fix
SURGICAL CONSULTATION REPORT	• A diagnosis but no recommendations	• Further investigations • Improper follow-up • Inaccurate expectations around recovery process • Missed opportunity to educate the physician	• Teach the learner how to incorporate continuing professional development into consultation letters (e.g. include relevant references, summary of clinical practice guidelines; incorporate education paragraphs about specific treatment, etc.)
DISCHARGE SUMMARIES	• Lack of a discharge plan, with far too much focus on the details of what transpired and little information on the next steps and who is responsible for following up on the issues identified • Delay in discharge note	• Patient safety is compromised • Confusion and frustration for the primary care physician and community services providing follow-up • Delay in needed services	• Tell the learner that it is critical to summarize major medical and surgical issues that transpired during the course of admission — it is easier to review the details if they are organized in a format that can be readily scanned (numbered list of issues, with bullet-point descriptions) • Explain that the discharge plan must be detailed enough to include the next steps post-discharge, who will do what, and what the patient has been told if the discharge plan isn't successful. Specifically, the discharge summary needs to clearly identify the expectations of the primary care provider • Provide clear guidelines for the completion and delivery of discharge notes

Communicator

© 2015 Royal College of Physicians and Surgeons of Canada

T8. SUMMARY SHEET FOR THE COMMUNICATOR ROLE

Created for the *CanMEDS Teaching and Assessment Tools Guide* by S Glover Takahashi. Reproduced with permission of the Royal College.

See Communicator Role teacher tips appendix for this teaching tool

COMMUNICATOR

Key features of a good communicator[a]
- Interactive
- Dynamic and responsive
- Reduces uncertainty
- Planned, purposeful
- Welcomes practice and feedback

Communication skills
- are skills that can be readily defined, taught, and assessed
- communication skills need to be intentionally developed and refined as all essential clinical skills
- need to actively engage in the development of their communication skills via deliberate practice

Non-verbal communication skills
- body posture
- eye contact
- touch
- smell
- facial expressions
- gestures
- space
- clothing

Paraverbal skills
- tone
- volume
- rhythm
- use of pauses
- pace
- pitch
- articulation

COMMUNICATION TASK[b]	PURPOSE
1. PROVIDING STRUCTURE (ONGOING)	• Making organization overt • Attending to flow
2. BUILDING THE RELATIONSHIP (ONGOING)	• Developing a therapeutic alliance • Involving the patient
3. INITIATING THE SESSION	• Establishing initial rapport • Identifying the reason for the visit
4. GATHERING INFO AND PHYSICAL EXAM	• Exploration of the patient problem to discover: Biomedical perspective (disease) Patient perspective (illness) Background information – context
5. CLOSING THE SESSION	• Forward planning • Ensuring appropriate point of closure
6. EXPLANATION AND PLANNING	• Providing the correct type and level of information • Aiding accurate recall and understanding • Achieving a shared understanding – incorporating the patient's perspective • Planning – shared decision-making

#	WRITTEN COMM skills task	When
1.	CONTENT (what is considered essential to include)	• Ongoing
2.	STYLE (visual layout)	• Ongoing
3.	Opening Statement – Reason for referral	• Beginning
4.	Presentation of Findings and Physical Exam	• Middle
5.	Opinion, Rationale, Recommendations and Planning	• End
6.	Closing Statement	• End

a Dojeiji S, 2015. Created for *CanMEDS Tools Guide*. Royal College.
b Kurtz S, Silverman J, Draper J. *Teaching and learning communication skills in medicine*. 2nd ed. London: Radcliffe Publishing. Copyright © 2005. Reproduced by permission of Taylor & Francis Books UK.

Communicator

T8. SUMMARY SHEET FOR THE COMMUNICATOR ROLE (continued)

CONSULT LETTER[c]	CONTENT	STYLE
PURPOSE: Communicates findings and opinions to the referring professional	**Referring physicians want:** • impressions (dx and answer referring question) • management plan (who will do what and when • medication changes • rationale for recommendations • who is providing ongoing care • guidance and education (articles, advice, guidelines) **Receiving physician want:** • history and physical exam info • context that enables interpretation of investigations • Proof the consultation actually occurred • A clear question	**Language:** • Simple language • No abbreviations, acronyms • Short words (less than three syllables) • Active vs. passive voice ("I saw Ms. X …" vs. "Ms. X was seen …") **Visual Display:** • Organized • Bullet points • Short sentences (one idea per sentence) • Short paragraphs (four to five sentences) • Section headings • Graphics • Right amount of information • Edited (Plan, Dictate, Edit)

HINTS

1. **Orient yourself to the patient.** Be situationally aware and oriented to the relationship with this patient — **aka patient-centred.**

   • WHO: Is there a prior patient-physician relationship? (Is this the first time you have had a conversation, or is this a follow-up visit? Or is this a long-standing patient-physician relationship? How have any past encounters proceeded?)

   • WHAT: type of problem does the patient have? (minor or serious); Nature of the patient's problem? (acute or chronic): particular needs of this patient? (e.g. health literacy, personality, age, gender)

   • WHERE will the communication take place? (e.g. office, clinic, emergency department, health facility)

   • HOW to orient to patient (e.g. charts, health care professional debriefing or handover information)

2. **Watch for signals and cues.** Pay attention to signals and cues that provide feedback about understanding, misunderstanding, or disagreement

   • signals of shared understanding (e.g. smiles, nods, relaxed or open body language) and

   • cues to misunderstanding or disagreement (e.g. looking away, shaking head, arms crossed, tensed muscles, silence, closed body language).

   • signals and cues vary by person, experience and culture

   • silence is not necessarily a sign of understanding and agreement. Seek confirmation frequently,

3. **Be careful about labels.** Avoid using labels such as 'minor' and 'mild'. What one person views as 'minor' and 'mild' may be perceived very differently by another who has different views and needs. For example, a 'minor' sprained ankle or 'mild' stroke may not be viewed as 'minor' or 'mild' by the patient.

   • Common/Repeated Communication Topics/Subjects

   • Challenging Communication Topics/Subjects

   • Available Resources and exemplars

---

c Keely E, Dojeiji S, Myers K. Writing effective consultation letters: 12 tips for teachers. *Med Teach.* 2002; 24(6):585-9.

© 2015 Royal College of Physicians and Surgeons of Canada

Communicator

A1. COMMUNICATION ASSESSMENT TOOL[a]

Communication with patients is a very important part of quality medical care.

We would like to know how you feel about the way your doctor communicated with you.
Your answers are confidential, so please be as open and honest as you can.

Your participation is completely voluntary and will not affect your medical treatment in any way.

Please rate the doctor's communication with you. Check your answer in each box below.

Doctor's Name: _____

#	The Doctor...	1 Poor	2 Fair	3 Good	4 Very good	5 Excellent
1.	Greeted me in a way that made me feel comfortable					
2.	Treated me with respect					
3.	Showed interest in my ideas about my health					
4.	Understood my main health concerns					
5.	Paid attention to me (looked at me, listened carefully)					
6.	Let me talk without interruptions					
7.	Gave me as much information as I wanted					
8.	Talked in terms I could understand					
9.	Checked to be sure I understood everything					
10.	Encouraged me to ask questions					
11.	Involved me in decisions as much as I wanted					
12.	Discussed next steps, including any follow-up plans					
13.	Showed care and concern					
14.	Spent the right amount of time with me					
15.	How would you rate the care provided by your doctor?					

Comments:

---

a   Makoul G, Krupat E, Chang CH. Measuring patient views of physician communication skills: development and testing of the communication assessment tool. *Patient Educ Couns.* 2007;67(3):333-42. Reproduced with permission.

Communicator

A2. CONSULTATION LETTER RATING SCALE[a]

See Communicator Role teacher tips appendix for this assessment tool

Instructions for Assessor:

- Communication competencies can be developed over time. Using the form below, please help this learner gain insight into his/her communication skills by providing valuable confidential feedback.

- This information will be shared with the learner in aggregate form and for the purposes of helping the learner improve.

- Please return this form in a confidential manner

  to _____

  by _____

- Circle your answer for each item.

Resident Name: _____

PGY Level: _____

Completed by: _____

Date: _____

CONTENT

1. HISTORY

- Identified chief problem/reason for referral
- Described the chief complaint
- Identified relevant past history
- Listed current medications, as appropriate
- Other history appropriate to presenting problem: Psychosocial history, functional history, family history, review of systems, etc.

POOR 1	BORDERLINE 2	ACCEPTABLE 3	GOOD 4	EXCELLENT 5
Missing relevant data		Most of relevant data present		All relevant data present

2. PHYSICAL EXAMINATION

- Described physical examination findings relevant to presenting problem

POOR 1	BORDERLINE 2	ACCEPTABLE 3	GOOD 4	EXCELLENT 5
Missing relevant physical exam		Most of relevant physical exam present		All relevant physical exam present

3. IMPRESSION AND PLAN

- Provided diagnosis and/or differential diagnosis
- Provided a management plan
- Provided a rationale for the management plan (education)
- Stated whether the management plan was discussed with patient
- Stated who would be responsible for elements of the management plan and follow-up
- Answered the referring physicians question (if present)

POOR 1	BORDERLINE 2	ACCEPTABLE 3	GOOD 4	EXCELLENT 5
Key issues not addressed. Did not answer referring physician's question. No rationale for recommendations. No education provided. No indication of who will do what.		Most key issues identified and addressed. Answered referring physician's question. Some rationale for recommendations. No education provided. Some indication of who is responsible for management plan elements and follow-up		All key issues identified and addressed. Answered referring physician's question. Provided rationale for recommendations made. Provided education. Clear plan for who will do what and who is responsible for follow-up. Noted what patient was told.

---

a Dojeiji S, Keely E, Myers K. Used with permission.

© 2015 Royal College of Physicians and Surgeons of Canada

A2. CONSULTATION LETTER RATING SCALE (continued)

Communicator

4. CLARITY AND BREVITY
- Words used:
  short (less than 3 syllables)
  active voice
  minimal medical jargon; minimal filler words/phrases
  no word or phrase repetition
- Length of sentences:
  one idea per sentence
  each sentence less than 3 lines long
- Length of paragraphs:
  one topic per paragraph
  each paragraph less than 4-5 sentences long

POOR 1	BORDERLINE 2	ACCEPTABLE 3	GOOD 4	EXCELLENT 5
Wordy. Message unclear Redundant words/phrases Lots of jargon and fillers. Mostly passive tone. Long sentences. Long paragraphs.		Concise. Minimal jargon and fillers. Some active tone. Some short sentences. Some sentences with one idea/sentence. Some short paragraphs.		Concise. Clear and organized. No redundant words/phrases. No jargon and fillers. Active tone primarily. Short sentences. One idea/sentence. Short paragraphs.

5. ORGANIZATION OF LETTER
- Use of headings
- Layout visually appealing with lots of white space
- Use of bulleted or numbered lists, tables, or graphics as appropriate
- Information easy to scan

POOR 1	BORDERLINE 2	ACCEPTABLE 3	GOOD 4	EXCELLENT 5
No headings. No white space. No bulleted or numbered lists. No tables. Difficult to scan.		Some headings used. Some white space. Some bulleted and numbered lists. Generally easy to scan. Most key info easy to find.		Headings clear and appropriate Lots of white space. Numbered and bulleted lists. Uses of graphics or tables. Very easy to scan.

OVERALL RATING OF LETTER

- Degree to which the letter is helpful to the referring physician

POOR 1	BORDERLINE 2	ACCEPTABLE 3	GOOD 4	EXCELLENT 5
Letter not helpful. Lacking key content. Lacking style elements to make the letter easy to scan Key info hard to find.		Generally helpful as key content available. Limited or no education incorporated. Some style elements incorporated. Most key information easy to find (impression and plan at a minimum).		Informative letter. Element of education incorporated. Key information easy to find.

Areas of strength	Areas for improvement
1.	1.
2.	2.
3.	3.

Comments:

© 2015 Royal College of Physicians and Surgeons of Canada

A3. WRITTEN QUESTIONS AND ANSWERS FOR THE COMMUNICATOR ROLE

Created for the *CanMEDS Teaching and Assessment Tools Guide* by J Sherbino and S Glover Takahashi. Reproduced with permission of the Royal College.

See Communicator Role teacher tips appendix for this assessment tool

Instructions for Learner:

Answer questions on your own in time allowed.

You have_____minutes to answer these questions.

Name:_____

Date:_____

1. Define a minimum of six communication terms from the list below.
    *   Categorization
    *   Chunking
    *   Common ground
    *   Difficult discussion
    *   Encounter
    *   Non-verbal communication skills
    *   Paraverbal communication
    *   Patient-centred approach
    *   Plain language
    *   Safety net
    *   Shared decision-making
    *   Signposting
    *   Therapeutic relationships

2. Complete the table below about verbal communication tasks. Identify the sequence, timing, and purposes of each of the communication skills tasks. ***Note: one task has been prefilled as an example.***

No.	Verbal communication skills task	When it takes place in encounter	Purpose(s) (Identify a minimum of two per task)
1.			
2.			
3.			
4.			
5.	Building the relationship	Ongoing	• Developing a therapeutic alliance • Involving the patient
6.			

© 2015 Royal College of Physicians and Surgeons of Canada

A3. WRITTEN QUESTIONS AND ANSWERS FOR THE COMMUNICATOR
ROLE (continued)

3. Complete the table below by listing some of the details you would include under each of these three parts of a written communication.

No.	Written communication skills task	Types of details to include
1.	History	
2.	Physician Exam Report (e.g. physical exam, interventions, plan, results)	
3.	Impression and Management	

4. Describe the purpose of a consult letter. List three or four things you would cover in the letter (content). List three style/ structure elements that you would incorporate into your letter.

_____

_____

_____

_____

5. Identify three impacts and/or outcomes of effective communication.

_____

_____

_____

_____

Communicator

A3. ANSWER KEY SHORT ANSWER QUESTIONS

1. **Define six of these Communicator terms***

- ***Categorization*** is a type of signposting that orients the patient to specific details about how information is going to be discussed. For example, "There are three important things I want to explain. First, I want to tell you what I think is going on; second, what tests I think would be …"

- ***Chunking and checking*** is an approach to giving the patient information in "pieces" then pausing to verify they understand before proceeding. It is a technique used to gauge how much information to give to a patient. This approach aids in achieving a shared understanding with the patient.

- ***Common ground*** provides a basis of mutual interest or agreement

- ***Difficult discussion*** refers to a patient-physician conversation related to the patient's health care preferences, needs, and values that can be challenging because of the high or intense emotion involved. The topics considered challenging or difficult vary on the basis of the patient's preferences, needs, and values; the physician's preferences, needs, values, and comfort level; and the environmental, cultural, and health care contexts.

- ***Empathy*** is a key skill in developing the physician-patient relationship. It has two parts: the understanding and sensitive appreciation of another's predicament or feeling; and the communication of that understanding back to the patient in a supportive way. It does not necessarily equate to agreeing with the patient's feelings. An example is "I can see that your husband's memory loss has been very difficult for you to cope with." Empathy is often confused with sympathy, which is feeling pity or concern from outside of the patient's perspective.

- ***Encounter*** refers to a purposeful patient-physician interaction.

- ***Non-verbal*** communication skills are the skills involved in transmitting information without the use of words. They include body language (e.g. facial expressions, eye contact, gestures), paraverbal skills (e.g. tone, pace, volume of speech), touch, space, smell, and clothing. Non-verbal communication is responsible for conveying most of our attitudes, emotions, and affect. Non-verbal communication can override what we actually say to patients.

- ***Paraverbal*** communication is what you convey in the characteristics of your words through your pace, tone, pitch, rhythm, volume, articulation, and use of pauses.

- ***Patient-centred*** approach is one providing care that is respectful of and responsive to individual patient preferences, needs, and values, and ensuring that patient values guide all clinical decisions.

- ***Plain language*** is the use of common words that are understandable by the patient. This may mean avoiding technical or medical terms unless they are carefully defined or described.

- ***Safety net*** means the set of contingency plans for the patient, which should be discussed at the end of the interview. Providing a safety net for the patient involves explaining what the patient should do if things do not go according to plan, telling them how they should contact you, and discussing what developments might require back-up.

- ***Shared decision-making*** is a communication approach where patients and their health care professionals, including their physician, make decisions following careful deliberation about the patient's preferences, needs, and values and with an understanding of the available options and evidence so that they can wisely choose the best action(s).

- ***Signposting*** is the use of bridging statements to alert patients that you are changing topics or direction in the encounter. Signposts help the patient to understand where the interview is going and why. They also help to provide structure to the interview and act as guide markers to keep you organized and patient focused. For example, "I have just finished getting a history of your stomach pain; now I would like to do a physical exam. Is that okay?"

- ***Therapeutic relationship*** is the working alliance between the physician and patient. Respect (i.e. unconditional positive regard), genuineness, and empathy have been correlated with good therapeutic outcomes.

---

* Refer to Communicator Key Terms in the Tools Guide for full definitions.

© 2015 Royal College of Physicians and Surgeons of Canada

A3. ANSWER KEY SHORT ANSWER QUESTIONS (continued)

2. Complete the table below about verbal communication task. Identify the sequence, timing, and purposes of each of the communication tasks.[a, b]

#	Verbal Communication COMMUNICATION TASK	Timing	PURPOSES (2-4 per task)
1.	INITIATING THE SESSION	Beginning	• Establishing initial rapport • Identifying the reason for the visit
2.	GATHERING INFO AND PHYSICAL EXAM	Middle	• Exploration of the patient problem to discover: • Biomedical perspective (disease) • Patient perspective (illness) • Background information – context
3.	EXPLANATION AND PLANNING	Middle	• Providing the correct type and level of information • Aiding accurate recall and understanding • Achieving a shared understanding – incorporating the patient's perspective • Planning – shared decision-making
4.	CLOSING THE SESSION	End	• Ensuring appropriate point of closure • Forward planning
5.	BUILDING THE RELATIONSHIP	Ongoing	• Developing a therapeutic alliance • Involving the patient
6.	PROVIDING STRUCTURE	Ongoing	• Making organization overt • Attending to flow

3. Complete the table below by listing some of the details you would include under each of these three parts of a written communication.

CONTENT		Sample details
1.	History	• Chief problem/reason for referral • Chief complaint • Relevant past history • Current medications, as appropriate • Other history appropriate to presenting problem: psychosocial history, functional history, family history, review of systems, etc.
2.	Physical Exam	• Physical examination findings relevant to presenting problem
3.	Impression and Management	• Diagnosis and/or differential diagnosis • Management plan • Rationale for the management plan (education) • Report on whether the management plan was discussed with patient • Notes who will be responsible for elements of the management plan and follow-up • Answer the referring physicians question (if present)

a   Kurtz SM, Silverman JD. The Calgary-Cambridge Referenced Observation Guides: an aid to defining the curriculum and organizing the teaching in communication training programmes. *Med Educ*. 1996 Mar; 30(2):83-9.

b   Silverman J, Kurtz S, Draper J. *Skills for communicating with patients*. 3rd ed. London: Radcliffe Publishing. Copyright © 2013. Reproduced by permission of Taylor & Francis Books UK.

A3. ANSWER KEY SHORT ANSWER QUESTIONS (continued)

4. Describe the purpose of a consult letter. List three or four things you would cover in the letter (content). List three style/structure elements that you would incorporate into your letter.

Written Communication	PURPOSE	CONTENT	STYLE
CONSULT LETTER	Communicates findings and opinions to the referring physician	**Referring physicians want:** • the consultants impressions (dx and answer to the referring question) • management plan (who will do what and when) • medication changes • rationale for recommendations • who is providing ongoing care • guidance and education (articles, advice, guidelines) **Consultants want:** • Record of the history and physical exam • Context that enables the interpretation of investigations • Proof the consultation actually occurred • A clear question	**Language** • Simple language • No abbreviations, acronyms • Short words (less than three syllables) • Active vs. passive voice ("I saw Ms. X …" vs. "Ms. X was seen …") **Visual display** • Organized • Bullet points • Short sentences (one idea per sentence) • Short paragraphs (four to five sentences) • Section headings • Graphics • Right amount of information • Edited (Plan, Dictate, Edit)

5. Identify three impacts/outcomes of effective communications.

#	Impacts/outcomes of effective communications.
1.	Increased accuracy, which improves patient understanding, recall, and compliance and increases efficiency for patients and physicians,
2.	Improved outcomes of care (physiological and psychological),
3.	Heightened perceptions by patients that they are supported by their physicians and improved relationships between patients and caregivers, resulting in higher satisfaction for patients and physicians,
4.	Reduced rates of adverse events/medical errors, and
5.	Better protection against complaints and malpractice claims.

© 2015 Royal College of Physicians and Surgeons of Canada

A4. OBJECTIVE STRUCTURED CLINICAL EXAM (OSCE) FOR THE COMMUNICATOR ROLE[a]

Created for the *CanMEDS Teaching and Assessment Tools Guide* by S Glover Takahashi. Reproduced with permission of the Royal College.

Instructions for Assessor:

- *Learning objectives:* OSCE assessments are an effective way to assess if all of your learners are at, above or below a common standard. They will also provide insight as to who is meeting or exceeding in their understanding and application of Communicator competencies, as well as who is falling behind.

- *How to adapt:*

  - Select from, modify, or add to the sample OSCE cases. Each case is designed as a 10-minute scenario.

  - Modify these cases to be 7- 8 minutes with the standardized patient (SP) and have two or three minutes of probing questions from faculty. The two to four probing questions within the scenario provide considerable additional insight into competence in the area.[25]

  - Combine a variety of different Roles in to the same exam.

  - Four to six cases is a reasonable number of cases for an in training program OSCE.

  - Consider using one scenario at a teaching session. Residents or SPs could do a demonstration.

  - Consider using a video recorded scenario for teaching purposes.

Scenario 1:

- A biopsy has come back for Teddy, a 23-year-old engineering student, showing osteosarcoma of the proximal tibia. Imaging shows that this tumour appears amenable to limb salvage with a tumour prosthesis. You have been asked to discuss the results with Teddy and his mother.

- Before this discussion, you speak to the orthopaedic oncologist, who indicates that current treatment for osteosarcoma, which consists of chemotherapy and surgery, is curative in 70%–80% of cases. Limb salvage is possible in 95% of cases. Most patients with a tumour prosthesis, however, lead relatively sedentary lives and are unable to participate in sporting activities.

- *You have <<XX (i.e. 8 or 10 minutes)>> to discuss the results with Teddy and his mother.*

Scenario 2:

- A 17-year-old girl, Casey, presents to the <emergency department, ambulatory pediatric clinic, family medicine clinic> with a soft tissue injury and abrasion to her forearm suffered when she fell off her bike.

- During your assessment it becomes apparent that she was not wearing her helmet because "helmets aren't cool."

- She is a goaltender for her soccer team and wants to play in two days.

- *You have <<XX (i.e. five, seven or ten minutes)>> for treatment planning with Casey.*

Scenario 3:

- Using the clinical information provided in the room, dictate a consultation letter.

- *You have <<XX (i.e. eight, ten or fifteen minutes)>> to create your letter.*

---

a Adapted from Glover Takahashi, Nayer, 2012, PGME, University of Toronto, ON. Reproduced with permission.

Communicator

A4. SCORING SHEET: SCENARIO 1 AND 2

Created for the *CanMEDS Teaching and Assessment Tools Guide* by S Glover Takahashi. Reproduced with permission of the Royal College.

Name:_____

Level:_____

Program:_____

COMMUNICATOR: 1. Provides structure and attends to the flow of the encounter

1 Needs significant improvement	2 Below expectations	3 Solid, competent performance	4 Exceeds expectations	5 Sophisticated, expert performance
Agenda setting not done. Few or confusing signposts and transitional statements. Sequence not organized. Either overly patient focused or overly physician focused. Encounter runs late, not achieving patient or physician goals.		Sets agenda. Signposts the key tasks, provides rationale for each task. Patient tells their story within a structured logical sequence. Completes encounter in reasonable time and with adequate efficiency.		Prepares for encounter. Sets agenda with patient. Signposts clearly and elegantly, ensuring patient understands each task and is engaged. Patient-centred while efficiently and effectively completing encounter.

COMMUNICATOR: 2. Develops a therapeutic alliance, involves the patient, and attends to, builds, and nurtures a trusting relationship with the patient

1 Needs significant improvement	2 Below expectations	3 Solid, competent performance	4 Exceeds expectations	5 Sophisticated, expert performance
Not attentive or responsive to the patient. Seems to be going through motions. Distracted (e.g. phone) or disinterested. Seems rushed. Seems to not listen. Does not appear interested or allow patient to share views, priorities, feelings, or concerns. Provides little opportunity for questions. Little or no attention to patient comfort, verbal or non-verbal cues, or safety needs. Does not share much information; what is shared is not really accurate.		Empathetically, non-judgmentally, and respectfully listens to understand the patient's feelings, concerns, views, and priorities. Attends to patient confidentiality, comfort, and safety. Verbally acknowledges patient's feelings and concerns. Shares accurate information. Shares power. Observes patient verbal and non-verbal cues, provides opportunity for questions, acknowledges cues.		Involves patient with ease. Skilled at building trust, listening attentively and anticipating needs and concerns. Enables patient to share views, priorities, feelings, and concerns with opportunities for questions. Anticipates patient comfort and safety needs. Shares accurate information in an efficient manner. Shares power with patient. Watches for and responds to patient's verbal and non-verbal cues.

Communicator

© 2015 Royal College of Physicians and Surgeons of Canada

A4. SCORING SHEET: SCENARIO 1 AND 2 (continued)

COMMUNICATOR: 3. Initiates the encounter, establishing initial rapport and identifying the reason for the visit

1 Needs significant improvement	2 Below expectations	3 Solid, competent performance	4 Exceeds expectations	5 Sophisticated, expert performance
Little or no eye contact, seems cold. No or unclear introduction. Seems distracted when patient talks, interrupts patient. Does not seem attentive or interested in patient's ideas, feelings, expectations, or concerns regarding the presenting issue(s) and its impact. Does not acknowledge patient or reflect understanding.		Makes eye contact, smiles, uses a warm tone, sits down. Introduces self (e.g. name, role, responsibility). Listens to the patient's opening statement without interrupting. Listens for and acknowledges patient's ideas, feelings, expectations, and concerns regarding the presenting issue(s) and its impact. Acknowledges understanding reason(s) for visit and reflects understanding. Uses semi-structured questions to clarify.		Centred and focused on the patient, engaging the patient with eye contact, smiles, a warm tone; sits down. Clearly introduces self. Rapport developed through attention to patient, listens without interrupting. Acknowledges patient's ideas, feelings, expectations, and concerns regarding the presenting issue(s) and its impact; reason(s) for visit; reflects understanding. Efficiently clarifies for shared meaning.

COMMUNICATOR: 4. Gathers information and explores the patient's problem to discover both the biomedical perspective (disease) and the patient's perspective (illness)

1 Needs significant improvement	2 Below expectations	3 Solid, competent performance	4 Exceeds expectations	5 Sophisticated, expert performance
Does not effectively gather information about both biomedical/disease and illness/patient perspective in a complete or sequenced manner. Not effective at integrating open, semi-structured, and closed-ended techniques.		Gathers biomedical/disease perspective in complete and sequenced manner using open, semi-structured, and closed-ended techniques, appropriately moving from one to the other. Gathers illness/patient perspective by active exploration of patient's ideas, feelings, expectations, and concerns of the presenting issue(s) and the impact of the issue(s) on the patient's life as the encounter unfolds.		Efficiently gathers and integrates both biomedical/disease and illness/patient information while effectively using open, semi-structured, and closed-ended techniques and attentive exploration of patient's ideas, feelings, expectations, and concerns of the presenting issue(s) and the impact of the issue(s) on the patient's life as the encounter unfolds.

A4. SCORING SHEET: SCENARIO 1 AND 2 (continued)

Communicator

COMMUNICATOR: 5. Explains and plans with a correct type and level of information, aiding accurate recall and understanding, achieving a shared understanding, and working toward shared planning

1 Needs significant improvement	2 Below expectations	3 Solid, competent performance	4 Exceeds expectations	5 Sophisticated, expert performance
Does not check for understanding, nor gives information in manageable chunks. Uses jargon. Indicates plan but is unclear or incomplete on rationale for investigations, medication choices, lifestyle changes. Little attention given to verbal and non-verbal cues. Presents plan as a 'run-on' sentence. Gives limited or no opportunity for questions and comments. Seems uninterested in patient perspective on the information provided or proposed management plan. Limits patient choices and decisions.		Checks understanding, gives information in manageable chunks. Uses simple terms, repetition, explicit categorization. Provides diagnosis and rationale for investigations (e.g. tests and referrals). Outlines medication choices, lifestyle changes. Observes verbal and non-verbal cues. Verbally encourages questions and comments. Elicits patient perspective on the information provided and proposed management plan. Offers choices and shares alternatives. Negotiates plan of action. Verbally encourages patient to make choices and decisions to the level that they wish.		Nuanced sharing of information in manageable chunks, ensuring shared understanding; uses lay terms, repetition, categorization. Clarity in providing diagnosis, rationale for investigations, medication choices, lifestyle changes. Responsive to verbal and non-verbal cues. Genuinely encourages questions, comments, patient perspective on the information provided and proposed management plan. Offers choices and shares alternatives. Verifies patient's understanding via patient repeating, handouts. Establishes shared plan of action with patient, enabling appropriate choices and decisions.

COMMUNICATOR: 6. Closes the session, ensuring appropriate closure and forward planning

1 Needs significant improvement	2 Below expectations	3 Solid, competent performance	4 Exceeds expectations	5 Sophisticated, expert performance
No summary or a confusing end to encounter. Not clear, or disagreement on plans and next steps. Omits or is unclear on safety net, next purpose, or process.		Summarizes session briefly and clarifies plan of care and clear plan of action. Establishes safety net, when and how to seek help.		Effectively, efficiently, and supportively ends the session, ensuring shared understanding of action plan, follow-up, and safety net if needed.

COMMUNICATOR: 7. Verbal communication skills

1 Needs significant improvement	2 Below expectations	3 Solid, competent performance	4 Exceeds expectations	5 Sophisticated, expert performance
Awkward phrasing (e.g. uses jargon, provides too much or too little information).		Clearly communicates information that is understood by an active listener. Encourages dialogue.		Exceptionally clear, comprehensive, easily understood explanations. Responds to patient's non-verbal cues. Deals with high emotions. Excellent command of expression (fluency, grammar, vocabulary, pronunciation).

© 2015 Royal College of Physicians and Surgeons of Canada

A4. SCORING SHEET: SCENARIO 1 AND 2 (continued)

COMMUNICATOR: 8. Non-verbal and paraverbal communication skills

1 Needs significant improvement	2 Below expectations	3 Solid, competent performance	4 Exceeds expectations	5 Sophisticated, expert performance
Distracting non-verbal behaviour that is disruptive (e.g. little or no eye contact; lack of control of facial expressions, gestures, vocalization, and tone; speech errors; inappropriate use of pauses or silence). Use of personal space inappropriate for patient care. Inappropriate grooming or dress.		Maintains appropriate eye contact. Exhibits enough control of non-verbal expression to engage listener. Demonstrates engagement through body language.		Is aware of and purposefully uses non-verbal behaviours and gestures to establish and maintain a relationship.

Communicator

OVERALL PERFORMANCE IN THIS SCENARIO

1 Needs significant improvement	2 Below expectations	3 Solid, competent performance	4 Exceeds expectations	5 Sophisticated, expert performance

PGY LEVEL OF PERFORMANCE[a] – What level of training was this performance?

B Below PGY1	1 Mid-PGY1	2 Mid-PGY2	3 Mid-PGY3	4 Mid-PGY4	5+ Mid-PGY5 or >

Areas of strength	Areas for improvement
1.	1.
2.	2.
3.	3.

Other comments:

---

a Programs that have moved to Competence By Design may want to modify these levels to the four parts of the resident competence continuum.

© 2015 Royal College of Physicians and Surgeons of Canada

A4. SCENARIO 3: SCORING SHEET

Created for the *CanMEDS Teaching and Assessment Tools Guide* by S Glover Takahashi. Reproduced with permission of the Royal College.

Name: _____

Level:[a] _____

Program: _____

COMMUNICATOR: 1. CONTENT includes what is considered essential, important, and relevant

1 Needs significant improvement	2 Below expectations	3 Solid, competent performance	4 Exceeds expectations	5 Sophisticated, expert performance
Missing or incomplete content about consultants impressions, management plan; any medication changes; rationale for recommendations; who is providing ongoing care; and provided/needed guidance and education.		Includes the key information about consultants impressions (dx and answer to the referring question), management plan (who will do what and when); any medication changes; rationale for recommendations; who is providing ongoing care; and provided/needed guidance and education.		Completely and efficiently includes all information which is essential, important and relevant to consultants management plan; any medication changes; rationale for recommendations; who is providing ongoing care; and provided/needed guidance and education (articles, advice, guidelines).

COMMUNICATOR: 2. STYLE visual layout helps with ease of reading and understanding

1 Needs significant improvement	2 Below expectations	3 Solid, competent performance	4 Exceeds expectations	5 Sophisticated, expert performance
Language is difficult to understand or comprehend. Many abbreviations or acronyms, some irregular or undefined. The content is disorganized with long run on sentences. There are typos and poor word choice.		Language is understandable and easy to comprehend. Some common abbreviations or acronyms that are defined. The content is organized in paragraphs. The sentences makes sense, there are no typos or mis-used words.		Language is very straightforward with elegance and efficiency of words, sentence and uses active voice. No abbreviations or acronyms. Visual display is organized, uses bullet points, section headings, short sentences and paragraphs. The content is 'tight' and edited.

COMMUNICATOR: 3. Opening statement provides reason for referral in clear, organized and complete manner.

1 Needs significant improvement	2 Below expectations	3 Solid, competent performance	4 Exceeds expectations	5 Sophisticated, expert performance
Purpose for consultation may not be expressly included. Doesn't orient reader to key information which informed consultation.		Clarifies the 'question' being answered the relevant context informing the consultation which occurred.		Clearly focuses reader to the consultations purpose providing key relevant contextual informing that guided/informed the consultation.

a Programs that have moved to Competence By Design may want to modify these levels to the four parts of the resident competence continuum.

© 2015 Royal College of Physicians and Surgeons of Canada

A4. SCENARIO 3: SCORING SHEET (continued)

COMMUNICATOR: 4. Presents findings incl physical exam in clear, organized and complete manner.

1 Needs significant improvement	2 Below expectations	3 Solid, competent performance	4 Exceeds expectations	5 Sophisticated, expert performance
Description of findings, poor, vague, variable inconclusive, lack of detail or overly detailed and technical for patient care, follow up or safety. Incorrect or incomplete procedure recorded.		Describes interventions and any findings with clarity and sufficient detail for patient care, follow up and safety. All needed pertinent information including complications or relevant incidents.		Organized, clear and complete description of intervention(s) and any findings. Specific commentary to inform patient care, follow up and safety. Attentive in commenting on risks, complications or relevant incidents.

COMMUNICATOR: 5. Provides opinion, rationale, recommendations, plans

1 Needs significant improvement	2 Below expectations	3 Solid, competent performance	4 Exceeds expectations	5 Sophisticated, expert performance
Inadequate synthesis of findings to formulate appropriate differential diagnosis, impression and management. Suggestions unclear. May include a diagnosis but no/unclear recommendations.		Adequate synthesis with differential diagnosis or to inform differential diagnosis or management. Provides rationale, options, patients response or choices. Writes to share opinion and effectively inform patient care. Risks, complications or relevant incidents noted.		Organized, clear and complete descriptions of synthesis with differential diagnosis or to inform differential diagnosis and management. Clarity about rationale, options, patients response or choices. Attentive in commenting on alternatives, options, risks, complications or relevant incidents.

COMMUNICATOR: 6. Closes the consultation with clarity including follow up.

1 Needs significant improvement	2 Below expectations	3 Solid, competent performance	4 Exceeds expectations	5 Sophisticated, expert performance
Lack of follow up, plan, with far too much focus on the details of what transpired and little information on the next steps and who is responsible for following up on the issues identified.		Comments on alternatives, options, next steps and follow up plan. Roles are commented on including next steps and who is responsible for following up on the issues identified.		Demonstrates collaborative approach with colleagues and effective communication with patient. Demonstrates commitment to shared care and clarity on next steps and who is responsible for following up on the issues identified.

Communicator

A4. SCENARIO 3: SCORING SHEET (continued)

OVERALL PERFORMANCE IN THIS SCENARIO

1 Needs significant improvement	2 Below expectations	3 Solid, competent performance	4 Exceeds expectations	5 Sophisticated, expert performance

PGY LEVEL OF PERFORMANCE[a] – What level of training was this performance?

B Below PGY1	1 Mid-PGY1	2 Mid-PGY2	3 Mid-PGY3	4 Mid-PGY4	5+ Mid-PGY5 or >

Areas of strength	Areas for improvement
1.	1.
2.	2.
3.	3.

Other comments:

© 2015 Royal College of Physicians and Surgeons of Canada

COMMUNICATOR ROLE TEACHER TIPS APPENDIX

T3 COMMUNICATION SCRIPTS

Instructions for Teacher:

- Setting and Audience: All learners.

- How to use: Plan for about 20 minutes for the worksheet.

  - Allow individuals to read the worksheet and spend about 5 minutes working on the answers.

  - Compare and discuss answers in small groups.

  - Reporting back by group.

  - Summary of key points by faculty.

- How to adapt:

  - You may wish to assign the worksheet as homework to be completed before the session or as a follow-up assignment.

  - Select only those questions that apply to your teaching. Modify questions as appropriate to match the specialty or the learners' practice context.

- Logistics:

  - Copies of worksheets, flip chart paper.

  - Extra pens for learners.

T8 SUMMARY SHEET FOR THE COMMUNICATOR ROLE

Instructions for Teacher:

- The summary sheet is intended to be a cheat sheet for the teacher as well as the learner. It is a one page resource on key concepts, frameworks and approaches.

A2 CONSULTATION RATING SCALE

Instructions for Teacher:

- Depending on the location and program, you may use this tool regularly for a particular learning experience (e.g. rotation, clinic) or from time to time across all locations (e.g. Block 8 every year)

- You will choose individuals to completes the form (e.g. all team members, physicians, nursing colleague, etc) and you will need to decide how you will collate the results (e.g. by site director, program administrator)

- Be transparent with your learner. Explain how you will administer the review and how you will integrate multiple views to provide feedback and coaching advice on areas of strength and areas for improvement.

- Plan to share the summary in written format as well as via face-to-face meetings to provide feedback and coaching advice on areas of strength and areas for improvement.

A3 WRITTEN QUESTIONS AND ANSWERS – COMMUNICATOR

Instructions for Assessor:

- *Learning objectives:* Written questions are an efficient way to assess if all of your learners are at, above or below a common standard. They will also provide insight as to who is meeting or exceeding expectations in their understanding and application of Communicator concepts as well as who is falling behind.

- *Audience:* All learners.

- *How to use:* Select from, modify, or add to the sample questions as appropriate. If selecting all of these questions, we suggest that you allow 30-45 minutes to complete.

- *How to adapt:* Add these or similar questions to a written test (e.g. on own or include in semi-annual program written exam). You may wish to assign as homework to be completed before the session or as a follow-up assignment.

- *Logistics:* Suggest you provide in similar format to specialty exam (i.e. if specialty exam is paper and pencil, suggest you use same. This will allow for some orientation/training for specialty exam)

- *Setting:* Classroom.

REFERENCES

1. Kurtz S, Silverman J, Draper J. *Teaching and learning communication skills in medicine.* 2nd ed. London: Radcliffe Publishing. Copyright © 2005. Reproduced by permission of Taylor & Francis Books UK.

2. Levinson W, Roter DL, Mullooly JP, Dull VT, Frankel RM. Physician-patient communication. The relationship with malpractice claims among primary care physicians and surgeons. *JAMA.*1997 277(7):553-9.

3. *Canadian framework for teamwork and communication Literature Review, Needs Assessment, Evaluation of Training Tools and Expert Consultations.* Edmonton: Canadian Patient Safety Institute; 2011. Last retrieved July 11, 2015 from http://www.patientsafetyinstitute.ca/english/toolsresources/teamworkcommunication/documents/canadian%20framework%20for%20teamwork%20and%20communications.pdf

4. Silverman J, Kurtz S, Draper J. *Skills for communicating with patients.* 3rd ed. London: Radcliffe Publishing. Copyright © 2013. Reproduced by permission of Taylor & Francis Books UK.

5. Coulehan JL, Block MR. *The Medical Interview: Mastering Skills for Clinical Practice.* 5th ed. Philadelphia: F.A. Davis Company; 2006.

6. Committee on Quality of Health Care in America, Institute of Medicine. 2001. Crossing the quality chasm: a new health system for the 21st century. Washington: National Academy Press. Last retrieved July 11, 2015, from http://iom.edu/Reports/2001/Crossing-the-Quality-Chasm-A-New-Health-System-for-the-21st-Century.aspx

7. Merriam Webster. Common ground. Last retrieved July 11, 2015, from http://www.merriam-webster.com/dictionary/common%20ground

8. Wikipedia. Shared decision-making. Last retrieved July 11, 2015, from https://en.wikipedia.org/wiki/Shared_decision-making

9. Kurtz SM, Silverman JD. The Calgary-Cambridge Referenced Observation Guides: an aid to defining the curriculum and organizing the teaching in communication training programmes. *Med Educ.* 1996 Mar; 30(2):83-9.

10. Keely E, Dojeiji S, Myers K. Writing effective consultation letters: 12 tips for teachers. *Med Teach.* 2002 Nov; 24(6):585-9.

Communicator

© 2015 Royal College of Physicians and Surgeons of Canada

HANDOVER
Cooperating RAPPORT
INTENTION AND IMPACT
DIFFERENCE Contributing
Team RELATIONSHIP-CENTRED CARE
COLLABORATOR
COMMUNICATING Building trust
INTERPROFESSIONAL COLLABORATION
RESPECTING Common ground
ACCOMMODATING
Situational awareness
DEBRIEFING
Process

Denyse Richardson

Dawn Martin

Susan Glover Takahashi

1. Why the Collaborator Role matters

Increasingly, health care is delivered in teams, but are our teams really effective? Most people recognize that collaboration in health care is a good and necessary thing for patients and clinicians. Evidence shows that effective collaboration improves patient care (e.g. patient outcomes,[1] patient safety,[2] patient satisfaction[3]); influences health professional practice (e.g. positive attitudes between and among professions,[4,5] clinician satisfaction, retention[6]); and enhances system efficiency (e.g. cost efficiency, access to care, wait times, coordination of care).[1] Despite this, opportunities for truly effective collaboration in day-to-day practice are often missed or underutilized.

In today's complex health care system no clinician, clinician educator, or clinical researcher works alone. Remember, collaboration involves only two or more people committed to a common purpose, performance goals and approach for which they hold themselves mutually accountable.[7] Collaboration can look and feel different depending on the context and the individuals involved. When individuals are learning to collaborate, there are established processes you can use to facilitate that learning. Our role as medical educators is to facilitate among our colleagues and learners the knowledge, skills and attitudes embedded in the Collaborator Role competencies to enable the delivery of the highest quality of patient care possible.

Healthy professional relationships are important to all of the 2015 CanMEDS Roles, for example:

- The Collaborator Role addresses the relationships between clinicians and colleagues in the health care professions.
- The Communicator Role focuses on the relationship(s) between physicians and patients and their families.[a]
- The Health Advocate Role covers physicians' relationships both with individual patients and with the community as they advocate with, and on behalf of, patients and populations.
- The Leader Role involves relationships related to managing people.
- The Professional Role covers relationships related to managing oneself.
- The Scholar Role addresses relationships related to research in teams.
- The Medical Expert Role covers relationships related to all Roles.

The following five points will help learners begin to appreciate the complexity and importance of the Collaborator Role.

Collaboration matters because:

1. Teams of clinicians with diverse knowledge and skill-sets assure the best health care and healthcare system.
2. Evidence shows that collaboration is good for patients and practitioners.
3. It can impact individuals, the dynamics of groups and their potential for high performance.
4. It provides opportunities to learn from one another.
5. Strong relationships affect the quality of patient care.

2. What the Collaborator Role looks like in daily practice

Effective collaborators look for opportunities to improve the efficiency and effectiveness of their work and the work of others. A high-functioning collaborator is one who feels personally accountable for his or her own behaviour, demonstrates respect, anticipates and prevents errors, and shares mutual accountability with the other members for the outcomes of the work.[8, 9]

Good collaborators:

- make an effort to build relationships
- assume others have good intentions
- respect time, expertise and contributions of others
- elicit input, actively seeking differences of opinions
- are genuinely curious about the perspectives of others
- authentically ask questions to clarify and promote understanding
- reframe problems to find common ground
- are receptive to feedback
- recognize their own limitations and blind spots
- are good listeners and good communicators
- transfer and share relevant information in an effective way
- aren't afraid to ask for help and always look for ways to be helpful

One way to help colleagues and learners make connections between their daily activities and the CanMEDS Collaborator Role is to familiarize them with key processes and content as outlined in the trigger words in Table COLL-1.

---

a Throughout the *CanMEDS 2015 Physician Competency Framework*, phrases such as "patients and their families" are intended to include all those who are personally significant to the patient and are concerned with his or her care, including, reference to the patient's family according to the patient's circumstances, family members, partners, caregivers, legal guardians, and substitute decision-makers.

© 2015 Royal College of Physicians and Surgeons of Canada

TABLE COLL-1. TRIGGER WORDS RELATING TO THE PROCESS AND CONTENT OF COLLABORATOR ROLE

Trigger words relating to the PROCESS of the Collaborator Role:		Trigger words relating to the CONTENT of the Collaborator Role:	
• Accommodating	• Engaging	• Common ground	• Organizational awareness
• Asking questions	• Helping	• Conflict resolution	• Power and Hierarchy
• Building trust	• Promoting understanding	• Debriefing	• Process
• Communicating	• Reframing	• Difference and Diversity	• Reflective practice
• Contributing	• Relationship building	• Disruptive behaviour	• Shared decision-making
• Cooperating	• Respecting	• Handover	• Situational awareness
• Embracing Diversity	• Sharing	• Intention and Impact	• Team development

Excerpt from the CanMEDS 2015 Physician Competency Framework[b]

DEFINITION

As Collaborators, physicians work effectively with other health care professionals to provide safe, high-quality, patient-centred care.

DESCRIPTION

Collaboration is essential for safe, high-quality, patient-centred care, and involves patients and their families,[a] physicians and other colleagues in the health care professions, community partners, and health system stakeholders.

Collaboration requires relationships based in trust, respect, and shared decision-making among a variety of individuals with complementary skills in multiple settings across the continuum of care. It involves sharing knowledge, perspectives, and responsibilities, and a willingness to learn together. This requires understanding the roles of others, pursuing common goals and outcomes, and managing differences.

Collaboration skills are broadly applicable to activities beyond clinical care, such as administration, education, advocacy, and scholarship.

KEY COMPETENCIES

Physicians are able to:

1. Work effectively with physicians and other colleagues in the health care professions

2. Work with physicians and other colleagues in the health care professions to promote understanding, manage differences, and resolve conflicts

3. Hand over the care of a patient to another health care professional to facilitate continuity of safe patient care

Collaborator

b Richardson D, Calder L, Dean H, Glover Takahashi S, Lebel P, Maniate J, Martin D, Nasmith L, Newton C, Steinert Y. Collaborator. In: Frank JR, Snell L, Sherbino J, editors. *CanMEDS 2015 Physician Competency Framework* Ottawa: Royal College of Physicians and Surgeons of Canada; 2015. Reproduced with permission.

© 2015 Royal College of Physicians and Surgeons of Canada

KEY TERMS OF THE COLLABORATOR ROLE

Collaboration is a way of working, organizing, and operating within a system or network that utilizes available resources effectively. It is a process in which **two or more people or organizations** work together toward common goals, by sharing knowledge, learning from one another, and building consensus.[1]

Collaboration in health care occurs across many areas, clinical care research, education, and administration. Directly or indirectly, the patient's voice is always part of the collaborative process.

Interprofessional collaboration is collaboration that involves more than one professional group (e.g. community professionals, laboratory technologists, nurses, pharmacists, physicians, surgeons, therapists).

Intraprofessional collaboration is collaboration that takes place amongst those of the same professional group (i.e. physicians working together - when an oncologist and neurologist collaborate in caring for the same patient).

Collaborative practice is collaboration occurring in the health care context to deliver the highest possible quality of care.[7]

Relationship-centred care is "an approach that recognizes the importance and uniqueness of each health care participant's relationship with every other, and considers these relationships to be central to supporting high-quality care, high-quality work environment, and superior organizational performance."[10]

In professional work relationships, individuals are familiar with each others' roles, trust each other, and demonstrate that they value, respect, appreciate, and support each other in their work.

Rapport[11] refers to a positive reciprocal connection shared by two or more people.

Shared decision-making[12] is a process whereby health care professionals, including physicians, make decisions about the best course of action. Direct patient care issues are informed by the patient's preferences, goals, needs, and values, as well as the available options and evidence.[13]

Misunderstanding is a failure to understand someone else's perspective correctly.[14]

Difference is a disparity in ideas, perspectives, priorities, preferences, beliefs, values, goals, or organizational structures, which might precipitate a transition from a disagreement to a conflict.[14]

Conflict is the interaction and clash of actions, goals, and/or desires.[15]

Disruptive Behaviour occurs when the use of inappropriate words, actions or inactions by a physician interferes with his or her ability to function well with others, to the extent that the behaviour interferes with, or is likely to interfere with, quality health care delivery.[16]

Impact is the consequence of actions on others whether it be intended or unintended.[17]

The concepts of position and interest are central to promote understandings, manage differences, and resolve conflicts.

* ***Positions*** are the suggestions or demands that an individual makes related to a difference or conflict. Position represents what a person says he or she wants.[18]

* ***Interests*** are the needs, concerns, and values that motivate an individual. Interests represent why a person wants what he or she wants.[18]

Organizational Awareness is a level of understanding of different aspects of the organization, including, structure, culture and political, social and economic issues affecting the organization.[19]

Handover (previously referred to as handoff), refers to the temporary or permanent transfer of responsibility and accountability for some or all aspects of care for a patient or group of patients.[20] Handovers occur within and across health care institutions, settings and health professionals. Handovers are high-risk points for patient safety incidents.[20]

© 2015 Royal College of Physicians and Surgeons of Canada

3. Preparing to teach the Collaborator Role

The Collaborator Role can be difficult for learners (and teachers) to learn, teach and assess. As someone who will be teaching the CanMEDS Collaborator Role, you should know that:

- Learners seem "open" to the notion of collaboration but often have a superficial appreciation of the value of collaborators and collaboration to patients and to themselves. For example, while research shows that residents feel that collaborative (team) practice is 'a good thing' it was noted that the concept of appropriate team behaviour was rudimentary (i.e. being a nice person).[21]

- Learners have reported receiving little formal education concerning the roles and responsibilities of other health professionals. The often overlooked simple acts of introducing oneself and clarifying one's role to others has been shown to have a significant impact on improving team function.[21]

- Learners need to develop collaboration competencies in addition to those of their professional identity. Look for a variety of diverse opportunities to incorporate a more contextualized understanding of their role and responsibilities in relation to others (e.g. early exposure to patient safety rounds, discharge planning, M&M rounds, quality improvement initiatives).

- Learners need to develop skills in managing the realities of collaboration in a busy workplace, including handling difference. Day-to-day practice presents multiple opportunities to help learners at different stages of training to develop skills in managing these realities, rather than being shielded or sheltered. Find ways for graduated participation in collaboration and conflict situations (e.g. explicitly label the skills and strategies you role modelled to manage shared decision-making for the more junior learner, provide nuanced feedback to the more experienced learner about workplace performance).

3.1 Common misconceptions to address with learners

Some people believe that collaboration and teamwork are synonymous. These words are frequently used interchangeably in the literature and in practice, which sometimes leads to confusion. In the CanMEDS 2015 Framework, the words 'team', 'teamwork' and 'collaboration' have very different meanings. CanMEDS highlights the distinction because some teams function without the characteristic interdependence that is essential for collaboration.

You can belong to a team but not work together. Teamwork can involve individuals contributing to the whole but not necessarily interacting or working together in a way that produces an outcome greater than the sum of all the individual contributions. By contrast, in a collaborative effort, the collaborators work interdependently and share decision-making, which improves the quality of the outcome. For example, as a clinical supervisor on the clinical teaching unit (CTU) you are part of a clinical teaching TEAM. As a team member you contribute to TEAMWORK through your individual supervision of learners while you are on service. In the role of supervisor on the CTU teaching team, you COLLABORATE with others by contributing your input and observations of the individual learners to aid in the process of shared decision-making regarding their performance assessments.

A second important misconception is the idea that collaboration requires face-to-face interactions among a large group of people in different professions. This viewpoint is limiting and misleading; the truth is that the principles of good collaboration should be used whether the situation involves two or many people, whether the collaborators are in the same or different locations and/or whether the collaborators are colleagues from different or the same profession.

Collaborator

Collaborator

Critical examples of collaboration opportunities that are currently underutilized in teaching include:

- A consultation/referral letter from one physician to another (not face-to-face and between only two colleagues);

- A referral to a professional resource (not face-to-face, and not co-located);

- Research study participation with others (not necessarily co-located or a large group);

- Phone conversations to clarify patient care, roles and responsibilities (not face-to-face, between only two people); and

- Handover of patient care for overnight call (between two colleagues).

Another point of confusion relates to people's perceptions that collaboration is always required. In reality, the degree of collaboration necessary is dependent on the complexity of the situation. Although factors such as team composition, purpose and organizational culture may influence the degree of collaboration possible, it is the situation that should determine the level of collaboration necessary. At times, a situation is not best served by multiple perspectives or skillsets — at times a more independent and autocratic approach is necessary. Collaboration is most needed in situations where diversity of opinion or expertise is required, which leads to better decisions.[22] For example, there is value to the input of health professionals and disciplines in the planning for and delivery of care to meet the needs of patients with complex problems such as planning for cancer care in the community, managing the chronic health needs of patients in underserved areas, or addressing child protection needs.

Finally, a related misconception is that collaborative decision-making is synonymous with a consensus-building approach. The emphasis in consensus building is on ensuring agreement, whereas the emphasis in collaborative decision-making is on actively sharing, soliciting and encouraging diverse perspectives so the best course of action can be deter-

mined. In this shared decision-making, differences of opinion and debate are encouraged and actively elicited. A consensus approach might be appropriate if the relationships in the group are more important than the outcome of the decision made by the group (e.g. staff party).

3.2 Use Collaborator Intelligence (CI) as a framework in the learning and assessment of collaborations

Collaboration in our health care system is complex partly because there are multiple factors that impact the ability to collaborate effectively. There are many different models and approaches for teaching and assessing these factors. One well known model is the Emotional Intelligence (EI) model.[23] EI influences participation and leadership in collaboration. EI is described as the ability to perceive, control and assess emotions.

Below we use the Collaborator Intelligence (CI) framework[c] to organize the key domains for learning, teaching and assessing the Collaborator Role. The four key domains are self, relationships, context and systems and each domain will benefit from development via targeted teaching and assessment. The CI domains include:

- Self (i.e. knowing one's strengths, values, limitations and managing one's own behaviour and emotions);

- Relationships (i.e. being able to use empathy to build relationships with others, including the patient);

- Context (i.e. demonstrating behaviours, actions that reflect and incorporate the awareness of the surrounding situations and circumstances); and

- System (i.e. recognizing and understanding of the aspects of health care organizations, including structures, operations and culture that influence the delivery of care across the continuum).

Table COLL-2 offers subdomains and examples for targeted teaching and assessment.

---

c   The Collaborator Intelligence (CI) framework described here outlines the domains for the learning and teaching of the Collaborator Role and is different than the organizational focus of the Collaborative Intelligence described by J. Richard Hackman, 2011.

   © 2015 Royal College of Physicians and Surgeons of Canada

TABLE COLL-2. RECOGNIZING AND DEVELOPING COLLABORATIVE INTELLIGENCE

Domain	SAMPLE subdomains
Self	• Professional Identity (i.e. scope of practice, self assessment) • Reflective Practice (i.e. emotional self-awareness, blind spots and triggers) • Self-Awareness (i.e. knowing limitations, values and beliefs, recognizing contribution)
Relationship	• Roles and responsibilities (i.e. intraprofessional, interprofessional) • Relationship Building (i.e. rapport, assumptions, intention and impact, conflict resolution) • Mutual Accountability (i.e. asking for, giving and receiving feedback)
Context	• Situational Awareness (i.e. team culture, process, protocols, physical environment) • Diversity (i.e. team development and dynamics, respectful culture, position and interests) • Transitions (i.e. content and process of communication)
System	• Organizational Awareness (i.e. political, social and economic culture, power hierarchy) • Collaborative Leadership (i.e. engagement, change, quality improvement) • Handover (i.e. continuum of care, content and process of communication)

3.3 Define the contexts in which collaboration is particularly important for *your* program, specialty or organization

As you prepare to teach the Collaborator Role consider orienting learners to specific examples in which collaboration is key for your program, specialty or organization. Real life examples that resonate with their own experiences will help clinicians and learners appreciate the value of collaboration and its potential for positively impacting patient outcomes.

As a starting point, consider the following three situations where collaboration is critical. These situations are virtually universal across specialties and therefore should be broadly applicable to all learners.

1. **Patient Handover** – Safe and efficient transfer of patient care is essential throughout all parts of our complex health care system. The institution of resident duty hours and the resulting increase in shiftwork seen over the past decade[24, 25] has accentuated the need for physicians to develop competence in the handover process, which includes the transfer of necessary clinical information and responsibility for patient care.

   Clinicians and learners readily accept handover as a time of risk; therefore they will generally acknowledge the value of investing in good collaboration to increase patient safety. Take time to determine when, where and how handover should occur in your specialty as this will provide many learning opportunities and may ultimately lead to better care.

Physicians should be able to utilize structured communication skills and employ strategies (i.e. effectively use written handover; verify roles and responsibilities; develop a shared understanding of the patient's condition, care plan, and anticipated problems and possible solutions) to reliably hand over patient care to colleagues.[26] There are a variety of structured tools for handover (e.g. I-PASS[27], ISBAR, iSoBAR[28]) that your program may consider using.

2. **Meetings** – Planning for and participating in meetings is another example of an activity that benefits from collaboration. Starting with something as simple as scheduling meetings at times that work for all, so you can efficiently share and exchange ideas is an important way to promote collaboration.

3. **Case management** – Care of a patient where multiple professionals are required is a perfect opportunity to help learners understand the roles of their colleagues (intraprofessional) and other health care professionals (interprofessional). It is an opportunity to learn how shared decisions are made and how goals of care are established when there are multiple viewpoints. As learners gain more experience and take on more of a leadership role, feedback on their ability to engage others and reframe problems to find solutions is important.

© 2015 Royal College of Physicians and Surgeons of Canada

3.4 Discuss how to establish and maintain positive relationships with colleagues in the health care professions

The quality of relationships between colleagues in the health care professions impacts quality of care and potentially patient safety.[36] Encourage learners to reflect on the consequences of both good and bad collaborative relationships. Help learners see that trusting relationships cultivate strong collaborations and that strong collaborations improve patient care and practitioner satisfaction. Trusting relationships allow for the kind of vigorous debate that challenging decisions demand. It is equally important for learners to understand the negative impact that poor relationships can have on patient care, the team's ability to function, and their own personal satisfaction.

Remind learners that relationships underpin the exchange of all forms of information, feelings, and concerns. If relationships are not founded in trust and respect, comments are more apt to be misinterpreted and motives questioned. Establishing positive professional relationships is both an important factor in the success of therapeutic regimens and an essential ingredient in collaborative relationships.[6]

In positive professional work relationships, individuals:

- are familiar with each others' roles and strengths,

- have rapport,

- trust each other, and

- demonstrate that they value, respect, appreciate, and support each other in the work (i.e. health care).

Chan et al found that the emergency department referral-consultation may be significantly altered by the familiarity and perceived trustworthiness of the referring and consulting physicians.[30]

Successful collaboration requires that individuals work interdependently. Interdependence involves an element of risk that may be unfamiliar to your learners: you may need to encourage them to trust team members who hold skill or knowledge sets different from their own. Trust is the starting point, not doubt or superiority. Emphasize to learners, that trust takes time to build, seconds to break and longer to rebuild.

Table COLL-3 provides some sample positive behaviour associated with relationship-centred care in the clinical environment. Share examples with learners from your program, specialty or organization. Explicitly draw attention to positive behaviours in day-to-day practice and encourage learners to reflect on the impact these positive behaviours have on:

- their own experience

- relationships

- quality of care provided

- culture

TABLE COLL-3. EXAMPLES OF POSITIVE BEHAVIOUR IN DEVELOPING RELATIONSHIP-CENTRED CARE

Scenario	Positive behaviour
Goals of care	No one person or profession/specialty dominates discussions. As goals of care are being developed, all relevant points of view are elicited, acknowledged and considered. A diversity of viewpoints is actively sought. Well-informed decisions, not only quick ones, are valued.
Meetings	Members have a rapport with one another. Members know and use one anothers' names and acknowledge one another both when they are in meetings and at other times (e.g. in the elevator, in the coffee line). Members participate and actively listen. Members demonstrate openness to all ideas. Engagement is demonstrated through eye contact and body posture. New members are introduced, oriented, and welcomed.
Handover	A back-and-forth dialogue/process between the sending and receiving members is demonstrated. Questions are encouraged. Clarifications are readily provided. The activity is efficient, yet not rushed. All participants feel comfortable and confident about the exchange.
Consultation letter	The consultant ensures the information needed is included in the consultation letter. Accessible language is used and explanations for abbreviations are provided. The letter is written in a tone of contribution to care, not being derogatory or authoritarian. The role of all MDs, including primary care providers, who care for the patient, is acknowledged and explicit. Physicians ensure that the relevant care providers are cc'ed. Contact information is provided for follow-up.

Collaborator

© 2015 Royal College of Physicians and Surgeons of Canada

ABOUT RELATIONSHIP-CENTRED CARE

Relationship-centred care is "an approach that recognizes the importance and uniqueness of each health care participant's relationship with every other, and considers these relationships to be central in supporting high-quality care, [a] high-quality work environment, and superior organizational performance."[10]

Relationship-centred care is not an alternative to patient-centred care. Rather, patient-centred care is an integral part of relationship-centred care. There are four dimensions of relationship-centred care:[31] namely the patient-clinician relationship, as well as the relationships of clinician-clinician, clinician-community, and clinician-self as foundational and intrinsic to health care.[31]

In the late 1960s and 1970s, the depersonalization of care that had taken place in the mid-20th century began to be challenged. The biomedical approach had grown to overshadow the lived experience of the patient. Health professionals and patients began to call for a bio-psychosocial model of care, which evolved into today's widely adopted patient-centred care model. In this model, patients are encouraged to participate actively in their care decisions, and those decisions reflect the patient's values and goals.

Although this patient-centred care model was an improvement over the preceding "doctor-centred" model, work in the last 20 years shows that the patient-centred approach may not fully reflect the process of care either. From that work has emerged a focus on the number of relationships that are needed to provide best care. The relationship between the patient and the clinician remains of paramount importance but there are three others that need to be recognized as significant. This model, called relationship-centred care, has had great impact on the success of care.[10]

Collaborator

RELATIONSHIP-CENTRED CARE

Patient-Centered Practice

Inter and Intraprofessional Practice

Patient – Clinician

Clinician – Clinician

Clinician – Self

Clinician – Community

Reflective Practice

Community-Based Practice

Pew-Fetzer Task Force (1994, 2000)

3.5 Explore the positive contribution that diversity and differences make to collaboration

Even though the system often creates silos so that people are isolated from others, clinicians and learners need to be encouraged to look for ways to build bridges. They need to consider "What do I have to offer that no one else can bring?" Remind learners it is the simple behaviours that build connections with others like:

- active listening
- acknowledging others' presence and perspective
- asking questions
- sharing information
- engaging with others
- being inclusive
- showing appreciation for contributions

It is the day-to-day practice of these behaviours that over time generates and sustains a positive, helpful culture, allowing the strength of diversity to flourish.

3.6 Help learners identify underlying concepts for understanding their own and deconstructing others' contributions in relationships

Health care systems can be stressful and complex. Conflict is more likely to occur when there is a high level of inter-dependence, differences of goals, scarce resources, stress and uncertainty in the environment.[14] Individuals with different professional socializations, experiences, personalities, respon-sibilities and attitudes must work together in often high emotion situations. As a result, anyone's good intentions can easily be misinterpreted as a result of ambiguity and uncer-tainty and lead to sub-optimal care for patients. Learners need a repertoire of strategies to help them identify, deconstruct and manage challenging situations.

Key concepts include:

- **Assumptions** – Assumptions help us ascribe our own meaning to events but are rarely accurate
- **Positions vs Interests** – Starting conversations from your own personal position of what you want with a predetermined solution is rarely helpful
- **Intention vs Impact** – Our words and behaviours do not necessarily have the impact intended

- **Curious stance** – Inquiring from a position of genuine interest furthers understanding, helps solve problem and is experienced as less threatening by others
- **90-10 rules:**
  - 90% of what you experience is related to how something is said and 10% is based on what is said;
  - 90% of what you experience is from the past expe-rience and 10% is based on the current moment;
  - 90% of life experience is from how you react and 10% is from what actually happens to you.[32]
- **Relationship vs Issues** – Determine in each instance whether defending the issue is more important than maintaining the relationship or vice versa.

3.7 Help learners understand the importance of identifying the source(s) and factor(s) leading to promote understanding or resolve conflict

Identify the source(s) of the misunderstanding or conflict – Recognizing the source(s) of the problem can help learners be more productive in finding appropriate solutions, which subsequently helps determine the strategies most likely to be effective. Use an acronym (PRIME) to help identify the possible factors related to misunderstanding or conflict:

PRIME[33, d] is an acronym that people can use to identify the possible factors that can lead to misunderstanding or conflict:

- *Personal, professional, and patient differences* (i.e. different personal histories or experiences that influence ideas, perspectives, priorities, preferences, beliefs, and values)
- *Role confusion* (i.e. ambiguity about roles, respon-sibilities, and goals)
- *Informational deficiencies* (i.e. a lack of correct, clear, adequate, or accessible information)
- *Methods* (i.e. differences in process and approach; ineffective or unacceptable methods)
- *Environmental stress* (i.e. stresses and uncertainty concerning organizational structures and changes in work environment, and stresses concerning time pressure, pace, change, and scarcity of resources)

Once the factor is identified then it is often easier to react appropriately.

---

d Richardson D, Wagner S. Collaborative Teams, Module 2, Educating health professionals in interprofessional care course (ehpic™), Module 2 – University of Toronto, 2013. Reproduced with permission.

© 2015 Royal College of Physicians and Surgeons of Canada

Collaborator

3.8 Provide learners with a process for engaging in challenging conversations and situations

Not everyone feels comfortable addressing differences or conflict directly. Here you will find three processes that may help learners engage in challenging conversations and situations where there are differences or conflict: 1) in the moment rules to ensure constructive approaches, 2) matching the approach to the situation, 3) using a stepwise approach to promote understanding.

You may find it helpful to provide learners with rules for conducting themselves in stressful and high emotion situations. Self-regulation in times of high emotion is very important and refreshing some general rules to respond 'in the moment' regulation at times of high emotion is worthwhile. (See Table COLL-4).

In challenging conversations and situations it is very important to match one's approach to the specific situation; not all situations are the same and therefore call for different approaches. Help learners to develop the ability to assess the situation and then to be flexible in their approach. Table COLL-5 outlines five approaches that apply to different situations.

Steps for promoting understanding: although these steps may seem basic, conversations or situations where there are differences or conflict are times of stress and high emotion and we often lose our way. Help learners understand and apply the steps necessary for holding helpful conversations. Table COLL-6 outlines the steps and provides sample tips and responses to promote understanding in managing differences and resolving conflicts. A more detailed coaching tool is found in the teaching tools section of this chapter (T7).

TABLE COLL-4. 'IN THE MOMENT' RULES

Rules	Behaviours	Impact
1. Stay calm	• Control the outward expression of emotions.	• Allows all to focus on issue (e.g. patient) rather than on an emotional response.
2. Stay focused	• Stay focused on the immediate problem. • Show flexibility in generating solutions.	• Prioritizes issues of concern first. • Focuses on immediate solutions. • System issues and solutions are viewed as secondary. Follow-up to prevent recurrence can occur later.
3. Slow down and talk to others	• Slow down and take time to talk aloud. Explain, listen and plan collectively.	• Enables shared understanding of problems and all involved in solutions.
4. Redirect others as needed	• Attend to distracting or destructive behaviour promptly. For example, "We are doing our best under the circumstances. Your shouting is rattling me and it is making the situation even more challenging."	• Clarifies expected behaviour.

TABLE COLL-5. SAMPLE APPROACHES TO APPLY TO DIFFERENT SITUATIONS[34, 35]

APPROACH	WHEN TO USE
DICTATE	• Quick, decisive action is vital • In acute situations where action needs to be taken immediately
AVOID	• Time is needed for people to cool down, reduce tension, regain perspective • Others can resolve the conflict more effectively
ACCOMMODATE	• The issue is more important to the other person • Preserving harmony is especially important
COMPROMISE	• A quick solution is needed under time pressure • Both parties willing to find common solution despite having different goals or perspectives
COLLABORATE	• Longer term solution needed that involves understanding the viewpoints of others • Buy-in, commitment and shared decision-making are important

Collaborator

TABLE COLL-6. STEPS AND HINTS TO PROMOTE UNDERSTANDING

Step	Hints	SAMPLE response to promotes collaboration
1. Identify the need for a conversation	Encourage the expression of concerns	"Help me to understand how you see the problem?"
2. Actively listen	Listen to understand different opinions and perspectives	"Tell me more"
3. Acknowledge others' points of view	Summarize your understanding of others' viewpoints before sharing your viewpoint or asking questions	"Let me see if I understand what you are saying…"
4. Share your viewpoint	Share all relevant information that is important to the situation	"Here's how I view the situation …"
5. Seek common ground	Highlight common interests and focus on solutions	"I think we can both agree that we are not happy with the current situation."
6. Reach agreement on next steps	Clarify who will develop and/or implement the move-forward plan and how and when this will be done	"So let's go over the plan to make sure we know who is doing what, when"

4. Hints, tips and tools for *teaching* the Collaborator Role

As a teacher the goal is to deliver the right content and in a way that helps residents learn. Sometimes this will involve teaching learners directly, while at other times, it may involve facilitating or supporting the teaching of others. There are parts of the Collaborator Role that can be especially difficult for learners to relate to and understand in the context of their work. For this reason, this section of the chapter includes a short menu of tips and tricks that are highly effective for teaching the Collaborator Role. You can treat the list as a buffet: pick and choose the tips that resonate most and that will work for you, your program and learners.

Teaching Tip 1.
Help learners recognize the value of integrating into a new context and how best to do that

Transitioning into new settings is an ongoing part of medical training. Learners are often pressed for time and overlook the importance of investing in their new setting and in new relationships. Learners need to be made aware that integration into a new setting takes effort on their part.

Clinical practice settings can be quite different from one to another, so learners need support to make a smooth transition to a new practice setting or context. The stress of adjusting to different practice contexts can interfere with time management, building relationships, patient care and of course, learning. In other words, the ability of learners to fully engage collaboratively from the outset can be limited.

Learners need strategies for quickly integrating into new settings. Here are five simple strategies that they can apply routinely, regardless of context:[36]

1. Clarifying clinical role responsibilities (e.g. on-call, consult)

2. Seeking to understand expectations (e.g. start time, dress code)

3. Introducing themselves to other health care professionals (e.g. name, role)

4. Reviewing setting protocols (e.g. scheduling, EMR, referral process)

5. Orienting themselves to the physical layout (e.g. lab requisitions, washroom, equipment)

Remind learners that as 'arriving guests' when they start a new rotation, they will benefit from being nimble, 'reading' the culture, and then quickly beginning to work as a helpful member of the new team.

Collaborator

© 2015 Royal College of Physicians and Surgeons of Canada

Teaching Tip 2.

Take advantage of day to day work-based opportunities (e.g. case presentations and rounds) to highlight opportunities for collaboration regardless of location

Collaboration lives in every interaction. Opportunities to collaborate exist despite the location, not because of it. It is about the quality of the interaction, not the location of the collaborators.

Collaborators may be co-located (i.e. working in the same place) or they may be reached by phone, email, or text. Table COLL-7 provides generic examples of collaboration occurring in a common location and at a distance. Substitute examples to highlight the same in your specialty.

Teaching Tip 3.

Support a culture that embraces collaboration, diversity and differences

Working with others is necessary, but to do it well, requires commitment and skills development.

Your role is to help learners appreciate collaboration, diversity and differences by role-modeling good collaborative behaviour. Remember to model the behaviours that support collaboration such as active listening, acknowledging others presence and perspective, asking questions, sharing information, engaging with others, being inclusive, and showing appreciation for contributions. Once learners experience the benefits of this kind of culture, give them an opportunity to practice the behaviour.

It is the day-to-day modelling and opportunities to practice these behaviours that over time generates and sustains learners' commitment to a positive, helpful culture, allowing the strength of diversity to flourish.

Collaborator

TABLE COLL-7. EXAMPLES OF COLLABORATION AT A SINGLE LOCATION AND AT A DISTANCE

Scenario	Collaboration at a single location	Collaboration at a distance
Goals of care	• Psychiatric team meet prior to a family meeting • Anaesthetist and Recovery Room RN discuss pain management	• Cardiologist discusses with the Charge nurse at a nursing home the cardiac status of a patient • Teleconference with community clinician and family to discuss care directives
Meetings	• Research colleagues meet to discuss a grant submission • Discharge planning meeting • MD and admin assistant meet to discuss office management	• Case conference by teleconference • The pathologist or radiologist helps a nurse practitioner in a northern town to sort out a diagnosis. • Video/web conferencing to join colleagues in a discussion
Handover	• Patient care handover to the on-call clinician • Paediatrician arranges transfer within children's tertiary hospital to a surgical colleague's care	• The surgeon transfers a patient to critical care colleagues for post-op care. • Discharge Planner assures all appropriate information is forwarded to CCAC/homecare for a patient being discharged
Written documentation	• Plan of care is updated • Clinician reviews the physio progress notes to inform next steps • Clinician writes summary of roles and responsibilities following a family meeting	• Physician calls pharmacist who has faxed information about a drug interaction to follow up on other options • Physician ensures all treating clinicians are cc'ed on consultation letter

Collaborator

Teaching Tip 4.

Incorporate handover into your curriculum and work-based teaching activities

Handover is an important activity that can have significant impact on a patient's care and outcomes. Patients receive care in multiple care settings and under multiple providers, and the increasingly fragmented nature of our health care system potentially threatens the quality and safety of care provided to patients at points of transition (e.g. transfer from the emergency department to the hospital ward, discharge from the acute care setting to the ambulatory care setting).[37,38,39] Learners need to develop competencies in working effectively and collaboratively with other physicians and colleagues in the health professions and with patients to maintain patient safety at these high-risk transition points.

While many of the concepts associated with handover (e.g. features of effective handover, handover tools, checklists) can be introduced around a seminar table, effective handover is best modelled, practiced and observed in day-to-day clinical activities. If learners can relate what they're learning to their daily work, they are more likely to develop a greater appreciation and understanding of these important concepts.

Practising handover and getting 'on the spot' coaching can significantly improve a learner's performance, especially, when there is an opportunity to incorporate the suggested improvements into action in subsequent encounters. Don't 'protect' learners from the messiness of when handover doesn't go well. Learners will benefit from seeing colleagues follow up to ensure that the needed patient care is provided. Learners need to be coached to take progressive responsibility for being active participants in appropriate follow-up activities, including identifying patterns of errors or omissions in handover that would be improved with systems solutions.

Sample teaching tools

You can use the sample *Teaching Tools for Collaborator* found at the end of this section as is, or you can modify or use them in various combinations to suit your objectives, time allocated, sequence within your residency program, and so on.

Easy-to-customize electronic versions of the *Teaching Tools for Collaborator* (in .doc, .ppt and .pdf formats) are found at: canmeds.royalcollege.ca

The tools provided are:

- T1 Lecture or Large Group Session: Foundations of the Collaborator Role

- T2 Presentation: Teaching the Collaborator Role

- T3 Case Report: Intention vs Impact

- T4 Case Report: PRIME factors to promote understanding, manage differences and resolve conflict

- T5 Guided Reflection and Discussion: Understanding the roles and responsibilities of others

- T6 Coaching: Handover in everyday practice

- T7 Coaching: Steps and hints for managing differences and resolving conflict

- T8 Tools and Strategies: Summary sheet for the Collaborator Role

© 2015 Royal College of Physicians and Surgeons of Canada

HANDOVER — PATIENT SAFETY ISSUES AND RISK REDUCTION THROUGH COLLABORATION

Effective handovers can enhance care and help to prevent harm to patients. When handovers go badly, care can be negatively impacted. Help learners develop competencies that will promote effective handovers.

Features of effective handovers[40]:

1. **Giving and receiving patient information**

   - Minimize or eliminate interruptions and distractions during transfer of information
   - Involves active listening and engaged discussion

2. **Utilizing standardized handover tools/procedures**

   - e.g. electronic handoff tools, formal checklists

3. **Preparation/training**

   - Provide nuanced feedback as learners practice handovers
   - Includes training of team as a whole (not simply individuals training separately)

RISK REDUCTION REMINDERS — FOR HANDOVER[20, e]

Remember that clarity is king in handover. The process for giving and receiving patient information should include steps that:

1. **CONFIRMation of WHY:**

   - When multiple health care professionals are involved in a case, confirm that the reason and rationale for the transfer of care is clear to all.

2. **CONFIRMation of WHO:**

   - Verify that the appropriate health professionals are aware of the patient's clinical condition and have agreed to accept the transfer of care.
   - Verify that the roles and responsibilities of each team member in the handover (i.e. sending and receiving) are clear to the patient and to the other health care professionals.

3. **STRUCTURE THE HOW:**

   - Consider using a structured tool for sharing information during handovers (e.g. I-PASS, ISoBar).
   - Follow the institution's protocols for patient handovers, including the transfer of care related to consultations, as well as responsibilities for treatment and discharge decisions.

4. **ENSURE UNDERSTANDING OF WHAT:**

   - Ensure sufficient patient information has been provided. Clarify, repeat back as needed.
   - Consider reconfirming the clinical history directly with the patient.

5. **DOCUMENT:**

   - Document relevant information when sending — for those assuming the care of the patient.
   - Document relevant information when receiving — entering key elements of handover information.

Collaborator

---

e CMPA Risk Fact Sheet. Patient Handover A1300-004-E © CMPA 2013. https://www.cmpa-acpm.ca/documents/10179/300031190/patient_handovers-e.pdf Reproduced with permission.

© 2015 Royal College of Physicians and Surgeons of Canada

5. Hints, tips and tools for *assessing* the Collaborator Role

Assessment Tip 1.
Assess in the clinical setting with the help of other colleagues in the health care professions

It's important for learners to receive feedback about their contributions and their impact on collaboration from their teachers, colleagues and other health care providers. Multiple assessments from multiple people improve the reliability and validity of the assessment. Assessment of the Collaborator Role lends itself to, and is not complete without, the input from different collaborators. Collaborators with different roles and responsibilities provide different viewpoints creating rich assessment and feedback.

Individuals often incorrectly assume that silence is approval. Not only should teachers be actively looking for moments to provide helpful feedback, learners should be comfortable with and responsible for seeking feedback. Everyone should be encouraged to create a culture of respectful feedback. Both successes and failures have lessons embedded, but these lessons need to be explicitly identified to ensure understanding of their relevance to collaboration.

Beyond your own observations, consider using multi-source feedback (MSF) forms or focused encounter forms. You can also ask others to provide input toward the interim or end-of-session in-training evaluation (ITER) form.

Assessment Tip 2.
Take advantage of day to day work-based opportunities (i.e. case presentations and rounds) to provide focused, timely feedback, coaching and formative assessment

Collaboration lives in every interaction. In some cases collaborators may be co-located while at others times collaborators may need to pick up the phone or send an email or text. In day-to-day practice, look for opportunities to provide learner's with nuanced, timely feedback, coaching, and formative assessment about their ability to build relationships, promote understanding and perform effective handover. Feedback in the moment from real life situations can be a powerful stimulus for further learning. Remember that it is often things like thanking someone, offering help and following up on a handover that make a difference, so try to make a point of noticing these things and encouraging the good behaviours.

Below is a list of example behaviours and SAMPLE QUESTIONS that can be assessed during case presentations, rounds etc. Does the learner:

- Share his/her thinking with team members?
- Make himself/herself available and approachable?
- Negotiate a plan of action including offering choices and sharing alternatives?
- Encourage others' viewpoints?
- Respond respectfully to others viewpoints?
- Reframe problems to find common ground?
- Seek feedback from collaborators?
- Ask for help appropriately?
- Identify key patient issues warranting transfer?
- Identify potential safety gaps?
- Document handover clearly, timely and accurately?

Assessment Tip 3.
Monitor and provide feedback on a learner's contribution to a culture of respect

For health care organizations to be collaborative places for patient-centered care, there needs to be a culture of respect for others' roles, responsibilities and viewpoints. While you and other faculty will encourage good collaboration you also need to be watchful for behaviours and attitudes that are not respectful, or that undermine positive relationships.

Your role is to assess your learner's behaviour and the impact of that behaviour on collaboration. Your feedback will prompt learners to explore how they interact with others and it should help them develop insight and improve their approach accordingly.

Assessment Tip 4.
Use realistic scenarios or simulations to assess learners', promote understanding, manage differences or resolve conflicts

Promoting understanding and resolving conflicts benefit from reflection, analysis and a supportive coaching relationship. One way to promote reflection and experimentation is to create a safe environment for the learning and assessment to occur. Consider having learners work through a typical scenario or a simulation to practise their conflict management skills in a low-stake situation (e.g. when patient care will not be impacted). This allows residents to order their thoughts, values and views, as they analyze the results of these low-stake scenarios or simulations.

© 2015 Royal College of Physicians and Surgeons of Canada

This reflection about collaboration can be captured during a formative discussion in the clinical environment, or submitted as an assigned case report (i.e. for marking against a standard rubric), integrated into a practice oral, written exam, or objective structured clinical exam (OSCE).

Sample assessment tools

You can use the sample *Assessment Tools for Collaborator* found at the end of the section as is, or you can modify or use them in various combinations to suit your objectives, the time allocated, the sequence within your residency program, and so on.

Easy-to-customize electronic versions of the *Assessment Tools for Collaborator* (in .doc, .ppt and .pdf formats) are found at: canmeds.royalcollege.ca

The tools provided are:

- A1 Multisource Feedback: Multisource feedback for Collaborator skills

- A2 Encounter Form: Collaborator Role encounter form

- A3 Encounter Form: Team meeting encounter form

- A4 Assignment: Collaborator quotient

- A5 Objective Structured Clinical Exam (OSCE): for the Collaborator Role

6. Suggested resources

- **Leasure EM, Jones RR, Meade LB, Sanger MI, Thomas KG, Tilden VP, Bowen JL, Warm EI. There is no "i" in teamwork in the patient-centered medical home: defining teamwork competencies for academic practice.** *Acad Med.* **2013;88(5):585-592.**

- **AHRQ. Patient Safety Network. Patient Safety Primers – handovers and signouts. Last retrieved July 12, 2015 from: http://psnet.ahrq.gov/primer.aspx?primerID=9** Accessible web site that includes foundational information about handover best practices. Also provides current literature and reports on topic. Includes link to full collection (i.e. 1000+) articles and reports on handover

VIDEOS

- **Just a routine operation**
  Collaboration gone awry at 'just a routine operation'
  https://www.youtube.com/watch?v=JzlvgtPIof4

- **Relationship-centred collaboration**
  Business leader Margaret Heffernan observes that it is social cohesion — built during every shared coffee break, and every time one team member asks another for help — that leads over time to great results. http://www.ted.com/talks/margaret_heffernan_why_it_s_time_to_forget_the_pecking_order_at_work?language=en

- **Dare to disagree**
  Margaret Heffernan shows us that disagreement is central to progress. and how great research teams, relationships and businesses allow people to deeply disagree. http://www.ted.com/talks/margaret_heffernan_dare_to_disagree?language=en

7. Other resources

- Fleming C. *It's the way you say it – becoming articulate, well-spoken and clear.* San Francisco: Berret Koehler Publishers; 2013.

- Covey S.M.R. *The speed of trust.* New York: Free Press; 2006.

- Heffernan M. Margaret Heffernan summarizes her recent book on the often-overlooked element necessary to build an effective, efficient organization: social capital. http://ideas.ted.com/the-secret-ingredient-that-makes-some-teams-better-than-others/

- Grant Halvorson H. *No one understands you and what to do about it.* Boston: Harvard Business Review Press; 2015.

- I-Pass website. Last retrieved Aug 25, 2015, from http://www.ipasshandoffstudy.com

- Hackman JR. *Collaborative intelligence using teams to solve hard problems.* San Francisco: Berret Koehler Publishers; 2011.

- Wiseman L. *Multipliers how the best leaders make everyone smarter.* New York: Harper Management; 2010.

- Schein EH. *Helping – how to offer, give and receive help.* San Francisco: Berret-Koehler Publishers; 2009.

- Stone D, Heen S. *Thanks for the feedback - the science and art of receiving feedback well.* New York: Viking Press; 2014.

- Stone D, Patton B. Heen S. *Difficult conversations – how to discuss what matters most.* New York: Penguin Books; 1999.

Collaborator

8. COLLABORATOR ROLE DIRECTORY OF TEACHING AND ASSESSMENT TOOLS

You can use the sample *teaching and assessment tools for the Collaborator Role* found in this section as is, or you can modify or use them in various combinations to suit your objectives, the time allocated, the sequence within your residency program, and so on. Tools are listed by number (e.g. T1), type (e.g. Lecture), and title (e.g. Foundations of the Collaborator Role).

Easy-to-customize electronic versions of the sample *teaching and assessment tools for the Collaborator Role* in .doc, .ppt and .pdf formats are found at: canmeds.royalcollege.ca

TEACHING TOOLS

ASSESSMENT TOOLS

Collaborator

© 2015 Royal College of Physicians and Surgeons of Canada

T1. FOUNDATIONS OF THE COLLABORATOR ROLE

Created for the *CanMEDS Teaching and Assessment Tools Guide* by S Glover Takahashi, D Richardson and D Martin. Reproduced with permission of the Royal College.

This learning activity includes:

1. Presentation: Teaching the Collaborator Role (T2)

2. Intention vs Impact (T3)

3. PRIME Factors to Promote Understanding, Manage Differences and Resolve Conflict (T4)

Instructions for Teacher:

Sample learning objectives

1. Recognize common words related to the process and content of Collaborator

2. Apply key Collaborator steps to examples from day-to-day practice

3. Develop a personal Collaborator resource for common patient needs

Audience: All learners

How to adapt:

- Consider whether your needs and goals match the sample objectives provided in this deck. If not, you can select from, modify, or add to the sample objectives as appropriate to your needs.

- The sample PowerPoint presentation is generic and foundational and tied to straightforward objectives. Consider whether you'll need additional slides to meet your own objectives. Modify, add or delete content as appropriate. You may want to include specific information related to your discipline and context.

- You may wish to review and customize the pocket card (i.e. most frequent collaborator needs in different locations or among different location) with learners as an additional teaching activity.

Logistics:

- Depending on how long you have for your session, you can select the activities for a given teaching session.

- Allocate about 20 minutes for each teaching activity: this time will be used for you to explain the activity and for learners to complete the activity individually, share their answers with their small group, discuss, prepare to report back to the whole group, and then deliver their small group's report to the whole group.

- Depending on the group and time available, you may wish to assign one or more activities as homework, to be completed before the session or as a follow-up assignment.

Setting:

- This teaching session is best done in a small-group format (i.e. less than 30 learners) if possible. It can also be done with a larger group if the room allows for learners to be at tables in groups of five or six. With larger groups, it is helpful to have additional teachers or facilitators available to answer questions arising from the activities.

Collaborator

© 2015 Royal College of Physicians and Surgeons of Canada

T2. TEACHING THE COLLABORATOR ROLE

Created for the *CanMEDS Teaching and Assessment Tools Guide* by S Glover Takahashi, D Richardson and D Martin. Reproduced with permission of the Royal College.

Instructions for Teacher:

- Setting and Audience: Faculty and all learners
- How to use: Use as an orientation to the Role
- How to adapt: Slides can be modified to match the specialty or the learners' practice context
- Logistics: Equipment – laptop, projector, and screen

Slide #	Words on slide		Notes to teachers
1.	Collaborator Role		• Add information about presenters and modify title
2.	**Objectives and agenda** 1. Recognize common words related to the process and content of Collaboration 2. Apply key Collaboration steps to examples from day to day practice 3. Develop personal collaboration resources for day to day practice		• SAMPLE goals and objectives of the session – revise as required. • CONSIDER doing a 'warm up activity' • Review/revise goals and objectives. • Insert agenda slide if desired
3.	**Why the Collaborator Role matters** • Professionals must work together • Collaboration improves patient care outcomes, patient safety, attitudes between practitioners, patient satisfactions, work systems, and clinical satisfaction. • Collaboration can look and feel different depending on the contest and individuals. • When collaboration is not working, there is an established process to improve it. • Collaboration also includes learning that occurs from the service provided.		• Reasons why this Role is important
4.	**The details: What is the Collaborator Role**[a] As Collaborators, physicians work effectively with other health care professionals to provide safe, high-quality, patient-centred care.		• Avoid including competencies for learners. • If using for teachers or planners may want to add that slide
5.	**Recognizing Collaborator process** • Accommodating • Asking questions • Building trust • Communicating • Contributing • Cooperating • Embracing Diversity	• Engaging • Helping • Promoting understanding • Reframing • Relationship building • Respecting • Sharing	• Trigger words relating to the process of Collaboration
6.	**Recognizing Collaborator content** • Common ground • Conflict resolution • Debriefing • Difference and Diversity • Disruptive behaviour • Handover • Intention and Impact	• Organizational awareness • Power and Hierarchy • Process • Reflective practice • Shared decision-making • Situational awareness • Team development	• Trigger words relating to the content of Collaboration

---

a Richardson D, Calder L, Dean H, Glover Takahashi S, Lebel P, Maniate J, Martin D, Nasmith L, Newton C, Steinert Y. Collaborator. In: Frank JR, Snell L, Sherbino J, editors. *CanMEDS 2015 Physician Competency Framework* Ottawa: Royal College of Physicians and Surgeons of Canada; 2015. Reproduced with permission.

© 2015 Royal College of Physicians and Surgeons of Canada

Collaborator

T2. TEACHING THE COLLABORATOR ROLE (continued)

Slide #	Words on slide	Notes to teachers
7.	**Good Collaborators** • make an effort to build relationships • assume others have good intentions • respect others time, expertise and contributions • elicit input, actively seeking differences of opinions • reframe problems to find common ground • are genuinely curious about others' perspectives • authentically ask questions to clarify and promote understanding • are receptive to feedback • recognize their own limitations and blind spots • are good listeners and good communicators • transfer and share relevant information in an effective way • aren't afraid to ask for help and always look for ways to be helpful	• Provide clinical and local examples
8.	**About Collaboration** • The 'team', 'teamwork' and 'collaboration' have different meanings. Collaboration is active, deliberate and relationship-centred. • Good collaboration is varied and involves two or more people, occurs in same or different locations and/or includes colleagues from different or same profession. • The degree of collaboration necessary is dependent on the complexity of the situation and based on patient (not practitioner) needs. • Collaborative decision-making includes actively sharing, soliciting and encouraging diverse perspectives so the best course of action can be determined	• Clarifies some misconceptions about collaboration
9.	**Collaborator Intelligence (CI)[b] key domains for learning, teaching and assessing the Collaborator Role.** • Self (i.e. knowing one's strengths, values, limitations and managing one's own behaviour and emotions), • Relationships (i.e. being able to use empathy to build relationships with others, including the patient), • Context (i.e. demonstrating behaviours, actions that reflect and incorporate the awareness of the surrounding situational and circumstances), and • System (i.e. recognizing and promote understanding the aspects of health care organizations, including structures, operations and culture that influence the delivery of care across the continuum).	• Provide clinical and local examples
10.	**Understanding collaboration in everyday care** 1. Draw learners attentions to context in which collaboration is particularly important for your specialty 2. Discuss how to establish and maintain positive relationships with colleagues 3. Explore the positive contribution that diversity and difference make to team effectiveness 4. Provide structures, approaches and processes to manage differences and resolve conflicts	• Provide clinical and local examples
11.	Relationship-centred care is "an approach that recognizes the importance and uniqueness of each health care participant's relationship with each other, and considers these relationships to be central in supporting high-quality care, high-quality work environment, and superior organizational performance.	

b The Collaborator Intelligence (CI) framework described here outlines the domains for the learning and teaching of the Collaborator Role and is different than the organizational focus of the Collaborative Intelligence described by J. Richard Hackman, 2011.

© 2015 Royal College of Physicians and Surgeons of Canada

Collaborator

T2. TEACHING THE COLLABORATOR ROLE (continued)

Slide #	Words on slide	Notes to teachers
12.	**HANDOVERS** – Effective handovers enhance care and help prevent harm to patients. Features of effective handovers:[c,d] • Focused on giving and receiving patient information (i.e. free of interruptions and distractions; active listening and clarifying when necessary. • Standardized handover tools for verbal communication, electronic handover tools, formal checklists • Teamwork training in handovers (i.e. not training of team members but actual teamwork training)	• Provide clinical and local examples
13.	**RISK REDUCTION REMINDERS**[d] 1. CONFIRM WHY: When multiple health professionals involved, confirm reason and rationale for transfer of care is clear to all. 2. CONFIRM WHO: Verify appropriate health professionals aware of patient's clinical condition and agreed to transfer of care. 3. Verify roles and responsibilities of each team member in handover is clearly given/received by patient and health professionals 4. STRUCTURE THE HOW: Structured communication tool and protocols are very helpful. Follow established processes each time. 5. ENSURE UNDERSTANDING OF WHAT: Ensure sufficient patient information is provided. Clarify and repeat back as needed. Valuable to reconfirm clinical history directly with patient 6. DOCUMENT: Document relevant information when sending—for those assuming the patient care. Document relevant information when receiving—entering key elements of handover information	• Provide clinical and local examples
14.	T3 – Intention vs Impact	• Do learning activity
15.	PRIME model[e] • **P**ersonal, professional, and patient differences • **R**ole confusion • **I**nformational deficiencies • **M**ethods • **E**nvironmental stress	• Do learning activity
16.	T4 – PRIME Factors	• Do learning activity
17.	**'In the moment'** rules for managing differences and conflict 1. Stay calm 2. Stay focused 3. Slow down and talk to others 4. Redirect others as needed	• Provide clinical and local examples
18.	**Approaches to apply to different situations**[f,g] DICTATE: • Quick, decisive action is vital • On important issues where unpopular action needed AVOID: • Time needed for reduced tension, regain perspective • Others can resolve the conflict more effectively ACCOMMODATE: • The issue is more important to the other person • Preserving harmony is especially important COMPROMISE: • A quick solution is needed under time pressure • Both parties have equal power and have different goals COLLABORATE: • Longer term solution and multiple viewpoints • Buy-in and shared decision-making are important	• Provide clinical and local examples

c AHRQ. Patient Safety Network. Patient Safety Primers – Handovers and signouts. http://psnet.ahrq.gov/primer.aspx?primerID=9
d CMPA Risk Fact Sheet- Patient handovers- A1300-004-E © CMPA 2013. https://www.cmpa-acpm.ca/documents/10179/300031190/patient_handovers-e.pdf Reproduced with permission.
e Richardson D, Wagner S. Collaborative Teams, Module 2, Educating health professionals in interprofessional care course (ehpic™), Module 2 – University of Toronto, 2013. Reproduced with permission.
f Thomas KW. Conflict and conflict management: Reflections and update. *J of Organ Behav.* 1992:13(3): 265-74.
g Shell, GR. Teaching Ideas: Bargaining Styles and Negotiation: TheThomas Kilmann Conflict Mode Instrument in Negotiation Training. *Negotiation J.* 2001;17(2):155-74.

© 2015 Royal College of Physicians and Surgeons of Canada

Collaborator

T2. TEACHING THE COLLABORATOR ROLE (continued)

Slide #	Words on slide	Notes to teachers
19.	**Steps and hints to promote understanding** 1. Identify the need for a conversation: Encourage the expression of concerns. 2. Actively listen: Listen to understand different opinions and perspectives. 3. Acknowledge others' points of view: Summarize understanding before sharing 4. Share your viewpoint: Share all relevant information that is important to the situation 5. Seek common ground: Highlight common interests and focus on solutions 6. Reach agreement on next steps: Clarify process and time for move-forward plan	• Provide clinical and local examples
20.	RECAP and revisiting objectives and next steps	• Revisit workshop goals and objectives

OTHER SLIDES

Slide #	Words on slide	Notes to teachers
21.	**Collaborator Key Competencies**[a] Physicians are able to: 1. Work effectively with physicians and other colleagues in the health care professions 2. Work with physicians and other colleagues in the health care professions to promote understanding, manage differences, and resolve conflicts 3. Hand over the care of a patient to another health care professional to facilitate continuity of safe patient care	• Use one slide for each key competency and associated enabling competencies

22.	**Collaborator Key Competency 1**[a]
	Physicians are able to:
	1. Work effectively with physicians and other colleagues in the health care professions
	  1.1 Establish and maintain positive relationships with physicians and other colleagues in the health care professions to support relationship-centred collaborative care
	  1.2 Negotiate overlapping and shared responsibilities with physicians and other colleagues in the health care professions in episodic and ongoing care
	  1.3 Engage in respectful shared decision-making with physicians and other colleagues in the health care professions	

23.	**Collaborator Key Competency 2**[a]
	Physicians are able to:
	2. Work with physicians and other colleagues in the health care professions to promote understanding, manage differences, and resolve conflicts
	  2.1 Show respect toward collaborators
	  2.2 Implement strategies to promote understanding, manage differences, and resolve conflicts in a manner that supports a collaborative culture	

24.	**Collaborator Key Competency 3**[a]
	Physicians are able to:
	3. Hand over the care of a patient to another health care professional to facilitate continuity of safe patient care
	  3.1 Determine when care should be transferred to another physician or health care professional
	  3.2 Demonstrate safe handover of care, using both verbal and written communication, during a patient transition to a different health care professional, setting, or stage of care	

T3. INTENTION VS IMPACT[a]

Instructions for Learner:

- Select a sample 'collaboration' scenario from the list below. If you prefer choose one from recent clinical practice

- You will be assigned a 'point of view'

- In a small group, choose a recorder and answer the questions below

- Identify the spokesperson to share observations with the larger group

SAMPLE scenarios:

- Resident from another program calls you to do a consult for a patient. The patients' needs/priority do not match your program or priorities

- Scheduling conflicts between residents

- Report from more senior resident and you do not agree with their findings

- Resident/Fellow confrontation over cases or procedures

- Being on call and being (over) paged for follow-up because other resident/service is not responding to inquiries

INTENTION, IMPACT AND ASSUMPTIONS

Completed by: _____

Questions	PROGRAM A Resident	PROGRAM B Resident
1. What assumptions do you think the physician has about the others' intentions?		
2. What intentions do you think the physician has personally?		
3. What impact does the physician's behaviour have on: • the patient? • themselves? • the health care team? • colleagues? • the health care system?		

Other notes:

---

a   Martin D, Glover Takahash S. International Resident Leadership Summit, Calgary, AB. 2013. Reproduced with permission.

© 2015 Royal College of Physicians and Surgeons of Canada

Collaborator

T4. PRIME FACTORS[a] TO PROMOTE UNDERSTANDING, MANAGE DIFFERENCES AND RESOLVE CONFLICT

Created for the *CanMEDS Teaching and Assessment Tools Guide* by S Glover Takahashi, D Richardson and D Martin. Reproduced with permission of the Royal College.

See Collaborator Role teacher tips appendix for this teaching tool

SAMPLE scenarios:

- Resident from another program calls you to do a consult for a patient. The patients' needs/priority do not match your program or priorities
- Scheduling conflict/needs
- Report from staff and you do not agree with their findings
- Resident/Fellow confrontations over cases or procedures
- Being on call and being (over) paged for follow up because other resident/service is not responding to inquiries

Completed by:_____

1. Choose one of the scenarios described above or describe your own experience where you and one or more colleagues experienced differences of opinion or a conflict.

_____

_____

_____

_____

_____

_____

_____

2. What are the **PRIME** factors that contributed to or caused the misunderstanding, difference or conflict?

_____

_____

_____

_____

_____

_____

_____

_____

_____

a   Richardson D, Wagner S. Collaborative Teams, Module 2, Educating health professionals in interprofessional care course (ehpic™), Module 2 – University of Toronto, 2013. Reproduced with permission.

© 2015 Royal College of Physicians and Surgeons of Canada

Collaborator

T4. PRIME FACTORS TO PROMOTE UNDERSTANDING, MANAGE DIFFERENCES AND RESOLVE CONFLICT (continued)

3. How would you solve the **PRIME** understanding, difference or conflict?

_____

_____

_____

_____

_____

_____

_____

4. Complete the table below:

What are some difficult situations from day-to-day practice that you have seen, heard or been engaged in?	What is/are the **PRIME** factor(s) that contributed to or caused the situation(s)?	What is/are the **PRIME** SOLUTIONS to Promoting Understanding, Managing Differences or Resolving Conflict for the situation(s)?

© 2015 Royal College of Physicians and Surgeons of Canada

T4. PRIME FACTORS TO PROMOTE UNDERSTANDING, MANAGE DIFFERENCES AND RESOLVE CONFLICT (continued)

BACKGROUND CONTENT FOR LEARNERS

CONTENT: Examples of analyzing what the problem is/are re: understanding, difference, and conflict

P ersonal, professional and patient differences (i.e. different personal histories or experiences that influence ideas, perspectives, priorities, preferences, beliefs and values)

R ole incompatibility (i.e. ambiguity about roles, responsibilities and goals)

I nformational deficiencies (i.e. a lack of correct, clear, adequate or accessible information)

M ethods (i.e. differences in process and approach; ineffective or unacceptable methods)

E nvironmental stress (i.e. stresses and uncertainty concerning organizational structures and changes in work environment, and stresses concerning time pressure, pace, change and scarcity)

PROCESS: Examples of applying the steps to promote understanding, manage difference and resolve conflict

Step	Notes on behaviours or attitudes	Sample response that promotes effective collaboration
1. Identify and clarify the information and interests	• Focus on issues, not personalities. • Use "I" statements rather than "you" statements when identifying an issue or stating your position (e.g. "I am frustrated with the timeline being suggested"). • Concentrate on data, facts, and objective criteria. • Encourage the expression of concerns. • Use PRIME to sort out the content issues. • Share all relevant information that people need. • Ask for help when you need it or are unsure. • Be respectful in your tone and manner. • Focus on interests, not positions.	"Help me to understand how you see the problem?" "Tell me more about what your concerns are?" I want us to work more effectively (or constructively, efficiently).
2. Listen actively	• Listen to understand different opinions and perspectives. • Do not interrupt when others are talking. • Respectfully acknowledge others' viewpoints.	Use nonverbal communication, such as eye contact and nodding, to show the speaker you are engaged.
3. Acknowledge others' viewpoints	• Summarize your understanding of others' viewpoints before sharing your viewpoint or asking questions.	"Let me see if I understand what you are saying…"
4. Seek common ground	• Take note of shared interests. • Look for potential solutions and possible barriers. • Confirm who/how decisions or directions will be made. • Be open to the possibility that you may be wrong. • Take time to reflect on your own actions and intentions. • Offer and accept apologies if appropriate. • There is always common ground; ask others to help find it if you are at an impasse.	"I think we can both agree that we are not happy with the current situation." "What can we agree to about this situation?"
5. Reach agreement on next steps	• Determine what information is still needed to reach a solution. • Clarify who will develop and/or implement the move-forward plan and how and when this will be done. • Establish who is responsible for follow-up steps.	"So we've agreed that before making a final decision we need more information. John, you are going to…" "Let's recap where we are."

Collaborator

T5. UNDERSTANDING THE ROLES AND RESPONSIBILITIES OF OTHERS[a]

To work effectively with physicians and other colleagues in the health professions, you need to understand and appreciate the professional roles and responsibilities of the people you work with. Many of the concerns underlying the "how to" of collaboration emerge from a lack of understanding of the professional roles and responsibilities of others. This exercise is designed to help you identify any gaps that you may have in your understanding.

Instructions for Learners:

- Mark an X beside the roles that you feel you understand well enough to explain to others.

- Add a description for each role, including the skills and expertise that individuals in this role contribute to patient care.

- Add clarifying notes if or how 'it depends' on the work place context.

- Reflect on the roles that have no X next to them. Is it important to your practice and to the care of your patient that you understand these roles? If so, make the time to find out.

ROLE	X	DESCRIPTION
PHYSICIANS		
Medical clerk		
Physician's assistant		
Resident		
Fellow		
Staff physician		
Family physician		
Specialist		
OTHER HEALTH CARE PROFESSIONALS		
Nurse practitioner		
Advanced practice nurse		
Registered nurse		
Registered nurse assistant		
Venipuncturist		
Charge nurse		
Nurse manager		
Triage officer		
Audiologist		
Chiropodist and podiatrist		
Chaplain		
Chiropractor		
Dental hygienist		
Dentist		
Denturist		

a Adapted from Richardson D, Martin D, Glover Takahashi S. Chapter 3. In *The CanMEDS Toolkit for Teaching and Assessing the Collaborator Role*. Ottawa: Royal College of Physicians and Surgeons of Canada; 2012. Reproduced with permission.

© 2015 Royal College of Physicians and Surgeons of Canada

Collaborator

T5. UNDERSTANDING THE ROLES AND RESPONSIBILITIES
OF OTHERS (continued)

ROLE	X	DESCRIPTION
OTHER HEALTH CARE PROFESSIONALS		
Dietician		
Kinesiologist		
Massage therapist		
Medical laboratory technologist		
Medical radiation technologist		
Midwife		
Occupational therapist		
Optician		
Optometrist		
Paramedic		
Pharmacist		
Physiotherapist		
Prosthetist		
Psychologist		
Respiratory therapist		
Social worker		
Speech pathologist		
Other		
Other		
COMMUNITY RESOURCES		
In-home patient care		
Community-based nursing care		
Other		
Other		
PRACTICE SUPPORT SERVICES		
Dietary service		
Housekeeping		
Security		
Volunteer		
Unit clerk		
Bed coordinator		
Health records		
Dictation/Transcription		
Central supply room (CSR) service		
Other		
Other		

Collaborator

T6. HANDOVER IN EVERYDAY PRACTICE

Created for the *CanMEDS Teaching and Assessment Tools Guide* by S Glover Takahashi. Reproduced with permission of the Royal College.

See Collaborator Role teacher tips appendix for this teaching tool

One of the key competencies of the CanMEDS 2015 Collaborator Role is to hand over the care of a patient to another health care professional to facilitate continuity of safe patient care. Effective handovers can enhance care and help to prevent harm to patients. When handovers go badly, care can be negatively impacted. The purpose of this exercise is for you to relate what you are learning about hand over to your daily work. In doing so, you may develop a greater appreciation and understanding of these important concepts.

Completed by:_____

A. Drawing from your clinical practice over the past four weeks, answer the following questions. Please be sure to use specific details.

1. Describe a situation where you led or participated in a handover that you were pleased with the process and outcomes. Include general details about the background context (patient types, type of service, your role and the situation). What, if any impact did the location and your role in that location have on the outcomes? What factors contributed to the outcome?

   _____

   _____

   _____

2. Describe a situation where you led or participated in a handover that you were not pleased with the process and outcomes. Include details about clinical location (patient types, type of service, your role in this location and situation). What, if any impact did the context and your role in that location have on the outcomes?

   _____

   _____

   _____

Based on ONE of the situations from above answer the following questions.

3a. **What aspects of handover did you do well in that situation?**

   _____

   _____

   _____

3b. **What would you do differently in future to achieve better process or outcome(s)?**

   _____

   _____

   _____

© 2015 Royal College of Physicians and Surgeons of Canada

Collaborator

T6. HANDOVER IN EVERYDAY PRACTICE (continued)

4. Review the tables below. Select and complete the tables below that apply to your 'selected' situation

HANDOVER[a] IN THIS CASE	Rate your approach IN THIS SITUATION. **Explain rating**						Areas or ideas for priority improvement?
	1 Very poor	**2** Poor	**3** Solid competent	**4** Very good	**5** Superb	Not applicable	
I focused on giving and receiving patient information (e.g. when necessary I removed distractions; I listened actively and engaged in discussions)							
I used standardized handover tools (e.g. for verbal communication, electronic handover tools, formal checklists)							
I leveraged experience from team-based training on handovers to handle this situation							
I confirmed the reason and rationale for the transfer of care. Ensured clarity for all							
I verified that appropriate health professionals were aware of the patient's clinical condition and that they agreed to accept the transfer of care							
I verified that the roles and responsibilities of each team member in handover were clear to the patient and to other colleagues in the health care professions							
I followed institution's protocols for patient handovers, including transfer of care related to consultations, as well as responsibilities for treatment and discharge decisions							
I ensured sufficient patient information has been provided to the team during the handover							
I clarified and repeated back as needed							
I documented relevant information including self-identification							
OVERALL							

---

a   Adapted from CMPA Risk Fact Sheet- Patient handovers- A1300-004-E © CMPA 2013. https://www.cmpa-acpm.ca/documents/10179/300031190/patient handovers-e.pdf Reproduced with permission.

T6. HANDOVER IN EVERYDAY PRACTICE (continued)

Other notes/reflection:

_____

_____

_____

_____

_____

_____

_____

B. Summary of current/new priorities for improvement of handover

- Based on your reflections above, complete the table below to help you make a learning plan around handover competencies.
- What aspects of handover can you do better?
- What are your goals and how will you know if you have been successful?

☐ APPLIES TO PERIOD: FROM _____ TO _____

#	HANDOVER SKILLS	Goal(s) including timeframe	Metrics or criteria for success	Key next steps, resources, supports for success
1.				
2.				

© 2015 Royal College of Physicians and Surgeons of Canada

T7. STEPS AND HINTS FOR MANAGING DIFFERENCES AND RESOLVING CONFLICT[a]

Created for the *CanMEDS Teaching and Assessment Tools Guide* by S Glover Takahashi, D Martin and D Richardson. Reproduced with permission of the Royal College.

Step	Process	HINTS	SAMPLE responses
1.	Identify the need for a conversation	**1A. Initiator** • Identify possible sources of misunderstanding and conflict. • Focus on issues, not personalities. • Think about timing. • Ask for help when you need it. **1B. Responder** • See Step 2	"I am having some difficulty interpreting how the schedule was made, can you help me understand?" "Help me to understand how you see ..." "I am frustrated with the timeline being suggested, what about yourself?" "I am curious about how you view ..." "Is this a good time to talk?" "Happy to talk"
2.	Actively listen	• Listen to understand other opinions and perspectives. • Use nonverbal communication, such as eye contact and nodding to show the speaker you are engaged. • Listening to others, helps them listen to you. • Listening authentically means you are genuinely curious and care, not just because you are supposed to. • Do not interrupt when others are talking, listen until they are finished. • Assume others have good intentions too. • Listen for potential solutions.	"Tell me more" "What else?" "Help me understand"
3.	Seek and acknowledge others' viewpoints	• Summarize your understanding of other viewpoints before sharing your viewpoint or asking questions. • Recognize viewpoints are not right or wrong, not better or worse, just different. • Watch personalizing others' viewpoints • Ask questions, before making assumptions about others intentions or motivations. • Watch your "blind spots" (your facial expression, tone, body posture. • Acknowledgement and understanding are not the same as agreement.	"Let me see if I understand what you are saying..." "Sounds like we agree that ..." "Help me understand why this is important to you" "Help me understand the sticking points for you"
4.	Share your viewpoint	• Present your concerns as your viewpoint, not the truth • Share what is important to you about your views, intentions, feelings and contributions • Take time to reflect on your own actions and contributions to the situation • Share all relevant information that is important to the situation • Be open to feedback	"Here's how I view the situation ..." "It was not my intention to ... it was my intention ..." "How can I rebuild trust?"
5.	Seek common ground	• Given what you have learned about the other person's story, how can you move forward together? • Highlight shared interests. • Reframe problems into potential solutions. • Mistakes should be acknowledged without shame or blame. • Be open to the possibility that you may be wrong. • Make others your partner in finding solutions. • Offer and accept apologies if appropriate. • There is always common ground; ask others to help find it if you are at an impasse.	"I think we can both agree that we are not happy with the current situation." "Who needs to benefit from this decision?" "What can we agree to about this situation?" "I am wondering if ...it would make sense, we could try, we should speak to,
6.	Reach agreement on next steps	• Determine what information is still needed to reach a solution. • Clarify who will develop and/or implement the move-forward plan and how and when this will be done. • Confirm who/how decisions or directions will be made. • Establish who is responsible for follow-up steps. • Solutions can involve accommodation and compromise.	"So we've agreed that before making a final decision we need more information. John, you are going to..." "Let us recap where we are."

a   Glover Takahashi, adapted from Rogers DA, Lingard L, Boehler ML. Espin S, Mellinger JD, Schindler N, Klingensmith M. Surgeons managing conflict in the operating room: defining the educational need and identifying effective behaviours. *Am J Surg*. 2013:205(2):15-30.

© 2015 Royal College of Physicians and Surgeons of Canada

T8. SUMMARY SHEET FOR THE COLLABORATOR ROLE

Created for the *CanMEDS Teaching and Assessment Tools Guide* by S Glover Takahashi, D Richardson and D Martin. Reproduced with permission of the Royal College.

See Collaborator Role teacher tips appendix for this teaching tool

COLLABORATOR

- The terms 'team', 'teamwork' and 'collaboration' have different meanings. Collaboration is active, deliberate and relationship-centred.

- Good collaboration is varied and involves two or more people, occurs in same or different locations and/or includes colleagues from different or same profession.

- The degree of collaboration necessary is dependent on the complexity of the situation and based on patient (not practitioner) needs.

- Collaborative decision-making includes actively sharing, soliciting and encouraging diverse perspectives so the best course of action can be determined.

RELATIONSHIP-CENTRED COLLABORATION[a]

Positive professional work relationships. Individuals:

- are familiar with each other
- have rapport
- trust each other, and
- demonstrate that they
  - value,
  - respect,
  - appreciate, and
  - support each other in the workplace

PROCESS of the Collaborator Role:

- Collaborating
- Compromising
- Conflicting
- Cooperating
- Resisting
- Resolving
- Respecting
- Sharing

CONTENT of the Collaborator Role: (The What)

- Collaboration
- Conflict, Conflict resolution
- Disruptive behaviour
- Diversity
- Handover
- Inter/Intra professional
- Rapport
- Shared decision-making
- Teams, teamwork

PRIME[b] – to identify the possible factors related to promoting understanding:

CONTENT of differences and conflicts	*PROCESS of differences and conflicts*
- **P**ersonal, professional, and patient differences	- Inventory and clarify the information and interests
- **R**ole incompatibility	- Listen actively
- **I**nformational deficiencies	- Acknowledge other viewpoints
- **M**ethods	- Seek common ground
- **E**nvironmental stress	- Reach agreement on next steps

HANDOVERS

Effective handovers enhance care and help prevent harm to patients.

Features of effective handovers:[c]

- Focusing on giving and receiving patient information (i.e. free of interruptions and distractions; active listening and clarifying when necessary

- Standardized handover tools for verbal communication, electronic handover tools, formal checklists

- Teamwork training in handovers (i.e. not training of team members but actual teamwork training)

---

a Beach MC, Inui T, the Relationship-Centered Care Research Network. Relationship-centered Care: A Constructive Reframing. *Journal of General Internal Medicine.* 2006;21(Suppl 1):S3-S8. doi:10.1111/j.1525-1497.2006.00302.x.

b Richardson D, Wagner S. Collaborative Teams, Module 2, Educating health professionals in interprofessional care course (ehpic™), Module 2 – University of Toronto, 2013. Reproduced with permission.

c AHRQ. Patient Safety Network. Patient Safety Primers – Handovers and signouts. http://psnet.ahrq.gov/primer.aspx?primerID=9

© 2015 Royal College of Physicians and Surgeons of Canada

Collaborator

T8. SUMMARY SHEET FOR THE COLLABORATOR ROLE (continued)

COLLABORATOR INTELLIGENCE (CI)

Key domains for learning, teaching and assessing the Collaborator Role:

- Self (i.e. knowing one's strengths, values, limitations and managing one's own behaviour and emotions)

- Relationships (i.e. being able to use empathy to build relationships with others, including the patient)

- Context (i.e. demonstrating behaviours, actions that reflect and incorporate the awareness of the surrounding situations and circumstances)

- System (i.e. recognizing and promote understanding of the aspects of health care organizations, including structures, operations and culture that influence the delivery of care across the continuum)

'In the moment' rules for managing differences and conflict

1. Stay calm
2. Stay focused
3. Slow down and talk to others
4. Redirect others as needed

Approaches to apply to different situations

DICTATE
- Quick, decisive action is vital
- On important issues where unpopular action is needed

AVOID
- Time needed to reduce tension, regain perspective
- Others can resolve the conflict more effectively

ACCOMMODATE
- The issue is more important to the other person
- Preserving harmony is especially important

COMPROMISE:
- A quick solution is needed under time pressure
- Both parties have equal power and have different goals

COLLABORATE
- Longer term solution and multiple viewpoints
- Buy-in and shared decision-making are important

RISK REDUCTION REMINDERS[b]

1. CONFIRM WHY: When multiple health professionals are involved, confirm that the reason and rationale for transfer of care is clear to all

2. CONFIRM WHO: Verify appropriate health professionals are aware of patient's clinical condition and agree to transfer of care

   Verify roles and responsibilities of each team member in handover is clearly given/received by the patient and health professionals

3. STRUCTURE THE HOW: Structured communication tool and protocols are very helpful. Follow established processes each time

4. ENSURE UNDERSTANDING OF WHAT: Ensure sufficient patient information is provided. Clarify and repeat back as needed. It is valuable to reconfirm clinical history directly with patient

5. DOCUMENT: Document relevant information when sending — for those assuming the patient care. Document relevant information when receiving — and entering key elements of handover information.

STEPS AND HINTS TO PROMOTE UNDERSTANDING

1. ***Identify the need for a conversation***
   Encourage the expression of concerns

2. ***Actively listen***
   Listen to understand different opinions and perspectives

3. ***Acknowledge others' points of view***
   Summarize understanding before sharing

4. ***Share your viewpoint***
   Share all relevant information that is important to the situation

5. ***Seek common ground***
   Highlight common interests and focus on solutions

6. ***Reach agreement on next steps***
   Clarify process and time for move-forward plan

A1. MULTISOURCE FEEDBACK FOR COLLABORATOR SKILLS[a]

See Collaborator Role teacher tips appendix for this assessment tool

Instructions for Assessor:

- Collaborator competencies can be developed over time. Using the form below, please help this learner gain insight into his/her skills by providing valuable confidential feedback.

- This information will be shared with the learner in aggregate form and for the purposes of helping the learner improve his/her competencies.

- Please return this form in a confidential manner

to _____

by _____

Learner's Name: _____

Postgraduate year (PGY): _____

Indicate ☑ all that apply. I am a:
- ☐ Health professional team member (including co-resident)
- ☐ Resident supervisor
- ☐ Faculty
- ☐ Other, please describe _____

Degree of Interaction
- ☐ I had considerable interaction with this learner
- ☐ I had occasional interaction with this learner

#	Area	1 Never or very poorly	2 Occasionally or needs to improve	3 Satisfactory	4 Consistently	5 Highly skilled	Not able to comment
1.	Listens respectfully to others' views						
2.	Approach contributes positively to the dynamics of collaboration						
3.	Engages and demonstrates appreciation for colleagues						
4.	Is available and approachable						
5.	Effective non verbal (e.g. eye contact, posture, expressions) and other verbal skills tone, pace, volume of speech, pauses						
6.	Negotiates overlapping and shared responsibilities for the benefit of patient care						
7.	Engages in shared decision-making approach includes finding common ground on needs, priorities, next steps; plan of action negotiated; offers choices and alternatives						
8.	Asks for feedback and incorporates feedback for improvement						

a Adapted from Glover Takahashi S, Martin D, Richardson D. Chapter 5 In *The CanMEDS Toolkit for Teaching and Assessing the Collaborator Role.* Ottawa: The Royal College of Physicians and Surgeons of Canada; 2012.

© 2015 Royal College of Physicians and Surgeons of Canada

Collaborator

A1. MULTISOURCE FEEDBACK FOR COLLABOROR SKILLS (continued)

Areas of strength	Areas for improvement
1.	1.
2.	2.
3.	3.

Comments:

_____

_____

_____

_____

_____

_____

_____

Please return this form to: _____

Collaborator

© 2015 Royal College of Physicians and Surgeons of Canada

A2. COLLABORATOR ROLE ENCOUNTER FORM

See Collaborator Role teacher tips appendix for this assessment tool

Instructions for Assessor:

- Collaborator competencies can be developed over time. Using the form below, please help this learner gain insight into his/her skills by completing this form

- Share your assessment and feedback in a timely manner

Name: _____ PGY: _____

Inter/Intra professional communication

1	2	3	4	5	n/a
Borders on rude. Authoritarian or differential in approach. Overly passive. Debates or is dismissive of feedback.		Respectful, clear and timely communication. Responsive to other's requests and feedback.		Skilfully works with others to coordinate patient's care.	

Collaboration with patient/family

1	2	3	4	5	n/a
Does not inform patient/family of plans. Does not elicit patient/family perspective. Provides misinformation.		Recognizes when to organize patient. Recognizes when to organize patient/family meetings. Encourages shared decision-making. Provides clear patient information patient/family meetings. Shared decision-making. Provides clear patient information.		Independently coordinates and leads patient/family meetings. Confidently negotiates and manages patient/family difference.	

Discharge planning

1	2	3	4	5	n/a
Passive. No initiative. Lacks awareness of appropriate team and community resources.		Actively seeks out appropriate resources and consults with patient/team/ community resources. Formulates a d/c plan.		Independently facilitates and coordinates a comprehensive discharge plan, including follow-up. Delegates responsibility.	

Team meeting

1	2	3	4	5	n/a
Consistently late or absent. Behaviour disruptive or non-contributory to team process.		Actively participates and contributes. Reliably performs assigned tasks. Able to co-chair or co-lead meetings.		Independently able to facilitate and coordinate meetings and follow-up. Actively moves meeting forward. Builds consensus, resolves differences, and provides direction.	

a   Adapted from Glover Takahashi S, Martin D, Richardson D. Chapter 5 In *The CanMEDS Toolkit for Teaching and Assessing the Collaborator Role*. Ottawa: The Royal College of Physicians and Surgeons of Canada; 2012. Reproduced with permission.

© 2015 Royal College of Physicians and Surgeons of Canada

Collaborator

A2. COLLABORATOR ROLE ENCOUNTER FORM (continued)

Management of difference and conflict

1	2	3	4	5	n/a
Argumentative. Lacks awareness of own personal contributions to difference or conflict. Debates feedback. Does not listen.		Identifies and manages differences constructively. Listens to understand and for common ground. Demonstrates a willingness to act upon feedback.		Proactively assists in subverting and resolving conflict with other team/ family members. Recognizes own role in contributing to differences and acts to professionally resolve.	

Handover

1	2	3	4	5	n/a
Disorganized or incomplete handover. Not attentive in giving and receiving patient information, does not clarify. Not efficient or effective in teamwork.		Provides needed patient information Competent approach or use of structured tool. Understands role of team members and competently collaborates in handover.		Attentive in giving and receiving patient info. Uses structured approach/tools with ease and efficiency. Is attentive to and enables effective team handover assisting if/as needed.	

OVERALL EVALUATION

1	2	3	4	5
Unsatisfactory		Solid performance		Superior
Below the minimally acceptable level for a trainee at specified training level.		Demonstrates a solid ability to perform competently. Does what is expected at the specified training level.		Significantly exceeds the benchmark for competence at the specified training level.

Describe STRENGTHS

Actions or areas for Improvement

Comments:

© 2015 Royal College of Physicians and Surgeons of Canada

Collaborator

A3. TEAM MEETING ENCOUNTER FORM[a]

See Collaborator Role teacher tips appendix for this assessment tool

Instructions for Assessor:

- Collaborator competencies can be developed over time. Using the form below, please help this learner gain insight into his/her skills by completing this form

- Share your assessment and feedback in a timely manner

Name:_____

Level of Evaluation is PGY: _____

DATE: _____

Evaluator: _____

Participation in team meetings

1	2	3	4	5	n/a
Consistently late or absent. Disruptive to process. Disrespectful to roles of others. Unprepared.		Reliably performs assigned tasks. Respects roles and opinions of others. Listens to understand and for common ground.		Behaviours consistently move meeting forward. Facilitates mutual accountability for shared decisions. Builds consensus, manages differences and resolves conflict.	

Communication in team meetings

1	2	3	4	5	n/a
Does not listen respectfully. Verbal and non verbal communication is disruptive to process.		Clearly and directly communicates. Uses reflective listening. Acknowledges and responds to others' questions, concerns and contributions.		Skilfully recognizes and manages communication challenges. Maintains and coordinates necessary communication outside of meeting.	

Leadership skills in team meetings

1	2	3	4	5	n/a
Consistently avoids or declines leadership responsibilities. Cannot follow others.		Values difference. Builds on others opinions. Supports consensus building efforts. Encourages multiple viewpoints.		Flexible approach and situationally aware. Respectfully delegates and shares power. Demonstrates followership when issue is better lead by another.	

---

a   Adapted from Glover Takahashi S, Martin D, Richardson D. Chapter 5 In *The CanMEDS Toolkit for Teaching and Assessing the Collaborator Role.* Ottawa: The Royal College of Physicians and Surgeons of Canada; 2012. Reproduced with permission.

© 2015 Royal College of Physicians and Surgeons of Canada

Collaborator

A3. TEAM MEETING ENCOUNTER FORM (continued)

Management of difference and conflict in team meetings

1	2	3	4	5	n/a
Argumentative. Lacks awareness of own personal contributions to difference or conflict. Debates feedback.		Identifies and manages differences constructively. Listens to understand, and for common ground. Demonstrates a willingness to act upon feedback.		Proactively assists in subverting and resolving conflict with team members regardless of context.	

OVERALL PERFORMANCE IN TEAM MEETINGS

1	2	3	4	5
Unsatisfactory		Solid performance		Superior
Below the minimally acceptable level for a trainee at specified training level.		Demonstrates a solid ability to perform competently. Does what is expected at the specified training level.		Significantly exceeds the benchmark for competence at the specified training level.

Describe STRENGTHS	Actions or areas for Improvement

Comments:

_____

_____

_____

_____

_____

_____

_____

_____

Collaborator

A4. COLLABORATOR QUOTIENT

Created for the *CanMEDS Teaching and Assessment Tools Guide* by S Glover Takahashi. Reproduced with permission of the Royal College.

Instructions for learners:

- The purpose of this exercise is to help you reflect on your impact on group dynamics in a recent situation or clinical setting.

- Thoughtful reflection can lead to improvement.

- Focus is not on 'correct' score, but to identify ways to improve you 'collaboration quotient'.

- Be prepared to discuss at next meeting.

Insert your name:_____

Describe your role/responsibilities in this location:

_____

_____

_____

_____

_____

_____

_____

Describe the Rotation/Site/Organization: (include details about when, where, how long, type of service)

_____

_____

_____

_____

_____

_____

_____

© 2015 Royal College of Physicians and Surgeons of Canada

Collaborator

A4. COLLABORATOR QUOTIENT (continued)

Collaborator Quotient: Calculate your personal "score"

Do you...	0 No or rarely	1 Occasionally or sometimes	2 Often or mostly	3 Always	Notes or examples
I genuinely appreciate the role and contribution of others.					
I demonstrate a respectful approach — even when things aren't going well or not going as I wish.					
I introduce myself to people.					
I clarify if I don't understand what is being said.					
I develop positive, trusting relationships.					
I work to be aware of the difference between myself/other's 'intention' and myself/other's 'impact'. I work to ensure the impact of my behaviour on others is aligned with my intentions.					
I apologize with ease and sincerity.					
I use both my preferred style to work in teams and flexibly use other styles if it is better suited to the situation.					
I ask for feedback regularly.					
I say please and thank you.					
YOUR TOTAL					

Areas for improvement

Area(s) for improvement over the next three to four weeks?

_____

_____

What will improvement look like?

_____

_____

Collaborator

© 2015 Royal College of Physicians and Surgeons of Canada

A5. OBJECTIVE STRUCTURED CLINICAL EXAM (OCSE) FOR THE COLLABORATOR ROLE

Created for the *CanMEDS Teaching and Assessment Tools Guide* by D Richardson and S Glover Takahashi. Reproduced with permission of the Royal College.

Instructions for Assessor:

- *Learning objectives:* OSCE assessments are an effective way to assess if all of your learners are at, above or below a common standard. They will also provide insight as to who is meeting or exceeding in their understanding and application of Collaborator competencies, as well as who is falling behind.

- *How to use adapt:*

  - Select from, modify, or add to the sample OSCE cases. Each case is designed as a ten-minute scenario.

  - Modify these cases to be seven to eight minutes with the standardized patient (SP) and have two to three minutes of probing questions from faculty. The two to four probing questions within the scenario provide considerable additional insight into competence in the area.

  - Combine a variety of different Roles into the same exam.

  - Four to six cases is a reasonable number of cases for an in training program OSCE.

  - Consider using one scenario at a teaching session. Residents or SPs could do a demonstration.

  - Consider using a video recorded scenario for teaching purposes.

Scenario #1:
Phone consultation of patient

You are on call. A resident from _____ program calls you to do a consult for a Patient AA. The patient needs/ priority for AA do not match your program or priorities. You go to see the resident to discuss.

TASK: Discuss patient needs and differing priorities with the other resident (who can be a standardized team member, fellow resident or faculty member playing that role.

Scenario #2:
Handover

You are doing handover from xx to your clinical area, yy. You review the available information and determine you need more information. You call the resident/staff from xx to get additional information. Take two to three minutes to review the handover documents from xx to yy and then call YY.

TASK: On the phone, discuss the handover information received and what is also needed with the sending team member.

NOTES:
1. Simulated 'incomplete' handover documents needs to be developed for this scenario.
2. Team member can be a standardized team member, fellow resident or faculty member.

Scenario #3:
Goals of care

There is a family meeting that includes the patient and their spouse. The patient is now palliative and she wants to go home as soon as possible. The home care planner dominates the discussion. Bed availability is low.

At the family meeting, there are comments indicating lack of agreement from the spouse (re: ability to cope), nurse (re: safety in ambulation, disorientation at night, help needed for personal care) and resident (re: trouble controlling pain at this time). The resident steps out to answer a page. As the resident returns to the family meeting, the home care planner announces that plans for discharge should proceed tomorrow to the patient's home while awaiting a hospice bed. Equipment will be ordered right away. The meeting is adjourned.

As the meeting adjourns, the social worker approaches the resident to sign the discharge orders.

TASK: Discuss discharge with the social worker.

© 2015 Royal College of Physicians and Surgeons of Canada

A5. OBJECTIVE STRUCTURED CLINICAL EXAM (OCSE) FOR THE COLLABORATOR ROLE (continued)

OSCE SCORING SHEET[a]

Name:_____

Program:_____

Collaborator: EFFECTIVE TEAM WORK

1	2	3	4	5
Unaware of need for communication with other health care providers.	Unable to integrate the provision of care by medical team with that provided by allied health professional.	Generally appropriate collaboration with allied health professional.	Appropriate collaboration with allied health professional.	Exceptional ability to elicit relevant detail with efficient use of time.

Collaborator: TEAM COMMUNICATION

1	2	3	4	5
Authoritarian or deferential in approach. Does not listen respectfully. Verbal and non-verbal communication is disruptive to process.	Actively listens and engages in meeting. Conveys information. Builds trust through actions.	Clearly and directly communicates. Uses reflective listening. Responsive to others requests and feedback.	Effectively and efficiently communicates relevant information, either verbal or written. Identifies communication barriers. Delegates responsibility appropriately and respectfully.	Skilfully recognizes and manages communication challenges. Maintains and coordinates necessary communication outside of meeting(s). Skilfully coordinates patient's care with others.

Collaborator: COLLABORATION ALONG PATIENT CARE CONTINUUM

1	2	3	4	5
Passive. No initiative. Lacks awareness of role and responsibility.	Contributes to the care plan. Able to identify team and community resources.	Actively seeks out appropriate resources and consults with patient/team/community resources. Formulates a care plan.	Synthesizes information from patient/team/community to formulate a comprehensive care plan.	Independently facilitates and coordinates a comprehensive care plan, including follow-up. Delegates responsibility.

Collaborator: HANDOVER

1	2	3	4	5
Disorganized or incomplete handover. Not attentive in giving and receiving patient information, does not clarify. Not efficient or effective in teamwork.	Poor skills in handover. Inattentive in giving or receiving handover leading to errors or delays. Is not team oriented.	Provides needed patient information. Competent approach or use of structured tool. Understands role of team members and competently collaborates in handover. Accurate documentation.	Strong skills in handover including effective clarification and documentation.	Superb handover including documentation and follow up. Uses structured approach or tools with ease and efficiency. Enables effectiveness of team assisting if/as needed.

a Adapted from Glover Takahashi S, Martin D, Richardson D. Chapter 5 In *The CanMEDS Toolkit for Teaching and Assessing the Collaborator Role*. Ottawa: The Royal College of Physicians and Surgeons of Canada; 2012.

Collaborator

© 2015 Royal College of Physicians and Surgeons of Canada

A5. OBJECTIVE STRUCTURED CLINICAL EXAM (OCSE) FOR THE COLLABORATOR ROLE (continued)

Collaborator: MANAGEMENT OF DIFFERENCE AND CONFLICT:

1	2	3	4	5
Argumentative, does not feel there are any concerns. Lacks awareness of own personal contributions to difference or conflict.	Acknowledges others viewpoints. Respectfully listens to feedback. Prevents misunderstanding by actively listening. Recognizes role and limitations.	Identifies and manages differences constructively. Listens to understand, and for common ground. Demonstrates a willingness to act upon feedback.	Recognizes own role in contributing to difference and acts to professionally resolve. Identifies potential problematic team dynamics. Reflects on actions.	Respectfully and skilfully manages differences and conflict. Resolves and gains consensus among team members.

OVERALL PERFORMANCE IN THIS SCENARIO

1	2	3	4	5
Needs significant improvement	Below expectations	Solid, competent performance	Exceeds expectations	Sophisticated, expert performance

PGY LEVEL OF PERFORMANCE[b] – At what level of training was this performance?

B	1	2	3	4	5+
Below PGY1	Mid-PGY1	Mid-PGY2	Mid-PGY3	Mid-PGY4	Mid-PGY5 or above

Areas of strength	Areas for improvement
1.	
2.	
3.	

---

b NOTE: Programs that have moved to Competence By Design may want to modify these levels to the four parts of the resident competence continuum.

© 2015 Royal College of Physicians and Surgeons of Canada

Collaborator

COLLABORATOR ROLE TEACHER TIPS APPENDIX

T4. PRIME FACTORS TO PROMOTE UNDERSTANDING, MANAGE DIFFERENCES AND RESOLVE CONFLICT

Instructions for Teacher:

- Introduce learners to the PRIME model.

- Give learners a scenario that includes a misunderstanding, difference or conflict OR work with them to select scenarios from their recent practice.

- Choose from the samples provided or create your own.

- If doing in a workshop or group setting, allocate about 20 minutes for each activity.

- Depending on the group and time available, you may wish to assign one or more worksheets as homework to be completed before the session, or as a follow-up assignment.

T6. HANDOVER IN EVERYDAY PRACTICE

One of the key competencies of the CanMEDS 2015 Collaborator Role is to hand over the care of a patient to another health care professional to facilitate continuity of safe patient care. Effective handovers can enhance care and help to prevent harm to patients. When handovers go badly, care can be negatively impacted. The purpose of this exercise is for your learners to relate what they are learning about hand over to their daily work. In doing so, they may develop a greater appreciation and understanding of these important concepts.

Instructions for Teacher:

- You can adapt this tool by assigning it as homework or by having learners discuss it with you and/or their peers.

- It could also be modified into an assessment tool by adding a scoring rubric.

T8. SUMMARY SHEET FOR THE COLLABORATOR ROLE

Instructions for Teacher:

- The summary sheet is intended to be a cheat sheet for the teacher as well as the learner. It is a one page resource on key concepts, frameworks and approaches.

A1. MULTISOURCE FEEDBACK FOR COLLABORATOR SKILLS

Instructions for Teacher:

- Modify the form by adding or removing criteria that do/ do not apply.

- To optimize learning and to protect the identity of those who provide feedback, be mindful of the size and composition of your data sample.

- Be sure to provide your 'assessors' with clear instructions and provide guidance on your rating scale.

- It is a good idea to notify your learners of your intention and rationale for collecting feedback on their CanMEDS Collaboration skills. Be clear about the timeframe when you will collect the data, how you will maintain confidentiality and how and when you will present the data back to the learner.

- Plan to share the summary of feedback with your learner in written format and in a face-to-face meeting. A meeting will allow for valuable coaching around areas of strength and areas for improvement.

A2 AND A3: ENCOUNTER FORMS

Instructions for Teacher:

- Depending on your location and program, you may use a tool like this regularly, for a particular learning experience or on an as needed basis.

- You will choose who should complete the form and how the results will be located.

© 2015 Royal College of Physicians and Surgeons of Canada

Collaborator

REFERENCES

1. Way D, Jones L, Busing N. *Implementation strategies. Collaboration in primary care: family doctors and nurse practitioners delivering shared care.* Toronto: Ontario College of Family Physicians; 2000.

2. Neily J, Mills PD, Young-Xu Y, Carney BT, West P, Berger DH, Mazzia LM, Paull DE, Bagian JP. Association between implementation of a medical team training program and surgical mortality. *JAMA.* 2010; 304(15):1693-700.

3. Clements D, Dault M, Priest A. Effective teamwork in healthcare: research and reality. *Healthc Pap.* 2007;7(Spec No):26-34.

4. Katz JS, Titaloye VM, Balogun JA. Physical and occupational therapy undergraduates' stereotypes of one another. *Percep Mot Skills.* 2001; 92(3 Pt 1):843-51.

5. McCallin A. Interdisciplinary practice--a matter of teamwork: an integrated literature review. *J Clin Nurs.* 2001;10(4):419-28.

6. Shamian J, El-Jardali F. Healthy workplaces for health workers in Canada: knowledge transfer and uptake in policy and practice. *Health Pap.* 2007;7(Spec No):6-25.

7. World Health Organization. *Framework for action on interprofessional education and collaborative practice.* Geneva: World Health Organization Press; 2010.

8. Leape LL, Shore MF, Dienstag JL, Mayer RJ, Edgman-Levitan S, Meyer GS, Healy GB. Perspective: a culture of respect, part 2: creating a culture of respect. *Acad Med.* 2012; 87(7):853-8.

9. Katzenbach R, Smith DK. *The wisdom of teams: Creating the high-performance organization.* Cambridge: Harvard Business Press; 1993.

10. Safran DG, Miller W, and Beckman H. Organizational dimensions of relationship-centered care. *J Gen Intern Med.* 2006;21 Suppl1:S9-15.

11. Adapted from www.skillsyouneed.com: Rapport. Last retrieved July 11, 2015, from http://www.skillsyouneed.com/ips/rapport.html

12. Adapted from Wikipedia: Shared decision-making. Last retrieved July 11, 2015, from http://en.wikipedia.org/wiki/Shared_decision-making

13. Kurtz S, Silverman J, Draper J. *Teaching and learning communication skills in medicine.* 2nd ed. London: Radcliffe Publishing; 2005.

14. Saltman DC, O'Dea NA, Kidd MR. Conflict management: a primer for doctors in training. *Postgrad Med J.* 2008;82(963);9-12.

15. Leslie K, Nasmith L. Approaches to conflict and differences. In Richardson D, Glover Takahashi S. Nasmith L, Leslie K, Bandiera G, Paterson M, et al. The CanMEDS train-the-trainer Collaborator faculty development program [PowerPoint slides]. Ottawa: Royal College of Physicians and Surgeons of Canada; 2007.

16. College of Physicians and Surgeons of Ontario. Guidebook for managing disruptive physician behaviour. Toronto: College of Physicians and Surgeons of Ontario; 2008. Available at http://www.cpso.on.ca/CPSO/media/uploadedfiles/CPSO_DPBI_Guidebook1.pdf

17. Stone D, Patton B, Heen S. *Difficult conversations: how to discuss what matters most.* New York: Penguin Books; 2000.

18. Fisher R, Ury WL. *Getting to yes. negotiating agreement without giving in.* Boston: Houghton Mifflin Company; 1981.

19. Competency: Organizational Awareness. State of California. 2011. Last retrieved July 12, 2015 from: http://www.dpa.ca.gov/training/analyst-virtual-help-desk/competency-guides/organizational-awareness.pdf

20. Canada Medical Protective Association. CMPA Risk Fact Sheet- Patient handovers-A1300-004-E © CMPA 2013 last retrieved July 12, 2015 from: https://www.cmpa-acpm.ca/documents/10179/300031190/patient_handovers-e.pdf

21. Russell L, Nyhof-Young J, Abosh B, Robinson S. An exploratory analysis of an interprofessional learning environment in two hospital clinical teaching units. *J Interprof Care.* 2006;10(1):29-39.

22. Postmes T, Spears R, Cihangir S. Quality of decision-making and group norms. *J Pers Soc Psychol.* 2001;80(6):918-30.

23. Goleman D. What makes a leader? *Harv Bus Rev.* 1998;76(6):93–102.

24. Okie S. An elusive balance—residents' work hours and the continuity of care. *N Engl J Med.* 2007; 356(26):2665-7.

25. Vidyarthi AR, Arora V, Schnipper JL, Wall SD, Wachter RM. Managing discontinuity in academic medical centres: strategies for a safe and effective resident sign-out. *J Hosp Med.* 2006;1(4):257-66.

26. Gordon M, Findley R. Educational interventions to improve handover in health care: a systematic review. *Med Educ.* 2011;45(11):1081-9.

Collaborator

© 2015 Royal College of Physicians and Surgeons of Canada

REFERENCES

27. I-PASS. Last retrieved July 12, 2015 from http://www. ipasshandoffstudy.com/about

28. ISoBAR. Last retrieved July 12, 2015 from https://www. mja.com.au/journal/2009/190/11/isobar-concept-and-handover-checklist-national-clinical-handover-initiative ALSO: *Porteous, J. et al MJA, Volume 190 Number 11, 1 June 2009.*

29. Tresolini CP, the Pew-Fetzer TaskForce. *Health professions education and relationship-centered care.* San Francisco: Pew Health Professions Commission; 1994, 2000.

30. Chan T, Sabir K, Sanhan S, Sherbino J. Understanding the impact of residents' interpersonal relationships during emergency department referrals and consultations. *J Grad Med Educ.* 2013;5(4):576-81.

31. Beach MC, Inui T, the Relationship-Centered Care Research Network. Relationship-centered care: a constructive reframing. *J Gen Intern Med.* 2006;21(Suppl1):S3-8.

32. Covey SR. *The 7 habits of highly effective people.* New York: Free Press; 1989, 2004.

33. Richardson D, Wagner S. Collaborative Teams, Module 2, Educating health professionals in interprofessional care course (ehpic™), Module 2 – University of Toronto, 2013.

34. Thomas KW. Conflict and conflict management: reflections and update. *J Organ Behav.* 1992;13(3):265-74.

35. Shell GR. Teaching ideas: bargaining styles and negotiation: the Thomas Kilmann conflict mode instrument in negotiation training. *Negotiation J.* 2001;17(2):155-74.

36. Martin D, Glover Takahashi S. Putting out the "Welcome Mat" for residents transitioning into Postgraduate Training. ICRE poster; 2011.

37. Coleman EA, Berenson RA. Lost in transition: challenges and opportunities for improving the quality of transitional care. *Ann Intern Med.* Oct 5 2004;141(7):533-536.

38. Forster AJ, Murff HJ, Peterson JF, Gandhi TK, Bates DW. The incidence and severity of adverse events affecting patients after discharge from hospital. *Ann Intern Med.* 2003 138(3):161-7.

39. Moore C, Wisnivesky J, Williams S, McGinn T. Medical errors related to discontinuity of care from an inpatient to an outpatient setting. *J Gen Intern Med.* 2003; 18(8):646-651.

40. AHRQ. Patient Safety Network. Patient Safety Primers – handovers and signouts. Last retrieved July 12, 2015 from: http://psnet.ahrq.gov/primer.aspx?primerID=9

Collaborator

© 2015 Royal College of Physicians and Surgeons of Canada

FOLLOWING
ORGANIZING
Quality improvement
TIME MANAGEMENT Changing
LEADING Patient safety
Systems thinking PRIORITIZING

LEADER

Safe Culture Managing
TRANSITIONING
Monitoring
EFFICIENCY Stewardship
DELEGATING
Continuously improving
Incident

Deepak Dath

Ming-Ka Chan

Brian Wong

Susan Glover Takahashi

1. Why the Leader Role matters

The CanMEDS Leader Role sets the expectation that physicians actively engage with patients, collaborators, and the health care system as leaders and managers in decision-making, in quality improvement and in patient safety within day-to-day operations and act as stewards of health care delivery at both a local and systems level.

Prior to the 2015 edition of the CanMEDS Framework, this role was called Manager, though leadership was inherent to the role in all of the earlier editions of the CanMEDS Framework. Research and consultations with stakeholders in the development of CanMEDS 2015 demonstrated a need for increased emphasis on leadership competencies while also maintaining important managerial competencies for 21st century health care.[1] These new competencies are grounded in an emerging, broader concept of the word "leader."

Getting oriented to the Leader Role will take effort for most of us. When introducing others to the Role, be sure to emphasize these four overarching themes:

- By engaging in processes of quality improvement, patient safety and resource stewardship, physician leaders play an important and influential part in the future of health care. An increasingly complex health care system needs the collaboration, leadership, and insight of physicians, other professionals and patients to identify when, where, and how improvements can be made.

- Collaborative leadership competencies help facilitate improvements that enhance patient outcomes.[2]

- The health care system depends on physicians taking responsibility for the stewardship of the system's finite resources.[3]

- Today's physicians face multiple personal and professional demands, a variety of career options, and an explosion of distractions. They must make personal management skills a high priority if they are to succeed.

2. What the Leader Role looks like in daily practice

It is common for people to associate physician leadership primarily with those who hold titled leadership positions. Help your learners see leadership through a different lens by pointing out your own leadership activities in your everyday work and by showing how physician leaders work in collaboration with other professionals within the health care system.

In day-to-day practice, the Leader Role is closely linked to Medical Expert, but it is also intertwined with the other six CanMEDS Roles because leadership influences various aspects of all the Roles. For example:

- As Leaders, physicians engage with others to contribute to a vision of a high-quality health care system and take responsibility for the delivery of excellent patient care through their activities as clinicians, administrators, scholars, or teachers. In these capacities, the Leader Role would be closely intertwined with Health Advocate, Medical Expert, and Collaborator.

- As Leaders managing health human resources in their practice, physicians also need to work effectively in the Communicator Role and Professional Role.

- The Leader Role is connected to the Scholar Role as it relates to being a lifelong learner and teacher who values both self-awareness and the giving and receiving of feedback to coach (or be coached).

If you find that some of your learners have trouble picking out the Leader Role in their daily activities, you can encourage them to listen for some of the words in Table L-1, which can be associated with the Leader Role in day-to-day practice. When they hear or use these trigger words and phrases, they can be relatively confident that they are functioning within the Leader Role of the CanMEDS Framework.

TABLE L-1. TRIGGER WORDS RELATING TO THE PROCESS AND CONTENT OF THE LEADER ROLE

Trigger words relating to the PROCESS of the Leader Role:		Trigger words relating to the CONTENT of the Leader Role:	
• Leading	• Organizing	• Culture	• Patient flow
• Changing	• Prioritizing	• Patient safety	• Resources (e.g. human, financial, equipment)
• Transitioning	• Scheduling	• Incident	
• Continuously improving	• Budgeting	• Quality improvement	• Time management
• Following	• Running a unit/ department/ service	• Systems thinking	• Workflow
• Managing		• Priorities	• Schedule
• Implementing	• Stewarding, Choosing wisely[4]	• Strategy	• Human resources
• Delegating		• Effectiveness	• Career planning
• Strategizing, Monitoring	• Utilizing technology	• Efficiency	• Integrity

© 2015 Royal College of Physicians and Surgeons of Canada

Leader

Excerpt from the CanMEDS 2015 Physician Competency Framework[a]

DEFINITION

As Leaders, physicians engage with others to contribute to a vision of a high-quality health care system and take responsibility for the delivery of excellent patient care through their activities as clinicians, administrators, scholars, or teachers.

DESCRIPTION

The CanMEDS Leader Role describes the engagement of all physicians in shared decision-making for the operation and ongoing evolution of the health care system. As a societal expectation, physicians demonstrate collaborative leadership and management within the health care system. At a system level, physicians contribute to the development and delivery of continuously improving health care and engage with others in working toward this goal. Physicians integrate their personal lives with their clinical, administrative, scholarly, and teaching responsibilities. They function as individual care providers, as members of teams, and as participants and leaders in the health care system locally, regionally, nationally, and globally.

KEY COMPETENCIES

Physicians are able to:

1. Contribute to the improvement of health care delivery in teams, organizations, and systems

2. Engage in the stewardship of health care resources

3. Demonstrate leadership in professional practice

4. Manage career planning, finances, and health human resources in a practice

KEY TERMS OF THE LEADER ROLE

To help your learners familiarize themselves with the Leader Role, have them review key terms that are important to the Leader Role.

Emotional intelligence[5] is a group of skills that leaders use to guide their thinking, behaviour, and outcomes. It includes the following:

- **Self-awareness** – knowing one's strengths, weaknesses, drivers, values, and impact on others

- **Self-regulation** – the ability to monitor and control one's own behaviour, emotions or thoughts, altering them in accordance with the demands of the situation. It includes the abilities to exhibit first responses, to resist interference from irrelevant stimulation and to persist on relevant tasks even when we don't enjoy them

- **Motivation** – a strong internal drive to pursue goals and achievement for reasons that are personally meaningful

- **Empathy** – considering others' feelings, values, and preferences

- **Social skill** – building rapport and relationships with others

Self-assessment refers to the monitoring of one's own performance. Much research suggests that we do this poorly when we rely on internal assessment alone and that guided self-assessment is better. Guided self-assessment is most effective using established criteria or metrics and with feedback or information collected from others,[6] especially mentors. For example, learners may self-assess their performance in leading team rounds by beginning with reflection and consideration of what worked (and what did not) at recent rounds and then seek further external guidance by incorporating the input of team feedback data, comments from peers and supervisors, and/or coaching advice from mentors.

Transitions[7] means the process or period of changing from one state or condition to another. In medical education, professional transitions include: medical school to residency; junior to senior; residency into practice; changes in practice; and transition out of practice.[8]

Health informatics encompasses a variety of tools, technologies, and techniques that inform health care and health care professionals to guide clinical processes and decision-making. Health informatic tools include computers, clinical guidelines, formal medical terminologies, and information and communication systems.[9]

Leader

---

a Dath D, Chan M-K, Anderson G, Burke A, Razack S, Lieff S, Moineau G, Chiu A, Ellison P. Leader. In: Frank JR, Snell L, Sherbino J, editors. *CanMEDS 2015 Physician Competency Framework*. Ottawa: Royal College of Physicians and Surgeons of Canada; 2015. Reproduced with permission.

Stewardship[10] of resources entails appropriate use of finite health care system resources. Activities related to stewardship can be done at the individual and/or the system level and include consideration of available evidence to guide appropriate use of tests and treatments, effective communication with patients and families to arrive at shared decisions, and system-level measurement and interventions to optimize quality and value.

Choosing Wisely Canada[4] (CWC) is a campaign focused on resource stewardship to raise awareness of the need to reduce unnecessary tests, treatments, and procedures, and to help physicians and patients make smart and effective choices to ensure high-quality care.

Six domains of health care quality:[11]
One of the most influential analytic frameworks for quality assessment is the framework put forth by the Institute of Medicine (IOM), which includes the following six aims for the health care system:

1. **Safe:** Avoiding harm to patients from the care that is intended to help them.

2. **Effective:** Providing services based on scientific knowledge to all who could benefit and refraining from providing services to those not likely to benefit (avoiding underuse and misuse, respectively).

3. **Patient-centred:** Providing care that is respectful of and responsive to individual patient preferences, needs and values, and ensuring that patient values guide all clinical decisions.

4. **Timely:** Improving access and reducing waits and sometimes harmful delays for those who require care.

5. **Efficient:** Avoiding waste, including waste of time, resources, equipment, supplies, and energy.

6. **Equitable:** Providing care that does not vary in quality because of personal characteristics such as gender, ethnicity, geographic location, and socioeconomic status.

Quality improvement is a structured "approach to the analysis of performance and systematic efforts to improve it."[12] One common approach, called the Model for Improvement,[13] has two parts. The first part consists of three organizing questions: What are we trying to accomplish? How will we know that a change is an improvement? What changes can we make that will result in improvement? The second part involves the Plan-Do-Study-Act (PDSA) cycle "to test and implement changes in real work settings."

PDSA stands for Plan-Do-Study-Act, and represents a common rapid-cycle change approach used for quality improvement (often referred to as a small test of change). These rapid cycles of change occur within the Model for Improvement, a commonly used framework for quality improvement. There are four steps:[14]

1. **Plan** – What small change would you like to test? What do you predict will happen when you put the change in place?

2. **Do** – Test the change on a small scale; test it against your prediction.

3. **Study** – Gather a small amount of data, or make some observations to see what happened with the change and reflect on what was learned. Did it confirm or refute your prediction?

4. **Act** – Based on your findings, decide what to do next, and plan your next change.

Patient safety is an attribute of health care systems that minimizes the incidence and impact of patient safety incidents and maximizes recovery from such incidents toward the goal of achieving a trustworthy system of health care delivery.[15, 16]

Safety culture[13] is a characteristic of an organization or system that demonstrates commitment to openness, honesty, fairness, and accountability. Safety culture supports opportunities for safety training and preparedness. It promotes understanding and learning, and strongly encourages individuals to report incidents and safety hazards to promote improvement. In a health care system, it "requires flexibility and resilience so that people, unexpected situations and priorities can be managed in a timely and effective manner" that consistently reflects the commitment to patient-centred care.

Just Culture is a culture in which individual practitioners and others are not punished for actions, errors, omissions or decisions which arise from system failures over which they have no control. A just culture also recognizes that many errors represent predictable interactions between human operators and the systems in which they work and also that competent professionals make mistakes. It acknowledges that even competent professionals may develop unhealthy habit, norms or shortcuts.[17, 18]

A *provider* is a physician, professional or non-professional staff member, or other person engaged in the delivery of health care services.[13]

© 2015 Royal College of Physicians and Surgeons of Canada

Incident analysis is a structured process that aims to identify what happened, how and why it happened, what can be done to reduce the risk of recurrence and make care safer, and what was learned from the incident. In most education programs, organizations, and systems, all learners and physicians would be expected to know their roles in, and responsibilities for, incident analysis. Below are two different types of incident analysis:

1. **Cause and Effect Analysis**[19] is a specific approach to incident analysis that uses a diagram-based technique and combines brainstorming to consider all the possible causes of a problem, rather than just the ones that are most obvious.

2. **Five Whys Analysis**[19] is a specific incident analysis process in which you repeatedly ask the question "Why?" (using five as a rule of thumb) so that you can peel away the layers of an issue, just like the layers of an onion, which can lead you to the root cause of a problem. You may need to ask the question fewer or more than five times before you get to the origin of a problem. The real key is to avoid assumptions and logic traps and to keep drilling down to the real root cause.

Incident management[13] consists of the various actions and processes that constitute the immediate and ongoing activities following an incident. Incident analysis is part of incident management. In most education programs, organizations, and systems, each learner and physician would be expected to know where to access incident management processes and who will conduct them.

A *patient safety incident*[13] is an event or circumstance that could have resulted, or did result, in unnecessary harm to a patient. There are three types of patient safety incidents:

- A **harmful incident** results in harm to the patient (previously called an adverse event, a sentinel event, or a critical incident). Harm is due to the medical care provided, not the underlying medical illness.

- A **no harm incident** reaches a patient but does not result in any discernible harm.

- A **near miss** does not reach the patient (previously termed a close call).

3. Preparing to teach the Leader Role

The Leader Role is one of the CanMEDS Roles where learners struggle to understand how it applies to their day-to-day practice, and even to their own personal development. There may be misconceptions about what leadership is all about and how they as individuals fit in — the word 'leader' is often associated with a title or an important position more than it is with a set of individual skills, for instance. Learners may also be uncomfortable with the uncertainty of part of the Leader Role, such as when decisions must be taken when not all of the facts are known. Time management may also be a challenge. In this section, we review common misconceptions about the Role, and suggest how to integrate the content and process of the Leader Role into practice.

3.1 Common misconceptions to address with learners

It is a common misconception that the word 'leader' means 'boss'.[20] Leadership in the CanMEDS Framework is not linked specifically to any job, title or position. **The Leader Role facilitates the expression of leadership no matter**

what title a physician may or may not hold. For example, leadership is more than being chief resident. Rather, leadership applies to the wide spectrum of clinical, academic, research and administrative functions that comprise a physician's everyday work.

A second misconception is that leaders always take charge. While it may be true that leaders do take charge when appropriate, it is also true that effective leaders know how to follow. Health care today requires leaders who ensure that the most capable and appropriate individual takes charge of a given situation in a given context. **Dynamic leaders know when and how to stand back, support and enable others to lead**, just as a dynamic follower knows how to share the leader's vision and contribute to its fruition.[21]

Another misconception is that there are no managerial competencies within the CanMEDS Leader Role. This is not the case. While there is increasing emphasis on leadership development, quality improvement, patient safety and resource stewardship within the Leader Role, **there is a very strong need for the teaching and assessment of the manager competencies such as the management of personal and professional practice.**

© 2015 Royal College of Physicians and Surgeons of Canada

Leader

3.2 Help learners build their leadership capabilities by embracing feedback

Prepare your learners to build their leadership capabilities by helping them to become more self-aware and to seek feedback.

Explain to them that self-awareness includes:

- in-the-moment awareness of personal emotional states, preferences, habits and biases;

- situational awareness of the learning and patient care environment you are in (including the perception of you by others); and

- deliberate attention to improving your behaviour and performance using feedback you have received from others.

Being self-aware is not an inherent trait, so it is important to teach your learners how to solicit feedback and how to learn from it. To help them along, share information on the science of emotional intelligence and alert them to the potential impact of self-awareness on a person's current ability and personal and professional satisfaction.[5] Learners also need to understand that in the absence of feedback and guidance, self-assessment has considerable limits.

No matter what your learners want to improve at, evidence suggests that they will get more out of it if they take charge of the learning opportunity. Recent research says that how we ask for, look for, receive, and integrate feedback may be as important as how it is given.[22] Guided self-assessment is most effective using established criteria or metrics and with feedback or information collected from others,[6] especially mentors. People who seek feedback, especially feedback that is corrective or instructive, are perceived to be more competent, settle into new responsibilities more quickly, and get better performance reviews.[23]

Encourage your learners to build and sustain a support team of people, in their personal and professional lives, who can provide affirmation, advice, and perspective to them.[24] This support team can also help them expand their perspective on the feedback they receive. To get the most from feedback, the receiver needs to see himself or herself as the key player in the feedback exchange. Since people tend to focus only on corrective components or to resist what they hear (and become defensive), you can help your learners listen for what they are doing well in addition to what they should change with the following tips (see Table L-2).

Finally, provide opportunities for your learners to safely become more self-aware and to seek and accept feedback. Residents are accomplished and high-achieving individuals who may have limited experience with failure, disappointment, and vulnerability. Some may be disinclined to speak openly about their limitations and biases. As such, you will need to provide opportunities for your learners to become more self-aware without feeling vulnerable by the feedback. Help them be open to the idea of errors as being 'opportunities' for learning and growth and to develop a willingness to seek and receive feedback.

You can help your learners see the value of self-awareness by breaking it down and making it real for them. Tell them how and where you continue to learn about your strengths and limitations, and how self-awareness assists you with your own problem solving.

Consider a combination of resources including:

- online or directed reading programs on topics such as leadership styles or emotional intelligence

- leadership training workshops or programs that focus on participant self-development

- learner retreats on topics like emotional intelligence, self-awareness etc.

- mentorship programs (formal and informal)

- small-group seminars or one-to-one coaching focused on leadership development and self-awareness

- development of learner and faculty skills on giving and receiving feedback.

3.3 Use coaching to help learners in leadership development

For learners who show a real interest and/or gap in their self-awareness, you may consider helping the learner connect with a coach who can help them do personalized development around self-awareness. Consider finding a coach to help your learners develop other leadership skills. A coach can work with them to identify areas of strength and weakness that they can build on and improve respectively.

Coaches are good observers who communicate well about what is working and what needs development. They draw out the knowledge and skill from their learners. They encourage and facilitate, provide excellent feedback, and enter into dialogue about performance. Coaches are best known in sports, music and dance where the learners use their help to improve skills that are used to perform.

© 2015 Royal College of Physicians and Surgeons of Canada

Leader

TABLE L-2. TIPS TO HELP LEARNERS PRACTICE ASKING FOR FEEDBACK[23, b]

1. **Ask someone who is willing and constructive.**

   - Be sure to ask them whether they have *time and interest* to provide feedback.

   - *Ask someone who has perspective.* Ask someone who sees you work. Even if you like someone and they like you, if they don't see you work, then they cannot help you improve. Ask a peer when you need peer feedback ("What more can I do to better organize our study group's sessions?"), and a supervisor when you need a supervisor's feedback ("How could I have improved the flow of this patient from the emergency to the inpatient unit?").

   - *Ask someone who is known to be direct* (or you might even consider asking someone with whom you have differences of opinion). You want feedback that is instructive and constructive. Ask this person to tell you one thing you are doing that is either helping or getting in the way of the performance you are interested in.

2. **Ask for specific feedback.**

   - *Avoid phrases like* "Do you have any feedback for me?" This question is too general for the assessor to formulate an actionable answer, and you leave yourself open to feedback that is not useful.

   - *Use prompts like*, "What is one thing you see me doing — or failing to do — that is getting in the way of my being more efficient at leading ward rounds?" This question directs the focus, asks for specific and constructive feedback, and gives the feedback provider permission to be honest.

3. **Listen and focus on what is helpful and specific.**

   - *Pay attention and avoid interrupting*, even if you feel defensive.

   - *Focus on feedback that is given in a helpful way.* If feedback does not make sense to you or is contrary to previous feedback in the same setting, then seek additional external perspectives and discuss further.

   - *Focus on what is helpful* in the feedback (i.e. behaviours to continue and behaviours to change).

4. **Thank your feedback providers for their input/help.**

   Remember: Those who get curious and ask for feedback can really accelerate their own learning

Performing as an effective leader involves development and integration of a complex group of skills that takes time to develop and is even more challenging to improve on your own — factors that make coaching an important consideration. Leaders who receive coaching report better skills and better outcomes.[25] Coaches are now becoming more common in leadership development where they may act as consultants to those who want to develop their leadership skills. The process is not yet common in medicine but is emerging.

3.4 Prepare your learners to be comfortable with ambiguity and uncertainty

Leaders work in complex, dynamic systems. They make decisions on incomplete and vague information. They have to seek out and assimilate relevant information before making judgments. Approaches to complex situations are similar in clinical and non-clinical decision-making. Your learners need to become competent and comfortable at addressing challenges without having 'all' of the evidence or information. Prepare your learners to accept ambiguity and uncertainty as part of everyday work and when and how to make decisions with 'enough' evidence or information.

- Teach them to avoid the indiscriminate application of evidence when they are faced with complex challenges. In the practice of medicine, evidence needs to be situated in the context and applied thoughtfully: "The practice of evidence-based medicine means integrating individual clinical expertise with the best available external clinical evidence from systematic research. By individual clinical expertise, we mean the proficiency and judgment that individual clinicians acquire through clinical experience and clinical practice.[26]"

b This chart is based on material in Stone D, Heen S. Thanks for the feedback: the science and art of receiving feedback well. New York: Penguin; 2014. Used with permission.

© 2015 Royal College of Physicians and Surgeons of Canada

Leader

- When making decisions, your learners will also need to weigh evidence with context, risks, benefits, resource availability and alignment with goals and objectives. Decision-making heuristics may be helpful techniques.[27, 28]

- Help your learners to organize what information they need to make decisions and to determine whether the information is easily available, obtainable and reliable. Use examples from your own practice to show how you find the facts you need, avoid information that you don't need and how you cope with uncertainty and the stress of decision-making — whether or not the decision works out well.

Learners need to be taught to seek instructive examples of both good and poor outcomes and to analyze how the decisions were made with the information that was available before the decision was made.[29] Your learners can become more skilful at applying evidence by asking those with more experience why certain choices were made when there was no obvious course of action. You can help provide examples by pointing out the leadership choices you make, both clinical and non-clinical, in your everyday practice.

3.5 Prepare your learners to analyze the quality of care delivery in their practice

Effective leaders get the right things done in the right way. To be more effective as leaders, your learners will benefit from employing a quality improvement framework to reflect on the quality of care delivery in their practice, such as the six domains of health care quality[11]. This framework can help you and your learners to brainstorm quality problems and discuss potential solutions using a quality lens. With such a framework, your learners can ask questions related to day-to-day practice (e.g. clinic running behind, test done in hospital that was not followed up, patient materials only in English when some patients do not understand English, hospital readmission). They can also use the framework to analyze their own 'practice'. Although examples can be found in all clinical settings, horizontal or longitudinal clinical experiences allow residents to reflect on quality problems over a longer period of time (e.g. flu shot completion rates, mammogram referrals, medication complications, infection rates). You can also think about using data that is available (e.g. public report cards, institutional performance measures, self audit). You and your residents can use this available data to analyze and discuss opportunities for improvement.

3.6 Prepare your learners to analyze the effectiveness of their leadership

Residents often undertake to 'practise' their leadership skills through activities that require complex leadership skills, such as introducing a new curriculum, planning a resident retreat or re-organizing resident responsibilities. Your residents will benefit from employing a structured process to guide their leadership activities. Using these structured processes can also be used to analyze your own techniques or skills as well as your leadership outcomes. Table L-3 shows how a structured process can be applied to a resident-led clinic, an example that is likely to resonate with your learners.[30]

3.7 Help your learners practise stewardship as it relates to your specialty, team, organization and system: Celebrate restraint[31]

Provide your learners with the information and decision-making criteria for how stewardship is practised in your specialty, team, organization, and/or system. Underscore that stewardship is about providing more value to health care delivery and not just about saving costs. Potential strategies to introduce these concepts include:

- In everyday patient case reports or discussions of treatment plans, help your learners understand the stewardship issues and options, including how and when different decisions were made based on individual patient needs, preferences, and values of the patient and organization.

- Look at guidelines to determine the appropriate use of testing.

- Consider "celebrating restraint"[31] by challenging learners to carefully consider why they are ordering tests. A useful question to ask learners is: "How will the result of this test influence our overall management plan?" If the test result has no bearing on the overall treatment plan, then it is likely of minimal benefit and should not be ordered.

- Positively reinforce learners' behaviours when they appropriately choose to order or to refrain from ordering tests. Learners sometimes order more tests to demonstrate their knowledge, and faculty need to make sure that learners know it's okay not to order tests if they are not warranted.

Choosing Wisely Canada[4] offers general information for physicians and patients to help them "engage in conversations about unnecessary tests, treatments, and procedures, and to help physicians and patients make smart and effective choices to ensure high-quality care."

© 2015 Royal College of Physicians and Surgeons of Canada

TABLE L-3. PROCESS FOR EFFECTIVE LEADERSHIP

Key steps[32]	Description	Purpose	EXAMPLE of leadership process steps: **Starting a resident-led clinic**
1. Ask what needs to be done	Gather information to decide on the vision, mission, reason for action	Gathering info	• Ground your idea in a strong need, not on what you want to do • Seek input from everybody — residents, nurses, hospital personnel, patients, chief of service, program director etc. • Clarify what needs to be done • State a rationale that everyone can stand behind
2. Ask what's right for the patient(s) and the organization	What will you be trying to achieve for the main benefactor?		• Describe how this will benefit your patients first, and how that will impact resident training, faculty supervision, a unit or hospital
3. Develop action plans	Organize all the big parts of your activity in sequence, with deadlines	Moving from information to action	• Break the project into parts by size, place, protocols, educational benefit etc. • Identify what you can and will do • Indicate who does what and specific timelines for action, or next steps
4. Take responsibility for decisions	Decide who makes decisions for the different parts and how decisions get made		• Identify who makes decisions (resource sharing, assessing learners, monitoring outcomes) on what criteria, shared with whom
5. Take responsibility for communications	Ensure bilateral communication exists between all interacting parties		• Identify what parts of the project need bilateral communication and how it is organized and monitored
6. Focus on opportunities rather than problems	Find new ways to solve problems		• For a new clinic being run in a new way, ask what good existing concepts can be borrowed and what new ways of doing things are necessary to deliver the outcome needed
7. Lead productive meetings	Ensure all meetings have stated purpose and assigned follow up tasks		• Identify how you can organize meetings and communication to maximize attendees' time and skill • Act on decisions made
8. Think and say "we" rather than "I"	Own responsibility, expect cooperation, share credit	Creating shared responsibility and accountability	• Create a collaborative culture • Accept and acknowledge your limits, failures and shortcomings • Celebrate and credit good outcomes to your team

Leader

3.8 Help your residents know how work is "usually" managed

As residents are paid for work, their role in managing within the health system is different than that of a medical student. Your residents will be better managers if they understand how they can satisfy these increased expectations and responsibilities. Help them to make the transition from working solo as a student to working as a health care professional within a team with multiple responsibilities.

A flow chart and high-level "job" description can be key tools to help your residents understand "standard" expectations of them, including what they need to do and when. Other documents that can clarify variations in expectations (e.g. for different levels of residents, for residents on different services, on-call expectations, expectations around exam times) will be helpful. If there are highly specific "rules" for specific locations, rotations, sites, or faculty members regarding organization of work tasks or patient flow, make those expectations known, so that such information is not hidden or available only through trial and error or by being "in the know."

Your learners can also make their own resources as they navigate new environments and become competent at functioning as working learners. Mnemonics, "cheat sheets" and to-do lists are useful to support learners' everyday decisions as they practise becoming good managers in their new, complex clinical settings.

Evaluate what aspects of management are key to your learners' managerial skills, especially as they transition from junior to senior learners. If you view scheduling rotations as a valuable activity for your learners because it requires leadership and negotiation with many people, consider what is needed to develop the necessary leadership and negotiation skills. If there are other ways to deliver on tasks that are highly administrative, they should consider who else might do it or how else that task can be done.

3.9 Help your learners work effectively by delegating to others

Learners need to understand that the goal is getting the work done, not doing all of the work themselves. Encourage your learners to perceive delegation as a skill that requires practice.

Effective delegation is essential to successful leadership and efficient management. Share the following steps with your learners:

- Organize so that you have a complete understanding of what needs to be done by what deadline.
- Identify the priority tasks.
- Establish the steps that are key to achieving the desired outcomes on time.

- Take time to inventory available resources and the competencies that reside in your collaborators (team).
- Assign people the authority and responsibility for important activities. Make assignments on the basis of (a) how well the person's competencies and strengths fit with the activity and/or (b) what activities the person needs to get more skilled at or what skills the person needs to develop.
- Monitor, communicate with, clarify expectations with, and support those to whom you delegate.
- Deploy or redeploy people to new, emerging, or challenging assignments to ensure that all elements needed for success are covered.

3.10 Encourage your learners to manage themselves

Self-management is a skill of leadership and one that needs to be learned, often with guidance from others. Teach your learners not only that they need to manage themselves (and to seek assistance in learning how) but also that struggling is not a badge of honour. Help your learners become better self-managers by teaching them organization and time management skills and offering them tools to do so. Help them see the value of being mindful and deliberate about managing their own busy schedules. Remind your learners that there is no magic solution that will work for everybody.

3.11 Help learners improve patient safety in daily practice including after critical incidents[13]

Patient safety is both a process and an outcome that needs to be integrated into daily practice. As a process, patient safety means promoting the welfare of your patients by pursuing the reduction and mitigation of unsafe acts within the health care system. As an outcome, patient safety means freedom from harm related to health care.

You can help your learners develop their capacity to anticipate and prevent incidents related to patient safety by encouraging mental rehearsal of how they would respond to a "what if" situation and by sharing real incidents and near misses. Your learners need to have an accurate picture of the threats and hazards to patient safety for their program, system, and organization so that they can anticipate them, learn to set barriers to prevent or mitigate patient safety incidents, learn to monitor for and respond to them when they occur, recover back to baseline smoothly and effectively, and reflect on the experience. Leadership from your learners, faculty, and team members is required at every step.

© 2015 Royal College of Physicians and Surgeons of Canada

HINTS TO EFFECTIVELY MANAGE YOUR TIME IN RESIDENCY:[33]

1. Training is a phase of your career when *you* **must learn to manage your time**. It is not the responsibility of others to manage your time. If others have assisted you in the past, medical school or residency is a good time for you to take control of managing your time.

2. **Keep a calendar.** It doesn't really matter whether it's paper or electronic; just make sure everything is in it. Pick a system to establish categories that you like (some people like colour coding; others detest it) and that you will keep up to date with ease and efficiency. If you like paper and highlighter and you find you can keep on time and organized with this system, stay with it.

3. **Keep notes.** Write down what you're going to do and when you'll do it. Follow the instructions on the notes, especially when you are tired or feeling overwhelmed. Think about tomorrow today.

4. (Re)-organize your tomorrows based on your yesterdays and todays. **Find or create wiggle room** in your calendar because something else will always come up. Looking ahead will reduce potential stress if and when detours arrive.

5. Develop, refresh, or revisit a **system to organize** yourself. Steven Covey[34] has a very good system that focuses on "first things first" and helps sort out the urgent from the important. There are other good systems. Choose a system and follow it.

6. Remember that **"no" is a complete sentence**. It should not be your first answer in all or even most circumstances, but the time will come when you have to learn (or relearn) how to say no because all of your time is spoken for. Keeping track of your schedule will allow you to know when you can say "no" with conviction.

7. **Avoid time-wasting activities**, but do not confuse time wasters with refreshing activities that feed your body, mind, heart, and soul. Sometimes planned time wasters can serve as rewards for staying on task.

8. You will never feel like you have enough time to **see your family and friends, exercise, relax, or do other important activities** like completing your taxes, seeing your family doctor, or going to the dentist. Schedule important, regular, predictable events like these and keep your scheduled appointments and commitments.

9. Studying is hard work. It takes "bum-in-chair time" when you are rested, focused, and productive. **Study smarter (when rested), not longer.**[35]

10. Multi-tasking interrupts the flow of good thinking, studying, and clinical practice. The literature tells us we are best when we **focus on one thing at a time**, regardless of which generation we were born in. Use social media in the service of making important decisions, learning, developing your professional network, engaging in a community-of-practice or doing high quality work[36, 37] instead of in a trivial capacity.

11. **Sleep, eat, and exercise.** These three ingredients will help you to manage yourself and will help you keep your sense of humour when things do not go as you wish or as you have planned.

Inventory the organization's resources for patient safety skills development and quality improvement skills development. Make a point to access your organization's information and/or people resources, which can make your preparation easier and ensure you are teaching the 'right stuff' that residents need to do for that workplace.

Specifically review and rehearse the key actions to follow when patient safety incidents occur:[13]

1. Meet the immediate and ongoing care needs of the patient (ensure the patient is clinically stable, correct the safety issue(s), limit further harm, and provide ongoing monitoring and care).

2. Explain to the patient what unexpected event or change happened; discuss the facts of the case and avoid speculation if details are not known.

3. Apologize that it happened.

4. Explain what will happen next, including explicitly discussing what will be done to avoid the incident recurring with future patients.

Your learners should know to contact their supervisor(s) and team members and report the incident using the appropriate mechanism to make sure that the proper process ensues when patient safety incidents occur. In addition, learners should know who or what resources to draw on.

You and your faculty sharing past experiences about past patient safety incidents can be beneficial to learners. In sharing, be sure to include how you coped with the emotional impact, and alert learners to where and how to get help for themselves. It is important to remind everyone to watch out for the effects of incidents on more junior learners, peers and other colleagues and to ensure that support is accessed when needed.

3.12 Help learners plan for the unexpected

Help your residents plan for the unexpected through rehearsal, review of past incidents, and knowledge of 'after care'. Teach your learners what the immediate response needs to be when things do not go as the team or their patients expected. The situation can take many different forms; for example, an unanticipated change in the patient's condition, a complication, an error, an oversight, a needle stick, a patient safety incident, a diagnosis of highly contagious infection or a case of "we just do not know right now."

3.13 Work with learners to rehearse apologies

Apologies take courage and some people struggle to be courageous in this way. People are often reluctant to apologize for a number of reasons, including feeling embarrassed or vulnerable, or thinking that apologies or explanations are just never made.

Often, the process of apologizing to patients and families needs to be carried out by the most responsible physician. However, taking responsibility for this process provides you with an opportunity to role model leadership for your learners as they accompany you. Set up the process and follow some simple guidelines for apologizing that will respect patients and their families. No matter how difficult it is to do, learners need to learn how to apologize effectively.

3.14 Help learners practise "systems thinking" and watch for needed improvements to health care delivery in teams, organizations and systems

You can talk about some of the situations where your patients have been victims of poorly designed systems or processes of care to explore "systems" thinking in more detail. Common examples of these situations include preventable readmissions and in-hospital complications such as delirium, falls, medication errors, failure of test follow-up, etc. These situations allow you and your learners to do an incident analysis to explore the individual factors (e.g. stress, fatigue) and system factors (e.g. interruptions, information technology problems, lack of care coordination) that contributed, using either the 5 Whys or Cause and Effect analysis to identify the following:

- What happened?
- How and *why* did it happen? In other words, what individual and system factors contributed to the incident?
- What can be done to reduce the likelihood of recurrence and make care safer?
- What was learned?

Your learners may notice differences in how departments adhere to an established patient care protocol, which may have implications for patient safety. Help your learners know that as leaders, they should not disregard their observations or assume that others have also noticed these situations. Teach them to speak up appropriately and work collaboratively to find ways to contribute to ongoing improvements.

Remember to orient your learners to improvements implemented in your program or organization over the past decade with the intention of improving reliability and safety. Examples may include operating room checklists, handover protocols, admission or discharge order processes, computerized provider order entry systems, and structured communication tools. Such everyday, practice-based solutions can have far-reaching benefits for patients, physicians, and health care systems.

4. Hints, tips and tools for *teaching* the Leader Role

As a teacher your goal is to deliver the right content and in a way that helps your residents learn. Sometimes you will teach directly. Other times you will facilitate and support the teaching of others. There are parts of the Leader Role that can be especially difficult for learners to relate to and understand in the context of their work. For this reason this section of the Tools Guide includes a short menu of tips and tricks that are highly effective for teaching the Leader Role. You can treat the list as a buffet: pick and choose the tips that resonate most and that will work for you, your program and your learners.

© 2015 Royal College of Physicians and Surgeons of Canada

WHY APOLOGIES ARE DIFFICULT

- Apologies take courage. Admitting that you were wrong puts you in a vulnerable position, which can open you up to attack or blame. Some people struggle to be courageous in this way.

- You may feel embarrassed or ashamed of your actions and you are struggling to face the other person.

- You may be following the advice "never apologize, never explain." Generally this is viewed as arrogant and as ineffective or unwise for leaders.

- Even if apologizing is difficult, you need to learn how to apologize effectively.

THREE RULES OF APOLOGIES[38, 13, c]

1. Be honest. To be effective, apologies need to be authentic.

2. Do not just explain. An explanation is not an apology and does not replace an apology. Sometimes an explanation is respectful after an apology. Use your judgment (e.g. provide explanation if they ask for it).

3. Do not use the word "but" while making an apology.

FOUR STEPS TO AN EFFECTIVE APOLOGY

1. **Express remorse** by saying, "I am sorry" or "I apologize." "I am sorry that your test was cancelled after you had completed your prep." Be sincere and authentic.

Timeliness is important. Apologize as soon as you are able.

2. **Take responsibility** for your actions or behaviour and acknowledge what you did. Empathize with the person wronged. "I am sure you are concerned—and I am too — about the risks with the medication you received in error. I checked and found out that the implications of you getting X in error are A, B, and C." If it was an error of omission, you could say: "the implications of you not getting the planned Y are L, M, and N."

3. **Make amends** for your actions to make the situation right. "I would like to offer you an opportunity to meet with the pharmacist or my supervisor to discuss the error" or "Is there someone you would like to speak to about this?" If unsure about this step, discuss with your faculty or senior resident. This needs to be appropriate and within your authority (i.e. you cannot promise more than you have authority for). Perhaps you need to say what the next steps are if you don't know the solutions. For example, "I am going to report this to my supervisor and the pharmacist and get their advice on future medication error prevention strategies."

4. **Rebuild trust.** Repair the relationship. "From now on, I will do Z to make sure that this does not happen to other patients in the future." Following up as indicated is important to rebuilding trust.

Leader

Teaching Tip 1.
Concentrate on specific Leader Role competencies that you will teach in your practice

Knowledge of terminology, models, and frameworks is essential when you are teaching the Leader Role (e.g. leadership styles, the management and delegating of patient priorities in clinical settings, techniques for leading a team, responses to patient safety incidents). Some of this may be new to you and your colleagues, as it may have never explicitly been taught to you. Acquaint yourself with the knowledge base and develop the capacity to discuss the Leader Role competencies with your learners by accessing faculty development resources (See key resources in sections six and seven of this chapter).

Teaching Tip 2.
Enable your learners to rehearse leadership skills in the workplace through practice opportunities and case discussions

Learners need plenty of opportunities for mental rehearsal of the issues and processes that physicians address as leaders in day-to-day practice. Leadership is ideally practised in the workplace.

As you navigate issues and problems, be explicit with your learners about your problem-solving process, clarifying the tensions and options deliberated and the rationale for the choices you make. There is also value in sharing the limits of and conditions for making similar choices (or not) when the same or different issues and problems recur in new situations.

c © Mind Tools Ltd, 1996-2015. All rights reserved. "Mind Tools" is a registered trademark of Mind Tools Ltd. Mind Tools. How to apologize: asking for forgiveness gracefully. www.mind-tools.com/pages.article/how-to-apologize.htm. Reproduced with permission.

Be explicit in your discussions. For example, during your workday, make learners aware of how you are exercising different competencies in the Leader Role (e.g. discussing with the charge nurse how to change practice to prevent drains and tubes being pulled by accident; re-organizing your schedule to make room for a meeting; contrasting how management of one situation may differ from another due to specific factors like resource availability; reflecting on a discussion with a colleague and how you were able to prevent a potential patient safety incident).

Teaching Tip 3.
Work with faculty, other team members and program training sites to promote a safety culture

You and your faculty enable a safety culture through

- the demonstration of honesty and transparency in everyday interactions,

- flatten or minimize hierarchy when appropriate, and

- by encouraging your learners to speak up when they are uncertain or concerned.

One of your goals as a teacher is to role model safe practice and to identify it for your learners so that they learn to recognize it in their daily experiences. Take the time to discuss what prompted your attention to safety in a particular situation, what factors you considered when making a decision and what skills you used to ensure patient safety.

Within the context of a safety culture, learners need to feel that it is safe to 'speak up' when they identify patient safety hazards. They can often feel anxious about the repercussions of flagging a safety hazard. Part of your role then, would be to encourage your learners to communicate their concerns and to support those who do speak up. Learners will take cues from you and your colleagues so it is important to make the environment one that values safety.[39]

Teaching Tip 4.
Provide explicit teaching on managing one's career and self

Managing one's career and self is hard work. It doesn't come naturally to everyone and there are factors, many of which are beyond your learners' control, which will make self-management extremely challenging. For this reason, you may want to bring in faculty guests to talk to your learners about self-management. Include people who are good at managing their careers and themselves, as well as people who struggle with it, but still manage to make it work. Ideally, the guests should be peers of your learners and they should be authentic about the tips and tricks that they use to manage themselves

Provide examples of people working in a variety of settings who demonstrate a variety of effective leadership approaches. Suggest physicians consider health providers who can serve as role models in such areas as clinical care management, practice management, and team leadership.

Sample teaching tools

You can use the sample **Teaching Tools for Leader** in this chapter as is, or you can modify or use them in various combinations to suit your objectives, time allocated, sequence within your residency program, and so on.

Easy-to-customize electronic versions of the **Teaching Tools for Leader** (in .doc, .ppt and .pdf formats) are found at: canmeds.royalcollege.ca

The tools provided are:

- T1 Lecture or Large Group Presentation: Foundations of the Leader Role

- T2 Presentation: Teaching the Leader Role

- T3 Small Group Teaching: Leading and managing in everyday practice

- T4 Coaching: Exploring and developing self-awareness

- T5 Case Report: Leader Role competencies

- T6 Morbidity and Mortality Rounds: Patient safety and quality improvement

- T7 Self-Directed Learning: Time management assignment – Where does the time go?

- T8 Tools and strategies: Summary sheet for the Leader Role

5. Hints, tips and tools for *assessing* the Leader Role

Assessment for learning is a major theme in this CanMEDS Tools Guide and a growing emphasis in medical education. You can and should use assessment as a strategy to inform a resident's learning plan (i.e. to alert or signpost to learners what is important to learn as well as what and how they will be assessed). This section offers a number of hints to help you develop a program of assessment that will ensure that both teachers and learners have a clear understanding of expectations, level of their performance and what needs improvement.

© 2015 Royal College of Physicians and Surgeons of Canada

Assessment Tip 1.
Assess your learners' leadership skills in 'real time' in the clinical setting

The CanMEDS Leader competencies are part of everyday practice. It is important to assess your learners early and throughout residency on such leadership competencies as their stewardship of health care resources (i.e. appropriate ordering of diagnostic tests), attentiveness to patient safety (i.e. responding to patient safety incidents), contributions to quality improvement (i.e. identifying and measuring problems of quality in their practice), leadership skills (i.e. asking for feedback to improve performance), team management (i.e. priority setting of clinical activities), management of people (i.e. delegation and supervision of others' work), and personal and career management (e.g. time management, vacation planning, electives planning).

Collect input and feedback from your learners' patients/ caregivers, peers, more junior learners, supervising residents, chief residents, faculty, or other health professional colleagues using multisource feedback (MSF) forms and session encounter forms or by asking for input for the interim or end-of-session in-training evaluation (ITER) form.

By asking questions during case reports or chart audits, you can assess stewardship in real time and gauge how your learners utilize human or health care resources (e.g. delegation and supervision of others, test ordering, medication prescribing).

Assessment Tip 2.
Include Leader Role process and content questions in case presentations, case reports, and rounds

In day-to-day cases, ask specific questions to gauge your learners' development as leaders:

- How did you think through which diagnostic tests/ interventions would make the most sense in this case? What did you consider and discard — why did you discard that option? What did you struggle with? (Assesses attention to stewardship and self-assessment)

- How did you respond when there was a patient safety incident? What was the type of patient incident? (Assesses patient safety and safety culture)

- What individual or system factors contributed to this patient safety incident? What feedback did you receive about your role as team leader today? (Assessing systems of care)

- As team leader, what went well today during rounds? Give me some ideas of what you could do differently next time. (Assesses leadership process)

- How might you introduce changes to your personal/ group's practice or to local processes of care to improve quality of care? For example, how could this patient's flow through the system be improved? (Assesses practice management and quality improvement)

- How did you sort out the patient care and team priorities for today? Did the sequence you planned work? What took longer than you expected? (Assesses priority setting of workplace activities and time management)

- How is your team functioning? Are there any differences or conflicts that you need to manage? How are you monitoring and supporting your team? What feedback did you give to or seek from your team today? (Assesses management of people)

- How did you sort out who would do what? How did you monitor and support their performance? Did you have to adjust any work? What time did everybody, including you, leave work? (Assesses delegation of work)

Assessment Tip 3.
Assess the Leader Role using a variety of formats

Use assessments to support the learning of Leader Role competencies. Your residents need to be able to use the language and models of leadership so they can interact effectively with the health care system and other colleagues in the health professions.

You can assess whether your learners know, can apply and communicate using leadership, management, quality improvement, stewardship, and patient safety 'language' in their everyday leadership and management of the health system. Assessing their understanding and use can be done using a variety of assessment tools such as case reports, reflection reports and multisource feedback assessments.

Leader

Sample assessment tools

You can use the sample *Assessment Tools for Leader* at the end of this chapter as is, or you can modify or use them in various combinations to suit your objectives, time allocated, sequence within your residency program, and so on. Easy-to-customize electronic versions of the *Assessment Tools for Leader* (in .doc, .ppt and .pdf formats) are found at: canmeds.royalcollege.ca

The tools provided are:

- A1 Multisource Feedback: Leadership skills in the CanMEDS Leader Role

- A2 Multisource Feedback: Managing people and resources in the CanMEDS Leader Role

- A3 Quality Improvement Project: Leader Role quality improvement project

- A4 Case Report: Leadership reflection

6. Suggested resources

LEADERSHIP

- **Canadian Medical Association–Physician Management Institute (PMI) Physician Leadership Courses.** Designed for physicians, these leadership courses are delivered in a variety of formats (i.e. face to face, in-house delivery or online). For more information see http://www. cma.ca/En/Pages/physician-leadership-institute.aspx (last retrieved July 2, 2015)

- **LEADS framework.** This is one of many leadership frameworks. It outlines key skills, abilities, and knowledge required to lead at all levels of an organization. This framework has been used in many parts of Canada's health sector as well as in other organizations. It aligns and consolidates the competency frameworks and leadership strategies. For more information see http://www. leadersforlife.ca/site/framework?nav=02 (last retrieved July 2, 2015)

- **Drucker PF, Goleman D, George WW.** *HBR's 10 Must Reads on Leadership.* **Boston: Harvard Business Review; 2011.** HBR articles on leadership are known for their deep and gripping messages about leadership. While the examples are not directly related to medical practice, they are very useful as guides and not recipes. These 10 easy-to-read articles look at different aspects of leadership that should resonate with all physicians whether or not they hold titled leadership positions.

TIME MANAGEMENT

- **Patel H, Puddester D.** *The time management guide: A practical handbook for physicians by physicians.* **Ottawa: Royal College of Physicians and Surgeons of Canada, 2012.** Written for physicians by physicians, this practical handbook offers easy, practical tips to enhance your abilities to make better use of your time and work better and smarter. For more information or for a sample chapter, see: http://www.royalcollege.ca/portal/page/ portal/rc/canmeds/resources/publications

STEWARDSHIP

- **QCV 100: An Introduction to Quality, Cost, and Value in Health Care.** (http://app.ihi.org/lms/coursedetailview. aspx?CourseGUID=5b730190-b61d-43d2-a05e-0afa3 2fc4178&CatalogGUID=6cb1c614-884b-43ef-9abd-d90849f183d4&LessonGUID=a6ded6a8-7ec1-4984-be0d-b2dd8fa7dc4b)

- **Choosing Wisely Canada.** Five things physicians and patients should question. A series of lists developed by specialties identify which commonly used tests, treatments or procedures are not supported by evidence, and/or could expose patients to unnecessary harm. Last retrieved July 2, 2015 from: http://www.choosingwisely-canada.org/recommendations/

PATIENT SAFETY

- **CMPA Good Practices Guide**. These online resources are designed by Canadian Medical Protective Associations to help physicians provide safe care to patients and reduce medico-legal risk. The Guide includes separate sections for learners and teachers. https://www.cmpa-acpm.ca/ serve/docs/ela/goodpracticesguide/pages/index/index. html (last retrieved July 2, 2015)

- **Agency for Healthcare Research and Quality.** *Patient safety network.* **Last retrieved July 4, 2015** from: http:// psnet.ahrq.gov/ Vast collection of very good patient safety cases with accompanying commentaries, and sometimes even slide decks with presentations.

- **AHRQ Morbidity and Mortality rounds on the web** http://webmm.ahrq.gov Cases, with commentaries and PPT slide presentations all free to access and download.

Leader

© 2015 Royal College of Physicians and Surgeons of Canada

- **I-PASS Handover curriculum**. The I-PASS Handoff Bundle is an endeavour of the I-PASS Institute to improve patient safety by standardizing communication during transitions of patient care.Last retrieved July 5, 2015 from: http://www.ipasshandoffstudy.com/

QUALITY IMPROVEMENT

- **Royal College publication Teaching Quality Improvement in Medical Education.** This resource provides an innovative curriculum to teach quality improvement to residents. This electronic publication covers topics such as setting learning objectives, assessing competencies, and curriculum evaluation from fundamentals to advanced quality improvement.

- **Wong, RY. Teaching Quality Improvement in Medical Education.** Ottawa: Royal College of Physicians and Surgeons; 2015. ePub.

- **IHI Open School modules.** Includes resources and online courses for use in different hospital settings and types of patient care handoffs and transitions. Last retrieved July 5, 2015 from: http://www.ihi.org/education/IHIOpenSchool/Courses/Pages/default.aspx

- **Health Quality Ontario Improvement Guide**. These guides, from Health Quality Ontario (HQO), are available for open use with proper attribution given to the appropriate source (i.e. Health Quality Ontario (April 2013). For example, in this guide, QI refers to a QI team, working towards a defined aim, gathering and reviewing frequent measures and implementing change http://www.hqontario.ca/portals/0/Documents/qi/qi-quality-improve-guide-2012-en.pdf

PRACTICE MANAGMENT

- **Resident focused resources for personal and professional management and financial planning.** https://www.cma.ca/En/Pages/practice-management-curriculum.aspx

- **These online learning modules provide a comprehensive and timely overview of the personal and professional issues that residents need to address to make the most of their practice.** https://www.cma.ca/En/Pages/pmc-modules.aspx

7. Other resources

- Busari JO, Berkenbosch L, Brouns JW. Physicians as managers of health care delivery and the implications for postgraduate medical training: a literature review. *Teach Learn Med.* 2011; Apr. 23(2):186-96.

- Frich JC, Brewster AL, Cherlin EJ, Bradley EH. Leadership development programs for physicians: a systematic review. *J Gen Intern Med.* 2015;30(5);656-74.

- Agency for Healthcare Research and Quality. Patient safety network. Last retrieved July 4, 2015 from: http://psnet.ahrq.gov/

VIDEOS ON LEADERSHIP

- "How to start a movement." Derek Sivers discusses what leaders need. http://www.ted.com/talks/derek_sivers_how_to_start_a_movement

- "What it takes to be a great leader." Roselinde Torres discusses what comes from studying great leaders all over the world. https://www.ted.com/talks/roselinde_torrves_what_it_takes_to_be_a_great_leader

- "Ten leadership theories in 5 minutes." Professor Michael Zigarelli presents leadership theories. https://www.youtube.com/watch?v=XKUPDUDQBVo

- "Inno-Versity Presents: Greatness." David Marquet, a retired US navy captain, discusses how great leadership involves letting go a little. https://www.youtube.com/watch?v=psAXMqxwol8

- "Brian Goldman: Doctors make mistakes. Can we talk about that?" It is Brian Goldman, White Coat, Black Art broadcaster on making medical mistakes and the need for change in medical culture; a just, caring supportive culture. https://www.youtube.com/watch?v=iUbfRzxNy20&feature=youtube

Leader

8. LEADER ROLE DIRECTORY OF TEACHING AND ASSESSMENT TOOLS

You can use the sample *teaching and assessment tools for the Leader Role* found in this section as is, or you can modify or use them in various combinations to suit your objectives, the time allocated, the sequence within your residency program, and so on. Tools are listed by number (e.g. T1), type (e.g. Lecture), and title (e.g. Foundations of the Leader Role).

Easy-to-customize electronic versions of the sample *teaching and assessment tools for the Leader Role* in .doc, .ppt and .pdf formats are found at: canmeds.royalcollege.ca

TEACHING TOOLS

ASSESSMENT TOOLS

© 2015 Royal College of Physicians and Surgeons of Canada

T1. FOUNDATIONS OF THE LEADER ROLE

Created for the *CanMEDS Teaching and Assessment Tools Guide* by S Glover Takahashi. Reproduced with permission of the Royal College.

This learning activity includes:

- Presentation: Foundations of the Leader Role (T2)

Suggested teaching activities

- Guided Reflection: Leading and managing in day-to-day practice (T3)
- Coaching: Exploring and developing self-awareness (T4)

Instructions for Teacher:

Sample learning objectives:

- Recognize common words related to the process and content of leadership
- Apply key leadership skills to examples from day-to-day practice
- Develop a personal leadership resource for day-to-day practice

Audience: All learners

How to adapt:

- Consider whether your session's objectives match the sample ones. Select from, modify, or add to the sample objectives as required.
- The sample PowerPoint presentation and activities are generic and foundational and tied to simple objectives. Consider whether you'll need additional slides to meet your objectives. Modify, add or delete content as required. You may want to include specific information related to your discipline and context.
- Depending on whether you are using these materials in one session (i.e. Leadership Basics Workshop) or a series of two to four academic half days will determine which activities you select and in what sequence.
- You may wish to review and customize the Leader Role Summary Sheet with your learners as an additional activity.

Logistics:

- Select one or two activities for each teaching session.
- Plan for about 20 minutes for each group activity: this time will be used for you to explain the activity and for your learners to complete the activity individually, share their answers with their small group, discuss, prepare to report back to the whole group, and then deliver their small group's report to the whole group.
- Allow individuals to read the worksheet and spend about five minutes working on the answers on their own before starting to work in groups. This format allows each person to develop his or her own understanding of the topic.
- Depending on the group and time available, you may wish to assign one or more worksheets as homework to be completed before the session or as a follow-up assignment.

Setting:

- This information is best taught in a small group format (i.e. less than 30 learners) if possible. It can also be effectively done with a larger group if the room allows for learners to be at tables in groups of five or six. With larger groups, it is helpful to have additional teachers or facilitators available to answer questions arising from the worksheet activities.

Leader

© 2015 Royal College of Physicians and Surgeons of Canada

T2. TEACHING THE LEADER ROLE

Created for the *CanMEDS Teaching and Assessment Tools Guide* by S Glover Takahashi. Reproduced with permission of the Royal College.

Instructions for Teacher:

- Setting and audience: Faculty and all learners
- How to adapt:
  - Select only those slides that apply to your teaching
  - Slides can be modified to match the specialty or the learner's practice context
- Logistics: Equipment – laptop, projector, screen

Slide #	Words on slide	Notes to teachers
1.	**CanMEDS Leader Role**	• Add information about presenters • Modify title as necessary
2.	**Objectives and agenda** 1. Recognize the process and content of leadership 2. Apply key leadership skills to examples from everyday practice 3. Develop a personal leadership resource for everyday practice	Sample goals and objectives of the section — revise as required • Consider doing a warm-up activity before or after slide 2 • Review/revise goals and objectives • Insert agenda slide if desired
3.	**Why the Leader Role matters** 1. Physician leaders play an important part in health care 2. Collaborative leadership competencies help facilitate improvements 3. The health care system depends on physicians taking responsibility for stewardship of finite resources 4. Physicians must make personal management skills a priority to manage competing demands	Reasons why this role is important
4.	**The details: What is the Leader Role**[a] As Leaders, physicians engage with others to contribute to a vision of a high-quality health care system and take responsibility for the delivery of excellent patient care·through their activities as clinicians, administrators, scholars, or teachers.	Definition from the *CanMEDS 2015 Physician Competency Framework* • Avoid including competencies for learners • If you are giving this presentation to teachers or planners you may want to add the competencies slides (provided below)
5.	**About the Leader Role** • The Leader Role facilitates the expression of leadership no matter what title a physician may or may not hold. • Dynamic leaders know when and how to stand back, support and enable others to lead • Leader Role continues to include important manager competencies (i.e. management of personal and professional practice)	Clarifying the misconceptions about Leader
6.	**Key terms for Leader** • *Stewardship* • *Quality improvement* • *Patient safety*	Define key terms from the Leader Role section

---

a   Dath D, Chan M-K, Anderson G, Burke A, Razack S, Lieff S, Moineau G, Chiu A, Ellison P. Leader. In: Frank JR, Snell L, Sherbino J, editors. *CanMEDS 2015 Physician Competency Framework*. Ottawa: Royal College of Physicians and Surgeons of Canada; 2015. Reproduced with permission.

© 2015 Royal College of Physicians and Surgeons of Canada

Leader

T2. TEACHING THE LEADER ROLE (continued)

Slide #	Words on slide		Notes to teachers
7.	**Recognizing leader process: (The how)** • Culture • Changing • Transitioning • Continuously improving • Following • Managing • Implementing • Delegating • Strategizing, Monitoring	• Organizing • Prioritizing • Scheduling • Budgeting • Running a team, unit, department, service • Stewarding, Choosing wisely[b] • Utilizing technology	Trigger words relating to the process of leadership
8.	**Recognizing leader content: (The what)** • Culture • Patient safety • Incident • Quality improvement • Systems thinking • Priorities • Strategy • Effectiveness • Efficiency	• Patient flow • Resources (e.g. human, financial, equipment) • Time management • Workflow • Schedule • Human resources • Career planning • Integrity	Trigger words relating to the content of leadership
9.	**Leadership improves with feedback[c]** 1. Ask someone who is willing and can be constructive 2. Ask for SPECIFIC feedback 3. Listen and focus on what is helpful and specific (i.e. Don't interrupt. Watch for resistance and defensiveness) 4. Say thank you for the input		
10.	**Analyse quality in day-to-day practice[d]** six domains of health care quality: 1. Safe 2. Effective 3. Patient-centred 4. Timely 5. Efficient 6. Equitable		• Illustrate these quality domains in day-to-day practice • How does this impact residents in day-to-day practice?
11.	**Quality improvement framework[e]** 1. What are we trying to accomplish? 2. How will we know that a change is an improvement? 3. What changes can we make that will result in improvement?		
12.	**PDSA Plan-Do-Study-Act** • Used to test and implement changes in practice		

Leader

---

b http://www.choosingwiselycanada.org
c Stone D, Heen S. *Thanks for the Feedback: the science and art of receiving feedback well.* New York: Viking; 2014.
d *Six Domains of Health Care Quality.* Consumer Assessment of Healthcare Providers and Systems (CAHPS) website. Last retrieved July 3, 2015 from: https://cahps.ahrq.gov/consumer-reporting/talkingquality/create/sixdomains.html.
e Langley GL, Nolan KM, Nolan TW, Norman CL, Provost LP. *The Improvement Guide: A Practical Approach to Enhancing Organizational Performance* 2nd Ed. Jossey Bass, San Francisco 2009. See more at (last retrieved July 3, 2015): http://www.institute.nhs.uk/quality_and_service_improvement_tools/quality_and_service_improvement_tools/plan_do_study_act.html.

© 2015 Royal College of Physicians and Surgeons of Canada

T2. TEACHING THE LEADER ROLE (continued)

Slide #	Words on slide	Notes to teachers
13.	**Stewardship of resources** • Be aware of stewardship issues, options, decisions based on individual patient needs, preferences, and values of the patient and organization. • Use guidelines to inform appropriate use of testing and get info from Choosing Wisely Canada[b] • Consider "How will the result of this test influence our overall management plan?" If no bearing on the overall treatment plan, then it is likely of minimal benefit and should not be ordered	Give EXAMPLES of how to do this in day-to-day What are common issues for your patients' problems re: stewardship
14.	**Patient safety** • Models a safety culture including demonstrating a commitment to openness, honesty, fairness and accountability • Expect the unexpected. Anticipation and prevention of errors is important as is vigilance and readiness ***Patient safety incident*** is an event or circumstance that could have resulted, or did result, in unnecessary harm to a patient. Harm is due to the medical care provided, not the underlying medical illness. Three types of patient safety incidents are: 1. A harmful incident results in harm to the patient, 2. A no harm incident reaches a patient but does not result in any discernible harm, 3. A near miss does not reach the patient	
15.	**Key actions when patient safety incidents occur** • Meet the immediate and ongoing care needs of the patient (ensure the patient is clinically stable, correct the safety issue(s), limit further harm, and provide ongoing monitoring and care). • Explain to the patient what unexpected event or change happened including who, how, what and prevention • Apologize that it happened • Explain what will happen next, including actions to avoid recurrence	
16.	**Manage career planning, finances, and health human resources** • Set priorities and manage time to integrate practice and personal life • Be mindful and deliberate about managing busy schedules • Use tools to get/stay organized	
17.	**Share the work** through **effective delegation** • Organize to ensure a complete understanding of what needs to be done by what deadline • Identify the priority tasks incl timelines • Establish the steps and sequence key to achieving the desired outcomes on time • Inventory available resources incl team member competencies • Assign people the authority and responsibility for important activities. Assign based on: (a) match/fit of competencies and strengths to activity and/or (b) needs for skill development • Monitor, communicate with, clarify expectations with, and coach delegates • Deploy or redeploy people to new, emerging, or challenging assignments as they arise	

Leader

© 2015 Royal College of Physicians and Surgeons of Canada

T2. TEACHING THE LEADER ROLE (continued)

Slide #	Words on slide	Notes to teachers
OTHER SLIDES		
18.	**Leader key competencies**[a] Physicians are able to: 1. Contribute to the improvement of health care delivery in teams, organizations, and systems 2. Engage in the stewardship of health care resources 3. Demonstrate leadership in professional practice 4. Manage career planning, finances, and health human resources in a practice	• Key competencies from the *CanMEDS 2015 Physician Competency Framework* • Avoid including competencies for learners • You may wish to use this slide if you are giving the presentation to teachers or planners
19.	**Leader key competency**[a] Physicians are able to: 1. Contribute to the improvement of health care delivery in teams, organizations, and systems 1.1 Apply the science of quality improvement to contribute to improving systems of patient care 1.2 Contribute to a culture that promotes patient safety 1.3 Analyze patient safety incidents to enhance systems of care 1.4 Use health informatics to improve the quality of patient care and optimize patient safety	• From *CanMEDS 2015 Framework* • Use one slide for each key competency and associated enabling competencies
20.	**Leader key competency**[a] Physicians are able to: 2. Engage in the stewardship of health care resources 2.1 Allocate health care resources for optimal patient care 2.2 Apply evidence and management processes to achieve cost-appropriate care	• From *CanMEDS 2015 Framework* • Use one slide for each key competency and associated enabling competencies
21.	**Leader key competency**[a] Physicians are able to: 3. Demonstrate leadership in professional practice 3.1 Demonstrate leadership skills to enhance health care 3.2 Facilitate change in health care to enhance services and outcomes	• From *CanMEDS 2015 Framework* • Use one slide for each key competency and associated enabling competencies
22.	**Leader key competency**[a] Physicians are able to: 4. Manage career planning, finances, and health human resources in a practice 4.1 Set priorities and manage time to integrate practice and personal life 4.2 Manage a career and a practice 4.3 Implement processes to ensure personal practice improvement	• From *CanMEDS 2015 Framework* • Use one slide for each key competency and associated enabling competencies
23.	**Effective leaders: Have courage and take responsibility for errors**[f] Three Rules of apologies: 1. Be honest and authentic 2. Do not explain 3. Do not use the word "but" Steps to an effective apology: 1. Express remorse: "I am sorry." 2. Take responsibility for actions or behaviour. 3. Make amends for your actions to make the situation right where appropriate and within your authority. 4. Rebuild trust. Repair the relationship.[f]	

f   © Mind Tools Ltd, 1996-2015. All rights reserved. "Mind Tools" is a registered trademark of Mind Tools Ltd. Mind Tools. How to apologize: asking for forgiveness gracefully. www.mind-tools.com/pages.article/how-to-apologize.htm. Reproduced with permission.

T3. LEADING AND MANAGING IN EVERYDAY PRACTICE

Created for the *CanMEDS Teaching and Assessment Tools Guide* by S Glover Takahashi, B Wong, M-K Chan, D Dath. Reproduced with permission of the Royal College.

See Leader Role teacher tips appendix for this teaching tool

Completed by: _____

INSTRUCTIONS FOR LEARNER

Draw from *your clinical practice over the past four weeks* to answer the following questions. Be sure to use specific details.

1. Describe a situation where you were a leader and you were pleased with the process and outcomes. Include details about clinical location/setting (patient types, type of service, your role in this location and situation). What, if any impact did the location/setting and your role in that location have on the outcomes?

   _____

   _____

   _____

2. Describe a situation where you were a leader and you were NOT pleased with the process and outcomes. Include details about clinical location (patient types, type of service, your role in this location and situation). What, if any impact did the location and your role in that location have on the outcomes?

   _____

   _____

   _____

3. Based on ONE of the situations from above answer the following questions.

   3a. What aspects of leadership (e.g. goal setting, accepting responsibility, delegation) did you do well in that situation?

   _____

   _____

   _____

   3b. What could you have done differently to achieve better outcome(s)?

   _____

   _____

   _____

Leader

© 2015 Royal College of Physicians and Surgeons of Canada

T3. LEADING AND MANAGING IN EVERYDAY PRACTICE (continued)

4. Review the tables below. Select and complete the tables below that apply to this situation

☐ **Leadership process applies to this situation**

☐ **Leadership process does not apply to this situation**

☐ Done

☐ Not done

☐ N/A

Leadership process IN THIS SITUATION	Rating			Comments	Areas or ideas for improvement?
	Done	Not done	Not applicable		
I asked what needed to be done					
I explicitly determined what was right for the patient(s), problem, organization etc.					
I developed and documented action plans					
I took responsibility for decisions					
I took responsibility for effective communications					
I found solutions and focused on opportunities rather than problems					
I lead productive meetings					
I demonstrated teamwork by thinking and saying "we" rather than "I"					

Other notes/reflections:

Leader

T3. LEADING AND MANAGING IN EVERYDAY PRACTICE (continued)

☐ **Managing people and resources applies to this situation**

☐ **Managing people and resources does not apply to this situation**

Managing people and resources IN THIS SITUATION	Rating			Comments	Areas or ideas for improvement?
	Done	Not done	Not applicable		
I ensured understanding of work and timelines					
I identified the priority tasks and timelines					
I established steps and sequence to deliver outcomes on time					
I shared the work through effective delegation					
I assigned people important activities					
I assigned tasks based on match/fit of competencies and strength					
I assigned tasks based on learning needs					
I monitored people's progress					
I communicated and clarified with people					
I supported peoples' progress and success					
I flexibly modified plans with new, emerging situations					
I deployed or redeployed people with new, emerging situations					
I integrated personal and professional priorities					
I used tools and resources effectively to achieve outcomes					

Other notes/reflections:

Leader

© 2015 Royal College of Physicians and Surgeons of Canada

T3. LEADING AND MANAGING IN EVERYDAY PRACTICE (continued)

☐ Stewardship process applies to this situation

☐ Stewardship process does not apply to this situation

Stewardship IN THIS SITUATION	Rating			Comments	Areas or ideas for improvement?
	Done	Not done	Not applicable		
I demonstrated careful consideration of the appropriate use of finite health care resources					
I demonstrated consideration of benefits and costs to the individual and the system					
I engaged patients in making informed decisions that reflect appropriate use of tests and treatments					
I applied evidence and processes to achieve high value care					
I supported others to make decisions that promote the appropriate use of finite health care resources					

Other notes/reflections:

Leader

T3. LEADING AND MANAGING IN EVERYDAY PRACTICE (continued)

☐ **Quality improvement applies to this situation**

☐ **Quality improvement does not apply to this situation**

Quality improvement IN THIS SITUATION	Rating			Comments	Areas or ideas for improvement?
	Done	Not done	Not applicable		
I identified an aspect of my practice or care setting that needed improvement, described as one or more of the six domains of quality (i.e. Safe, Effective, Patient-centred, Timely, Efficient, Equitable)					
I clarified what needed to be accomplished from an improvement standpoint					
I reviewed quality improvement measures (i.e. outcome, process, balancing measures) that help to determine 1) the extent of the quality problem; or 2) whether a change resulted in an improvement					
I used process tools (i.e. process mapping, Cause and Effect analysis, 5 Whys) to better understand what changes need to be made (or where opportunities for improvement exist)					
I identified the changes that could be implemented to result in improvement?					
I used rapid-cycle change methods, such as a PDSA cycle, to carry out a small test of change					

Other notes/reflections:

© 2015 Royal College of Physicians and Surgeons of Canada

T3. LEADING AND MANAGING IN EVERYDAY PRACTICE (CONTINUED)

☐ **Patient safety applies to this situation**

☐ **Patient safety does not apply to this situation**

Patient Safety **IN THIS SITUATION**	Rating			Comments	Areas or ideas for improvement?
	Done	Not done	Not applicable		
I recognized the patient safety incident, and was able to classify it as: 1) A **harmful incident** results in harm to the patient, Harm occurred due to medical care as opposed to underlying medical condition 2) A **no harm incident** reaches a patient but does not result in any discernible harm 3) A **near miss** does not reach the patient					
I contributed to a safety culture including demonstrating commitment to openness, honesty, fairness, and accountability. Include examples of how.					
I reported the incident(s) and safety hazard(s) and/ or notified my supervisor. Include who, how and when.					
I met the immediate and ongoing care needs of the patient, limited further harm, and provided ongoing monitoring and care.					
I explained to the patient what unexpected event or change happened. Include who, how and when.					
I apologized that it happened. Include who, how and when.					
I explained what would happen next including explicitly discussing prevention with future patients. Include who, how and when.					
I/we analyzed the patient safety incident(s) to enhance systems of care. Include who, how and when.					
I/we planned a debriefing to manage the emotional impact. Include who, how and when.					
OTHER:					

Other notes/reflections:

T3. LEADING AND MANAGING IN EVERYDAY PRACTICE (continued)

5. Summarize your TOP two or three areas of strength.

_____

_____

_____

_____

_____

6. Planning for improvement

#	Summarize your TOP two or three personal areas for improvement over the next four to eight weeks?	How are you going to work on your personal improvement priorities over the next four to eight weeks?	How will you know that you have achieved the needed improvement in your personal priority areas?
1.			
2.			
3.			

© 2015 Royal College of Physicians and Surgeons of Canada

Leader

T4. EXPLORING AND DEVELOPING SELF-AWARENESS

Created for the *CanMEDS Teaching and Assessment Tools Guide* by S Glover Takahashi.
Reproduced with permission of the Royal College.

See Leader Role teacher tips appendix for this teaching tool

Completed by: _____

A. LEADERSHIP INVENTORY

1. BASED on your awareness of yourself personally and professionally, complete the following table:

My ***personal strengths*** are:	What informs your view of your personal strengths?	Which strength needs further development? Why? How? When?	List one or two ways you will you use this strength to improve your practice over the next two to four weeks.
My ***professional strengths*** are:	What informs your view of your professional strengths?	Which strength needs further development? Why? How? When?	List one or two ways you will you use this strength to improve your practice over the next one or two weeks.
My ***personal areas for improvements*** are:	What informs your view of your personal areas for improvement?	Which areas need further development? Why? How? When?	List two ways you will address the areas to improve your practice over the next one or two weeks.
My ***professional areas for improvement*** are:	What informs your view of your professional areas for improvement?	Which areas need further development? Why? How? When?	List two ways you will address the areas to improve your practice over the next one or two weeks.

Other notes/reflections:

Leader

T4. EXPLORING AND DEVELOPING SELF-AWARENESS (continued)

B. VALUES INVENTORY[a]

2. Complete the table below about your values.

   Consider your personal list of core values.

   A *sample* list of values is found below the table to assist you in 'labelling' your core values.
   Feel free to use your own/preferred list of core values.

   Try and assign a rank to them with 1 being the most important value.

Rank	Value	Brief explanation (i.e. what does this value mean to you?)	How do your values motivate you? (i.e. guide and inform choices, priorities, actions)

Independence	Spirituality	Dignity	Courage	Loyalty	Risk-taking
Longevity	Wellness	Equality	Family	Friendship	Happiness
Wealth	Power	Integrity	Autonomy	Health	Vitality
Self-reliance	Authenticity	Challenge	Empathy	Honour	Hard Work
Perfection	Curiosity	Respect	Fairness	Truthfulness	Clear-mindedness
Status	Love	Balance	Physical strength	Other _____	

a Incardona N, Wanger F. University of Toronto 2014. Adapted for the healthcare context from the *Center for Ethical Leadership Self Guided Core Values Assessment,* 2002. www.ethicalleadership.org. Reproduced with permission.

© 2015 Royal College of Physicians and Surgeons of Canada

Leader

T4. EXPLORING AND DEVELOPING SELF-AWARENESS (continued)

3. In the last 4 weeks, how well have your life and work and your core values aligned?

_____

_____

_____

_____

_____

_____

4. Is the past 4 weeks 'typical' of how well your life and work align with your core values?

_____

_____

_____

_____

_____

_____

_____

5. If you find there is a disconnect between your values and their relative influence on your work, you may consider how to create better alignment. People are generally more satisfied and productive when their work and core values are well-aligned.

   If needed, list 1-2 ways you will improve alignment of life and values this week/month?

_____

_____

_____

_____

_____

_____

Leader

© 2015 Royal College of Physicians and Surgeons of Canada

T5. LEADER ROLE COMPETENCIES

Created for the *CanMEDS Teaching and Assessment Tools Guide* by S Glover Takahashi, M-K Chan, D Dath. Reproduced with permission of the Royal College.

See Leader Role teacher tips appendix for this teaching tool

Instructions for Learner:

- Observe and take (non-identifying) notes on your Leader Role activities in day-to-day practice

- Remember to be cautious about confidentiality when taking notes

- Review with faculty as arranged or initiate a review of your case reports to get feedback

Resident name: _____

Resident role in this location: _____

Rotation/Site/Organization: (include details about when, where, how long, type of service)

_____

_____

_____

_____

_____

_____

_____

A. RESOURCES FOR THIS ROTATION/SITE/ORGANIZATION

1. List the KEY resources, guidelines, policies and protocols that you used to understand your role and responsibilities. (i.e. job description, on call responsibility phone contact list)

2. List OTHER key sources for information/assistance that were available for this Rotation/Site/Organization? Are there gaps?

_____

_____

_____

_____

© 2015 Royal College of Physicians and Surgeons of Canada

Leader

T5. LEADER ROLE COMPETENCIES (continued)

3. Rate your approach to those elements of leadership that apply *in this case that you are reporting on* (e.g. leadership process, management, stewardship, quality improvement, patient safety). Rate your approach by including your own viewpoint and remember to include the feedback of others to inform your ratings. List important areas or ideas for improvement that are priorities for you.

A. Leadership process IN THIS CASE[a]	Rate your approach IN THIS SITUATION. **Explain rating**						Areas or ideas for priority improvement?
	1 Very poor	**2** Poor	**3** Solid competent	**4** Very good	**5** Superb	Not applicable	
Asks what needs to be done							
Asks what is right for the patient(s), problem, organization etc.							
Develops action plans							
Takes responsibility for decisions							
Takes responsibility for communications							
Focuses on opportunities rather than problems							
Leads productive meetings							
Thinks and says "we" rather than "I"							

Other notes/reflections:

---

a Drucker PF. *What makes an effective executive? Harv Bus Rev.* 2004;82(6):58-63-136.

Leader

T5. LEADER ROLE COMPETENCIES (continued)

B. Management process IN THIS CASE	Rate your approach IN THIS SITUATION. **Explain rating**						Areas or ideas for priority improvement?
	1 Very poor	**2** Poor	**3** Solid competent	**4** Very good	**5** Superb	Not applicable	
Ensures understanding of work and timelines							
Identifies the priority tasks and timelines							
Establishes steps and sequence to deliver outcomes on time							
Shares work through effective delegation							
Assigns people important activities							
Assigns tasks based on match/fit of competencies and strength							
Assigns tasks based on learning needs							
Monitors people's progress							
Communicates and clarifies with people							
Coaches peoples' progress and success							
Flexibly modifies plans with new, emerging situations							
Deploys people with new, emerging situations							
Integrates personal and professional priorities							
Uses tools and resources effectively to achieve outcomes							

Other notes/reflections:

© 2015 Royal College of Physicians and Surgeons of Canada

T5. LEADER ROLE COMPETENCIES (continued)

4. Summarize your TOP two or three areas of strength

_____

_____

_____

_____

_____

_____

_____

5. Planning for improvement

#	Summarize your TOP two or three areas that need priority improvement over the next four to eight weeks.	How are you going to work on your priorities over the next four to eight weeks?	How will you know that you have achieved the needed improvement in your priority areas?
1.			
2.			
3.			

Leader

T6. PATIENT SAFETY AND QUALITY IMPROVEMENT

Created for the *CanMEDS Teaching and Assessment Tools Guide* by B Wong, S Glover Takahashi.
Reproduced with permission of the Royal College.

See Leader Role teacher tips appendix for this teaching tool

Instructions for Learner:

• Observe and take (non-identifying) notes on your Leader Role activities in day-to-day practice

• Remember to be cautious about confidentiality when taking notes

• Review with faculty as arranged or initiate a review of your case reports to get feedback

Completed by: _____

Case report ID: _____

1. Provide an overview of this case (i.e. summary)

_____

_____

_____

_____

2. Describe the setting: *Workplace*

    ☐ Ward   ☐ Clinic   ☐ OR   ☐ ER   ☐ Other: _____

3. Outline any other relevant information about this case and/or organization and/or team.

_____

_____

_____

_____

4. What quality gaps, safety gaps or stewardship gaps were identified?

_____

_____

_____

_____

© 2015 Royal College of Physicians and Surgeons of Canada

Leader

T6. PATIENT SAFETY AND QUALITY IMPROVEMENT (continued)

5. What were the contributing factors to the safety, quality, or stewardship problem?

_____

_____

_____

6. What could be done to improve things?

_____

_____

_____

7. What was the patient and family's perspective?

_____

_____

_____

8. What did you learn from this that you will take into your future practice?

_____

_____

_____

9. What is KNOWN (in literature) about this problem? Possible solutions?

_____

_____

_____

10. How did this case affect you personally?

_____

_____

_____

11. What are the TOP two or three 'take home points' from this case?

_____

_____

_____

Leader

© 2015 Royal College of Physicians and Surgeons of Canada

T6. PATIENT SAFETY AND QUALITY IMPROVEMENT (continued)

12. What can be done?

    a. What can you do?

    b. What can others do?

_____

_____

_____

13. Planning for improvement

#	Top areas for improvement identified in this case	Who is responsible for improvements?	What can be done?
1.			
2.			
3.			

Other notes/reflections:

© 2015 Royal College of Physicians and Surgeons of Canada

T7. TIME MANAGEMENT ASSIGNMENT – WHERE DOES THE TIME GO?[a]

Objectives:

- Accurately assessing your actual time use is essential to managing your time more effectively.

- Consider your time wishes: What do you want more time for?

- Use a prospective time diary to take stock of your time use.

- Categorize and prioritize your activities.

- Assess whether the time spent on different activities is in alignment with your values and goals.

Few physicians would disagree that time is one of their most precious assets. But do they truly value and respect their own time? One way to judge this in your own case is to reflect on how your style of dealing with time affects others.

1. Self-assessment: time and action

- Do you frequently interrupt others?

- Do you often keep others waiting?

- Do you frequently miss agreed deadlines?

- Are you always running a few minutes (or more!) late?

- Do you often find yourself making excuses for being late?

When we repeatedly waste other people's time, we are sending them a message that we do not think their time is valuable. We may be unaware of habits that encroach on others' time, or we just do not stop to consider the implications. Sometimes the root of the problem goes even deeper than a lack of consideration for others: it reflects a feeling of powerlessness with regard to time. To claim ownership of your time, it is crucial to first take stock of it, examining what you spend time on, what you would like to have more time for, and whether the way you spend your time reflects your values and goals. Is there a gap between the time you have and the time you would like to have—in other words, between how you spend your time and what you really want to be doing and achieving?

Time wishes

Spend a few minutes to consider this question: What do you want more time for? What are the first things that jump to mind? Take a few moments to consider your time wishes, both personal and professional. They are both important.

Self-assessment: time wishes

Three things I would do if I had more personal time, or that I wish I had more time for, are:

1. _____

_____

_____

2. _____

_____

_____

3. _____

_____

_____

Three things I would do if I had more professional time, or that I wish I had more time for, are:

1. _____

_____

_____

2. _____

_____

_____

3. _____

_____

_____

The activities that are most important to you are likely those that came to mind first. There are no right or wrong answers. The fact that the number of minutes in the day is finite means that, to attain any of these wishes, you will need to eliminate another current activity—hopefully, a time-waster.

a   Patel H, Puddester D. *The time management guide: a practical handbook for physician by physicians.* Ottawa: Royal College of Physicians and Surgeons of Canada; 2012. Reproduced with permission.

© 2015 Royal College of Physicians and Surgeons of Canada

Leader

T7. TIME MANAGEMENT ASSIGNMENT – WHERE DOES THE TIME GO?[a]

(continued)

Time-wasters

Now try to identify habits, actions, and responsibilities that waste your time. What we are really talking about are undesired, possibly unproductive, activities. Take a few moments to jot down the top five things that you would rather do less often or not at all.

Self-assessment: time-wasters

Three things that waste my time or that I'd rather stop doing are:

1._____
_____
_____

2._____
_____
_____

3._____
_____
_____

Time-wasters come in two forms: the obvious and the not-so-obvious that are contextual and highly personal. Physicians often say that their time is wasted by email, paperwork, administrative tasks, and unimportant interruptions. On the home front, housework, the Internet, and television are frequently cited.

The not-so-obvious time-wasters are the dangerous ones, for they can siphon away our time without us even noticing. Procrastination is a good example of an occult time-waster. Chit-chat, the social glue that helps hold teams together, can insidiously move from team builder to time-waster. But the most dangerous time-waster is a lack of personal direction. See Chapter three of Patel H, Puddester D. *The time management guide: A practical handbook for physicians by physicians*. Ottawa: Royal College of Physicians and Surgeons; 2012, for tips to develop personal direction.

2. **Keeping a time diary**

   Much like a budget helps us with financial planning we need to draw up a "budget" for allocating our time. First, consider how your time is being spent currently. There are retrospective and prospective approaches to this task.

A retrospective accounting

A retrospective review of recent activities using your agenda, calendar, or planner can help you assess how you are spending your time. If you don't have a paper or electronic agenda, this approach won't work. If you do use an agenda, can you see how your time was spent in blocks of 30 minutes or less? Is it clear what you intended to accomplish on any given day? Did you succeed? Do you know where last week went? Are you able to identify any specific time-wasting activities? On the positive side, what desired tasks were you able to complete?

A prospective diary

Keeping a prospective time log or diary is the single best way to determine your actual time use. The quickest and easiest way to do this is with pen and paper.

1. Method one: Create a grid (with 15- or 30-minute time slots on a sheet of paper. Fold the paper up and carry it in your pocket with a pen. Write down your main activity in every block of time.

2. Method two: Record your time use with dictation or by using a mobile device. You will need to transcribe the results, as opposed to doing a quick overview on paper.

3. Method three: Keep a small pad of Post-it notes in your pocket and write the time and activity down every 30 minutes.

   You will learn a lot from recording a day's worth of activities, and even more by looking at a series of days, especially if your daily tasks vary significantly through the week. It is crucial to record activities as they truly happen, even when they are unexpected.

   When you try the time diary, you may find that the process of keeping a record is itself therapeutic. Just by being aware of your time, you will start to see your management of it in a different light. You may even find yourself making modifications through the course of the day in response to what you are noticing. It is similar to when we ask patients with chronic conditions such as headaches to keep diaries to help identify patterns and triggers. Diaries work well when self-reflection and behaviour modification are a key part of the intervention.

© 2015 Royal College of Physicians and Surgeons of Canada

Leader

T7. TIME MANAGEMENT ASSIGNMENT – WHERE DOES THE TIME GO?[a]

(continued)

3. Analyzing your time use

- Once you have collected some real data from your time diary, you will be ready to do some analysis. To borrow some advice from the business literature on time management, it's time to see whether your "commitments match your convictions."[b]

- Consider how you are spending your time now. What proportion of your day is spent doing the things that you want to do? Are you comfortable with this balance? Look through the activities recorded in your time diary and jot down whether this matches your goals.

- You are most likely to be effective in reaching your goals when you invest time in planning and preparation. Spend as little as possible on unimportant tasks and as much as possible on non-urgent but important tasks.

Other resources for time management:

One of the best-known ways to start working on this is to apply Stephen R. Covey's Time Management Matrix.[c] Developed decades ago, this model is still useful. Steven Covey suggests that we organize our activities and align our time so that we don't confuse urgency with importance, and short term with longer term outcomes.

There are, of course, other models for categorizing time use. All are based on the prioritization of tasks. For example, Brian Tracy, in his highly readable book *Eat That Frog!*,[d] describes a system in which, on a given day, "A" tasks must be done, "B" tasks should be done, "C" tasks could be done, "D" tasks could be delegated to someone else, and "E" tasks could be eliminated.

In a similar vein, David Sackett, in a series of articles on time management for clinical scientists,[e] suggests that all tasks be divided into: (a) items that the individual is doing and wants to keep doing; (b) items that the individual is doing and wants to stop; (c) items that the individual is not doing and wants to start; and (d) strategies that can be used to improve the balance between these categories. No matter which system you use, the key elements in analyzing your time are the same: taking stock of your actual time use, categorizing your activities with respect to priorities, and considering to what extent the proportion of time you spend on different types of activities matches your real values, objectives, and aspirations.

---

b Sull DN, Houlder D. *Do your commitments match your convictions?* Boston: Harvard Business Press; 2005.
c Covey SR. *The 7 habits of highly effective people.* New York: Free Press; 1989.
d Tracy B. *Eat that frog!* 2nd ed. San Francisco: Berrett-Koehler Publishers; 2006. p 37–40. www.briantracy.com
e Sackett DL. Clinician-trialist rounds: 3. Priority setting for academic success. *Clin Trials.* 2011;8(2):235–7. Permission to use provided by Sage Publications Ltd. www.sage.pub.co.uk

Leader

© 2015 Royal College of Physicians and Surgeons of Canada

T8. SUMMARY SHEET FOR THE LEADER ROLE

Created for the *CanMEDS Teaching and Assessment Tools Guide* by S Glover Takahashi, M-K Chan, B Wong, D Dath. Reproduced with permission of the Royal College.

See Leader Role teacher tips appendix for this teaching tool

LEADER

- The Leader Role facilitates the expression of leadership no matter what title a physician may or may not hold
- Dynamic leaders know when and how to stand back, support and enable others to lead
- Leader Role includes important manager competencies (i.e. management of personal and professional practice)

Effective leaders have:
EMOTIONAL INTELLIGENCE:[a]

- *Self-awareness* – knowing one's strengths, weaknesses, drivers, values, and impact on others
- *Self-regulation* – monitor and control own behaviour
- *Motivation* – internal drive and personally meaningful
- *Empathy* – considering others' feelings, values, and preferences
- *Social skill* – building rapport and relationships with others

Effective leaders demonstrate:
Stewardship of resources

- Be aware of stewardship issues, options, decisions based on individual patient needs, preferences, and values of the patient and organization.
- Use guidelines to inform appropriate use of testing and get info from Choosing Wisely Canada[b]
- Consider "How will the result of this test influence our overall management plan?" If no bearing on the overall treatment plan, then it is likely of minimal benefit and should not be ordered.

FEEDBACK[c]

Leadership improves with feedback:

1. Ask someone who is willing and can be constructive
2. Ask for SPECIFIC feedback
3. Listen and focus on what is helpful and specific (i.e. Do not interrupt. Watch for resistance and defensiveness)
4. Say thank you for the input

PROCESS FOR EFFECTIVE LEADERSHIP[d]

Key steps	Purpose
1. Ask what needs to be done	*Gathering info*
2. Ask what is right for the patient(s), problem, organization etc.	
3. Develop action plans	*Moving from information to action*
4. Take responsibility for decisions	
5. Take responsibility for communications	
6. Focus on opportunities rather than problems	
7. Lead productive meetings	*Creating shared responsibility and accountability*
8. Think and say "we" rather than "I"	

Effective leaders enable **Patient safety**
- Model a *safe culture* including demo commitment to openness, honesty, fairness, accountability
- *Patient safety incident* is an event or circumstance that could have resulted, or did result, in unnecessary harm to a patient. Three types of patient safety incidents: 1) A harmful incident results in harm to the patient, 2) A no harm incident reaches a patient but does not result in any discernible harm, 3) A near miss does not reach the patient
- Expect the unexpected. Anticipation and prevention of errors is important as is vigilance and readiness
- Contribute to a safety culture including demonstrating commitment to openness, honesty, fairness, and accountability
- Report incidents and safety hazards to promote improvement
- Analyze patient safety incidents to enhance systems of care
  - i.e. 1. *Cause and Effect Analysis* diagram-based technique and combines brainstorming with a type of mind map that stimulates consideration of all possible causes of a problem, rather than just the ones that are most obvious. And/or 2. *Five Whys Analysis* where you repeatedly ask the question "Why?" (Use five as a rule of thumb) so that you can peel away the layers of an issue, just like the layers of an onion, which can lead you to the root cause of a problem

---

a Goleman D. What makes a leader? *Harv Bus Rev.* 1998;76(6):93–102.
b http://www.choosingwiselycanada.org
c This chart is based on material in Stone D, Heen S. *Thanks for the feedback: the science and art of receiving feedback well.* New York: Penguin; 2014. Used with permission
d Drucker PF. What makes an effective executive? *Harv Bus Rev.* 2004; 82(6): 58-63,136.

© 2015 Royal College of Physicians and Surgeons of Canada

Leader

T8. SUMMARY SHEET FOR THE LEADER ROLE (continued)

Effective leaders: **Have courage and take responsibility for errors**

Three Rules of apologies:[e]
1. Be honest and authentic
2. Do not just explain
3. Do not use the word "but"

Steps to an effective apology:
1. **Express remorse:** "I am sorry"
2. **Take responsibility** for actions or behaviour
3. **Make amends** for your actions to make the situation right (i.e. be appropriate and within your authority)
4. **Rebuild trust.** Repair the relationship

Effective leaders contribute to:
QUALITY IMPROVEMENT of health care delivery in teams, organizations and systems

- **Quality improvement:** structured approach to the analysis of performance and systematic efforts to improve it.

Six domains of health care quality:[f]
1. Safe
2. Effective
3. Patient Centred
4. Timely
5. Efficient
6. Equitable

- **Model for Improvement,** has two parts:
  1) **Three Qs:** What are we trying to accomplish? How will we know that a change is an improvement? What changes can we make that will result in improvement?
  2) **Plan-Do-Study-Act (PDSA)** cycle "to test and implement changes in real work settings.

Key actions when patient safety incidents occur:[g]
1. Meet the immediate and ongoing care needs of the patient (ensure the patient is clinically stable, correct the safety issue(s), limit further harm, and provide ongoing monitoring and care).
2. Explain to the patient what unexpected event or change happened including who, how, what and prevention.
3. Apologize that it happened.
4. Explain what will happen next, including explicitly discussing prevention.

ALSO:
- Contact supervisor(s), team members
- Initiate any needed organizational systems
- Access personal support resources
- Plan a debriefing to manage the emotional impact

Effective leaders are **EFFECTIVE MANAGERS**.

Manage career planning, finances, and health human resources
- Set priorities and manage time to integrate practice and personal life
- Be mindful and deliberate about managing busy schedules.
- Use tools to get/stay organized
- **Share the work** through effective **delegation**
  - Organize to ensure a complete understanding of what needs to be done by what deadline
  - Identify the priority tasks including timelines
  - Establish the steps and sequence key to achieving the desired outcomes on time
  - Inventory available resources incl team member competencies
  - Assign people the authority and responsibility for important activities. Assign based on: (a) match/fit of competencies and strengths to activity and/or (b) needs for skill development
  - Monitor, communicate with, clarify expectations with, and coach delegates.
  - Deploy or redeploy people to new, emerging, or challenging assignments as they arise.

PERSONAL NOTES

KEY Guidelines/Policies/Protocols re: stewardship of resources, roles, responsibilities **for this Rotation/Site/Organization**

_____

Personal notes/inventory on SPECIFIC leadership, stewardship, managerial notes **for this Rotation/Site/Organization**

_____

Personal notes/inventory on Who/how to call/contact **for this Rotation/Site/Organization**

- Patient safety questions or incidents: _____

- Quality improvement questions or scenarios: _____

- Stewardship questions or scenarios: _____

- Management questions or scenarios: _____

- Leadership questions or scenarios: _____

e © Mind Tools Ltd, 1996-2015. All rights reserved. "Mind Tools" is a registered trademark of Mind Tools Ltd. Mind Tools. How to apologize: asking for forgiveness gracefully. www.mind-tools.com/pages.article/how-to-apologize.htm. Reproduced with permission.
f *Six Domains of Health Care Quality.* Consumer Assessment of Healthcare Providers and Systems (CAHPS) website. Last Retrieved July 3, 2015 from: https://cahps.ahrq.gov/consumer-reporting/talkingquality/create/sixdomains.html. Reproduced with permission.
g *Incident Analysis Collaborating Parties. Canadian Incident Analysis Framework.* Edmonton: Canadian Patient Safety Institute; 2012.

Leader

A1. LEADERSHIP SKILLS IN THE CANMEDS LEADER ROLE

Created for the *CanMEDS Teaching and Assessment Tools Guide* by S Glover Takahashi, M-K Chan, D Dath and B Wong. Reproduced with permission of the Royal College.

See Leader Role teacher tips appendix for this assessment tool

Instructions for Assessor:

- Leadership competencies can be developed over time. Using the form below, please help this LEARNER gain insight into his/her leadership skills by providing valuable confidential feedback.

- This information will be shared with the learner in aggregate form and for the purposes of helping the learner improve his/her leadership competencies.

- Please return this form in a confidential manner

to _____

by _____

Learner's Name: _____

Postgraduate year (PGY): _____

Place a check mark in your answer for each item.

Indicate ☑ all that apply. I am a:
- ☐ Health professional team member (including co-resident)
- ☐ Resident supervisor
- ☐ Faculty
- ☐ Other, please describe _____

Degree of Interaction
- ☐ I had considerable interaction with this learner
- ☐ I had occasional interaction with this learner

ASSESSMENT TOOL: RESIDENT LEADERSHIP SKILLS

#	The learner...	1 Never or very poorly	2 Occasionally or needs to improve	3 Satisfactory	4 Consistently	5 Highly skilled	Not able to comment
1.	Asks what needs to be done and makes an effort to be helpful						
2.	Demonstrates commitment to the patient(s)						
3.	Demonstrates commitment to the organization and program						
4.	Demonstrates effective planning						
5.	Takes responsibility for decisions						
6.	Takes responsibility for communications						
7.	Focuses on opportunities rather than problems						
8.	Leads productive meetings						
9.	Demonstrates commitment to team rather than self						
10.	Builds and maintains my trust						
11.	Works to develop rapport with me						
12.	Empathetic to my feelings, values, preferences						
13.	Asks for and welcomes my questions						
14.	Asks for and welcomes my feedback						

Leader

© 2015 Royal College of Physicians and Surgeons of Canada

A1. LEADERSHIP SKILLS IN THE CANMEDS LEADER ROLE (continued)

Overall rating on Leadership	1 Very poor leader	2 Weak leader	3 Competent leader	4 Strong leader	5 Highly skilled leader

Areas of strength	Areas for improvement
1.	1.
2.	2.
3.	3.

Comments:

_____

_____

_____

_____

_____

_____

_____

_____

_____

_____

_____

Please return this form to: _____

Leader

© 2015 Royal College of Physicians and Surgeons of Canada

A2. MANAGING PEOPLE AND RESOURCES IN THE CANMEDS LEADER ROLE

Created for the *CanMEDS Teaching and Assessment Tools Guide* by S Glover Takahashi, M-K Chan, D Dath and B Wong. Reproduced with permission of the Royal College.

See Leader Role teacher tips appendix for this assessment tool

Instructions for Assessor:

- As Leaders, physicians engage in the stewardship and management of health care people and resources. With practice and feedback these competencies can be developed over time.

- Using the form below, please help this resident physician gain insight into his/her skills by providing valuable confidential feedback.

- Rest assured this information will be shared with the physician in aggregate form and for the purposes of helping the physician improve his/her leadership competencies.

- Please return this form in a confidential manner

  to_____

Place a check mark in your answer for each item.

Learner's Name:_____

Postgraduate year (PGY): _____

Indicate ☑ all that apply. I am a:

- ☐ Health professional team member (including co-resident)
- ☐ Resident supervisor
- ☐ Faculty
- ☐ Other, please describe_____

Degree of Interaction
- ☐ I had considerable interaction with this learner
- ☐ I had occasional interaction with this learner

FEEDBACK FORM – MANAGING PEOPLE AND RESOURCES

#	The resident...	1 Never or very poorly	2 Occasionally or needs to improve	3 Satisfactory	4 Consistently	5 Highly skilled	Not able to comment
1.	Ensures his/her understanding of work and timelines						
2.	Identifies the priority tasks and timelines						
3.	Establishes steps and sequence to deliver needed outcomes on time						
4.	Shares work through effective delegation						
5.	Assigns people important activities						
6.	Communicates and clarifies with people about progress						
7.	Coaches peoples' progress and supports success						
8.	Flexibly modifies plans with new, emerging situations						
9.	Deploys or redeploys people with new, emerging situations						
10.	Uses tools and resources effectively to achieve outcomes						
11.	Demonstrates careful consideration of effects and efficient use of limited system resources						
12.	Demonstrates consideration of benefits and costs to the individual, system, risk management						
13.	Explains and engages patient in decisions that reflect stewardship						
14.	Applies evidence and processes to achieve cost appropriate care						
15.	Supports others in their stewardship decisions						

© 2015 Royal College of Physicians and Surgeons of Canada

A2. MANAGING PEOPLE AND RESOURCES IN THE CANMEDS LEADER ROLE (continued)

Overall rating	1 Very poor leader	2 Weak leader	3 Competent leader	4 Strong leader	5 Highly skilled leader

Areas of strength	Areas for improvement
1.	1.
2.	2.
3.	3.

Comments:

_____

_____

_____

_____

_____

_____

_____

_____

_____

_____

Please return this form to: _____

Leader

© 2015 Royal College of Physicians and Surgeons of Canada

A3. LEADER ROLE QUALITY IMPROVEMENT PROJECT

Created for the *CanMEDS Teaching and Assessment Tools Guide* by S Glover Takahashi, M-K Chan, D Dath and B Wong. Reproduced with permission of the Royal College.

See Leader Role teacher tips appendix for this assessment tool

Prepare a six to eight page summary report describing your quality improvement project.

Consider the following points:

• Describe your clinical experience, including details about the clinical context and type(s) of service.

• Reflect use of the QI core concepts, principles, QI methodology.

• Consider the following structure to organize your QI project report:
  1. Background and project rationale
  2. Aim statement
  3. Process analysis and changes tested
  4. Improvement results (if available)
  5. Lessons learned
  6. Next steps

• Please return this form in a confidential manner

  to_____

Learner's Name:_____

Postgraduate year (PGY): _____

Place a check mark in your answer for each item.

Indicate ☑ all that apply. I am a:
- ☐ Health professional team member (including co-resident)
- ☐ Resident supervisor
- ☐ Faculty
- ☐ Other, please describe_____

Degree of Interaction
- ☐ I had considerable interaction with this learner
- ☐ I had occasional interaction with this learner

Deadlines
• A 1-page (i.e. 250-word) abstract is due

  by_____
  (i.e. one month before the final deadline)

• The paper is due via email

  by/before_____

QUALITY IMPROVEMENT PROJECT: SAMPLE ASSESSMENT FORM[a]

1. MEDICAL EXPERT	1 Unsatisfactory	2 Needs improvement	3 Meets expectations	4 Exceeds expectations	5 Outstanding	Not able to comment
Demonstrates knowledge of basic QI principles (i.e. six aims of quality)						
Distinguish between measurement for QI as compared to evaluative research						
Identifies important quality gaps in their clinical environment as opportunities for improvement						
2. COLLABORATOR						
Contributes meaningfully to QI project and fulfills duties responsibly						
Collaborates effectively with other members of QI team and faculty						

a Quality Improvement In-training Evaluation Report Developed by: Alexander Lo, Rory McQuillan, Kieran McIntyre, Lisa Hicks, Jerome Leis, Geetha Mukerji, Adam Weizman, Jeannette Goguen, Brian Wong. University of Toronto Co-Learning Curriculum in Quality Improvement. Reproduced with permission.

© 2015 Royal College of Physicians and Surgeons of Canada

A3. LEADER ROLE QUALITY IMPROVEMENT PROJECT (continued)

3. LEADER	1 Unsatisfactory	2 Needs improvement	3 Meets expectations	4 Exceeds expectations	5 Outstanding	Not able to comment
Engages relevant stakeholders effectively and appropriately						
Employs a systems-based approach to address QI and patient safety issues						
Demonstrates commitment to improving health care quality and patient safety						
Applies QI tools (i.e. Fishbone, process mapping, PDSA cycles) appropriately to identify gaps in patient care and develop possible solutions						
4. SCHOLAR						
Critically appraises relevant medical and QI literature						
Uses appropriate methods for data collection and analysis (e.g. gap analysis, run or control charts)						
Clearly and effectively presents the QI project in oral and/or written format (including mid-year and final project presentations)						
Recognizes and addresses research ethics issues appropriately						
OVERALL RATING						

Two or three areas of strength _____

_____

_____

_____

Two or three areas for improvement _____

_____

_____

_____

Assessment date: _____

Completion by: _____

© 2015 Royal College of Physicians and Surgeons of Canada

Leader

A4. LEADERSHIP REFLECTION

Created for the *CanMEDS Teaching and Assessment Tools Guide* by M-K Chan. and S Glover Takahashi. Reproduced with permission of the Royal College.

See Leader Role teacher tips appendix for this assessment tool

Instructions for Learner:

- Observe, reflect and take (non-identifying) notes on your Leader Role activities in day-to-day practice.

- Remember to be cautious about confidentiality when taking notes

- Review with faculty as arranged or initiate a review of your case reports to get feedback

NAME:

PGY:

DATE OF LEADERSHIP ACTIVITY:

DATES OF PREVIOUS LEADERSHIP REFLECTION REPORTS:

-
-

CURRENT REPORTING PERIOD: FROM   TO

REFLECTION REPORT REVIEW MEETING
DATE:
REVIEWER:

Comments from Reviewer

REVIEW OF PAST PRIORITIES LEADERSHIP COMPETENICES (if applicable)

☐   Not applicable

☐   PAST REPORTING PERIOD: FROM _____ TO _____

#	Leadership area (e.g. leadership skills, managing self, engaging others, QI, stewardship, patient safety)	Past goal including timeframe	Identified metrics or criteria for success	Notes on progress, outcomes, completion
1.				
2.				
3.				

© 2015 Royal College of Physicians and Surgeons of Canada

Leader

A4. LEADERSHIP REFLECTION (continued)

SUMMARY OF CURRENT/NEW PRIORITIES FOR IMPROVEMENT OF LEADERSHIP COMPETENCIES

☐ APPLIES TO PERIOD: FROM _____ TO _____

#	Leadership area (e.g. leadership skills, managing self, engaging others, QI, stewardship, patient safety)	Goal(s) including timeframe	Metrics or criteria for success	Key next steps, resources, supports for success
1.				
2.				
3.				

Other notes:

_____

_____

_____

_____

_____

_____

_____

Leader

© 2015 Royal College of Physicians and Surgeons of Canada

LEADER ROLE TEACHER TIPS APPENDIX

T3 LEADING AND MANAGING IN EVERYDAY PRACTICE

Instructions for Teacher:

- This activity is quite versatile, it can be done as a small group activity at a workshop, or as an individual 'assignment' for discussion at a one-on-one meeting or even as part of a portfolio.

- Establish with your learner how you will discuss or debrief these reports (e.g. at one-to-one meeting, in small groups, via academic half day, via portfolio review, based on a summary paper or report)

T4 EXPLORING AND DEVELOPING SELF-AWARENESS

Instructions for Teacher:

- This tool is designed to help your learners explore and develop self-awareness. This exercise can be done as an individual assignment or small group activity at a workshop.

- Some learners will find this exercise challenging or uncomfortable. For this reason, you may choose to spend some time upfront to help learners see the value of and need for self-awareness.

- For learners who are struggling you may consider connecting them with a mentor or coach who can provide additional support and direction in improving self-awareness.

- Establish how you will discuss or debrief these reports (e.g. at one-to-one meeting, in small groups, via academic half day, via semi-annual meeting with program director, as part of portfolio review).

- These topics can be quite personal so group discussions may be most productive if kept general. Focus on the general benefits of self-awareness and some of the typical problems that can occur when someone is not self-aware (try to use examples of general behaviours/issues that your learners will relate to from your own work setting). Your learners will probably appreciate you addressing the types of things they can and should do if they find, for instance, that their values and work do not align. Consider providing a list of resources that your learners can refer to for further reading if they choose.

T5 LEADER ROLE COMPETENCIES AND T6 PATIENT SAFETY AND QUALITY IMPROVEMENT

Instructions for Teacher:

- These tools can be assigned for completion during a clinical experience, such as on one or more days or during a rotation.

- This tool could also be used as a portfolio submission.

- When assigning the work, indicate the number of case reports to be completed and if the case reports are to be done in the same location or during the same rotation.

- The deadline for completion should be established and circulated (i.e. posted in resident physical or virtual bulletin board).

- Reminders are helpful to ensure completion.

- The 'Summary Sheet for the Leader Role' would be important background materials to complete this assignment.

- After the case reports are completed and submitted, it is important to review and debrief, reinforce learning, focus areas for clarification or improvement.

T8 SUMMARY SHEET FOR THE LEADER ROLE

Instructions for Teacher:

- The summary sheet is intended to be a cheat sheet for the teacher as well as the learner. It is a one page resource on key concepts, frameworks and approaches.

A1 LEADERSHIP SKILLS AND A2 MANAGING PEOPLE AND RESOURCES

Instructions for Teacher:

- Modify the form by adding or removing criteria that do/ do not apply.

- To optimize learning and to protect the identity of those who provide feedback, be mindful of the size and composition of your data sample.

- Be sure to provide your 'assessors' with clear instructions and provide guidance on your rating scale.

- It is a good idea to notify your learners of your intention and rationale for collecting feedback on their CanMEDS Leader Role skills. Be clear about the timeframe when you will collect the data, how you will maintain confidentiality and how and when you will present the data back to the learner.

Leader

© 2015 Royal College of Physicians and Surgeons of Canada

LEADER ROLE TEACHER TIPS APPENDIX (continued)

- Plan to share the summary of feedback with your learner in written format and in a face-to-face meeting. A meeting will allow for valuable coaching around areas of strength and areas for improvement.

A3 LEADER ROLE QUALITY IMPROVEMENT PROJECT

Instructions for Teacher:

- *Audience:* All learners

- *How to use:* Select from, modify, or add to the essay assignment as appropriate.

- *How to adapt:* Could be a project done in pairs or small groups (i.e. three learners). Add a 10 minute presentation of their abstract with focused discussion at a teaching session so all learners can benefit from the diversity of assignments and topics.

- *Logistics:* Provide instructions and rubric in writing. Orient learners to the assignment. Allow eight weeks to complete with abstract due in 4 weeks. That will allow for sufficient time to organize and complete a high quality assignment. Completion of the abstract/preview of paper is an important opportunity for feedback and focusing of learners. Also provides insight into who may need additional support (i.e. 2nd draft of abstract) to ensure they are on track.

- *Setting:* Classroom. Can be done via phone meetings or video classroom. Consider taking a flipped-classroom approach to introducing the core concepts and principles.

  - There are many online modules (e.g. the IHI Open School modules) and written materials that can be used to introduce the core principles of QI methodology.

  - Learners can be asked to review these materials before attending the face-to-face meetings with their faculty/advisor and spend the in-person time discussing how they might apply these concepts in their project work.

A4 LEADERSHIP REFLECTION

Instructions for *Assessor:*

- You can assign this tool for completion during a clinical experience, such as on one or more days or during a rotation.

- This tool can also be used as a portfolio submission.

- Indicate the number of reflection reports to be completed and if the case reports are to be done in the same location or during the same rotation.

- The deadline for completion should be established and circulated (i.e. posted in resident physical or virtual bulletin board).

- Reminders are helpful to ensure completion.

- The 'Summary Sheet' (T8) information would be important background materials to complete this assignment.

- After the reflection reports are completed and submitted, it is important to review and debrief, reinforce learning, focus areas for clarification or improvement

- Learners can do a reflection report about faculty or peer example of leadership and/or on their own case(s).

Leader

© 2015 Royal College of Physicians and Surgeons of Canada

REFERENCES

1. What we heard: sharing the results of the CanMEDS 2015 Series I and II consultations. Ottawa: Royal College of Physicians and Surgeons of Canada. 2014. http://www.royalcollege.ca/portal/page/portal/rc/common/documents/canmeds/framework/canmeds2015_consultations_results_e.pdf

2. Zafar MA, Diers T, Schauer DP, Warm EJ. Connecting resident education to patient outcomes: the evolution of a quality improvement curriculum in an internal medicine residency. *Acad Med.* 2014;89(10):1341–7.

3. Jansen LA. Between beneficence and justice: the ethics of stewardship in medicine. *J Med Philos.* 2013; 38(1):50–63.

4. Choosing Wisely Canada. What is CWC? Last retrieved July 3, 2015, from http://www.choosingwiselycanada.org/about/what-is-cwc/

5. Goleman D. What makes a leader? *Harv Bus Rev.* 1998;76(6):93–102.

6. Eva KW, Regehr G, Gruppen LD. Blinded by "Insight": Self-Assessment and Its Role in Performance Improvement. In Hodges BD, Lingard L, editors. *The question of competence: reconsidering medical education in the twenty-first century.* Ithaca: Cornel University Press; 2014.

7. Oxford Dictionaries. Transition. Last retrieved April 21, 2015, from http://www.oxforddictionaries.com/definition/english/transition

8. Association of Faculties of Medicine of Canada. *Future of medical education in Canada: a collective vision for postgraduate medical education in Canada.* Ottawa. 2012. Last retrieved July 3, 2015 from: https://www.afmc.ca/future-of-medical-education-in-canada/postgraduate-project/pdf/FMEC_PG_Final-Report_EN.pdf

9. Mettler T, Raptis DA. What constitutes the field of health information systems? Fostering a systematic framework and research agenda. *Health Informatics J.* 2012;18(2):147–56.

10. Cowing M, Davino-Ramaya CM, Ramaya K, Szmerekovsky J. Health care delivery performance: service, outcomes, and resource stewardship. *Perm J.* 2009;13(4): 72–8.

11. Six Domains of Health Care Quality. Consumer Assessment of Healthcare Providers and Systems (CAHPS) website. Last retrieved July 3, 2015 https://cahps.ahrq.gov/consumer-reporting/talkingquality/create/sixdomains.html. The TalkingQuality website is a resource that supports public and private sector efforts aimed at improving the communication of health care quality information to consumers. TalkingQuality is a product of the Consumer Assessment of Healthcare Providers and Systems (CAHPS®) program funded by the Agency for Healthcare Quality and Research, United States Department of Health and Human Services. Reproduced with permission.

12. Department of Community and Family Medicine, Duke University Medical Center. Patient Safety–Quality Improvement. Introduction: what is QI? Last retrieved July 3, 2015, from http://patientsafetyed.duhs.duke.edu/module_a/introduction/introduction.html

13. Incident Analysis Collaborating Parties. *Canadian Incident Analysis Framework.* Edmonton: Canadian Patient Safety Institute; 2012.

14. Langley GL, Nolan KM, Nolan TW, Norman CL, Provost LP, *The Improvement Guide: A Practical Approach to Enhancing Organizational Performance 2nd Ed.* Jossey Bass, San Francisco; 2009. See more at (last retrieved July 3, 2015): http://www.institute.nhs.uk/quality_and_service_improvement_tools/quality_and_service_improvement_tools/plan_do_study_act.html

15. Berwick DM. A primer on leading the improvement of systems. *BMJ.* 1996; 312(7031): 619–22.

16. Emanuel L, Berwick D, Conway J, Combes J, Hatlie M, Leape L, Reason J, Schyve P, Vincent C, Walton M. What exactly is patient safety? In Henriksen K, Battles JB, Keyes MA, Grady ML, editors. *Advances in patient safety: new directions and alternative approaches (Vol. 1: Assessment).* Rockville (MD): Agency for Healthcare Research and Quality; 2008 1-18.

17. Eurocontrol website. Just culture. Last retrieved August 2015, from http://www.eurocontrol.int/articles/just-culture

18. Meyer GS, Edward P Lawrence Centre for Quality and Safety. Just culture: the key to quality and safety (PPT). Last retrieved August 2015, from https://www.partners.org/Assets/Documents/Graduate-Medical-Education/10_09_27_Just%20Culture.pdf

© 2015 Royal College of Physicians and Surgeons of Canada

Leader

REFERENCES (continued)

19. NHS Institute for Innovation and Improvement. Quality and service improvement tools: cause and effect (Fishbone). Last retrieved July 3, 2015, from http://www.institute.nhs.uk/quality_and_service_improvement_tools/quality_and_service_improvement_tools/cause_and_effect.html

20. Dath D, Chan M-K, Abbott C. CanMEDS 2015: From Manager to Leader. Ottawa: Royal College of Physicians and Surgeons of Canada;2015 March. See http://www.royalcollege.ca/portal/page/portal/rc/common/documents/canmeds/framework/canmeds2015_manager_to_leader_e.pdf (last retrieved July 7, 2015).

21. Baker SD. Followership: the theoretical foundation of a contemporary construct. *J. Leadersh. Organ. Stud.* 2007;14(1):50–60.

22. Watling C, Driessen E, van der Vleuten CP, Lingard L. Learning from clinical work: the roles of learning cues and credibility judgments. *Med Educ.* 2012;46(2):192–200.

23. Stone D, Heen S. *Thanks for the feedback: the science and art of receiving feedback well.* New York: Viking; 2014.

24. George B, Sims P, McLean AN, Mayer D. Discovering your authentic leadership. *Harv Bus Rev.* 2007;85(2):129–30,132-8,157.

25. Grant AM, Curtayne L, Burton G. Executive coaching enhances goal attainment, resilience and workplace well-being: a randomised controlled study. *J Posit Psychol.* 2009;4(5):396-407.

26. Sackett DL, Rosenberg WMC, Muir Gray JA, Haynes RB, Richardson WS. Evidence-based medicine: what it is and what it isn't. *BMJ.* 1996;312:71.

27. Busemeyer JR. Cognitive science contributions to decision science. *Cognition.* 2015;135:43-6.

28. Snowden DJ, Boone ME. A Leader's Framework for Decision Making. *Harv Bus Rev.* 2007;85(11):68-76.

29. Kahneman D. *Thinking, Fast and Slow.* New York: Farrar, Straus and Giroux; 2011.

30. Starmer AJ, Spector ND, Srivastava R, Allen AD, Landrigan CP, Sectish TC, I-PASS Study Group. I-pass, a mnemonic to standardize verbal handoffs. Pediatrics. 2012;129(2):201–4.

31. Detsky AS, Verma AA. A new model for medical education: celebrating restraint. *JAMA.* 2012;308(13):1329–30.

32. Drucker PF. What makes an effective executive? *Harv Bus Rev.* 2004;82(6):58-63,136.

33. Glover Takahashi S. 2015 adapted from Patel H, Puddester D. *The Time Management Guide: A Practical Handbook for Physicians by Physicians.* Ottawa: Royal College of Physicians and Surgeons of Canada; 2012.

34. Covey SR, Merrill AR, Merrill RR. *First things first: to live, to love, to learn, to leave a legacy.* New York: Simon and Schuster; 1994.

35. Brown PC, Roediger III HL, McDaniel MA. *Make it stick: the science of successful learning.* Cambridge: Harvard University Press; 2014.

36. Mind Tools. Minimizing distractions: managing your work environment. Last retrieved April 23, 2015, from http://www.mindtools.com/pages/article/distractions.html

37. Hallowell EM. Driven to distraction at work: how to focus and be more productive. Boston: *Harvard Business Review* Press; 2015.

38. Mind Tools. How to apologize: asking for forgiveness gracefully. Last retrieved July 3, 2015, from http://www.mindtools.com/pages/article/how-to-apologize.html

39. Bould MD, Sutherland S, Sydor DT, Naik V, Friedman Z. Residents' reluctance to challenge negative hierarchy in the operating room: A qualitative study. *Can J Anaesth.* 2015;62(2): 576-86.

© 2015 Royal College of Physicians and Surgeons of Canada

Leader

© 2015 Royal College of Physicians and Surgeons of Canada

HEALTH ADVOCATE

ADVISE Policy

JUSTIFY Health literacy

INFLUENCE

Prevention Health promotion

Poverty RECOMMEND

Access Risk factor modification

NEGOTIATE Barriers

Social environment ASSIST

FACILITATE Surveillance

Competing needs

Safety LIAISE

Jonathan Sherbino

Maria Hubinette

Brigitte Côté

Susan Glover Takahashi

1. Why the Health Advocate Role matters

It can be difficult for some learners to buy into the Health Advocate Role. This is often because they misunderstand it or think it means that they have to work to change the health care system singlehandedly. Trainees tell us that they have had few role models in Health Advocacy. For this reason, when you introduce your learners to the Role, be sure to cover these points:

- Advocacy happens all the time during patient care. Health advocacy is about working with patients' health care preferences, needs, and values (i.e. it is patient-centred).

- Health advocacy is a team sport.[1] Physicians, patients, other health care professionals, and community organizations, among others, work together to enhance care for individuals and populations. Physicians have a special responsibility to use their medical expertise and unique position in the health care system to advocate for change.

- Effective medical care requires disease prevention, health promotion, health protection, and the promotion of health equity (e.g. helping people to achieve their full health potential without being disadvantaged by socio-economic factors). Ill health starts long before an individual sees a physician. The most sophisticated diagnostic test or therapeutic intervention will have minimal impact if adverse living and working conditions are not addressed. Attention to patterns of ill health among patients and to issues in communities or populations helps identify factors that influence health.

2. What the Health Advocate Role looks like in daily practice

In day-to-day practice, the Health Advocate Role closely supports the Medical Expert Role. These two roles are intertwined, which can make the Health Advocate Role difficult to recognize.

Explain to your learners that it is often during the one-on-one conversation with a patient about issues related to assessments and therapies that the physician can learn about the patient's needs and also strengths (important to look from a strength model rather than always from a place of deficit- this makes things easier), and the impact of these needs on their health. Health advocacy begins when a physician and a patient work together to identify the gap between the patient's health goals and the patient's current situation.

If your learners are struggling to grasp some of these concepts, encourage them to listen for some of the words in Table HA-1, which can be associated with being a health advocate and with demonstrating health advocacy in day-to-day practice.

When they hear or use these words and phrases, they can be relatively confident that they are functioning within the Health Advocate Role of the CanMEDS Framework.

TABLE HA-1. TRIGGER WORDS RELATING TO THE CONTENT AND PROCESS OF THE HEALTH ADVOCATE ROLE

Trigger words relating to the PROCESS of the Health Advocate Role:		Trigger words relating to the CONTENT of the Health Advocate Role:	
• Advise	• Justify	• Access	• Policy
• Assist	• Liaise	• Barriers	• Poverty
• Empower	• Navigate	• Competing needs	• Prevention
• Encourage	• Negotiate	• Health behaviours	• Risk factor modification
• Facilitate	• Recommend	• Health literacy	• Safety
• Influence	• Support	• Health promotion	• Social environment
		• Literacy	• Surveillance

© 2015 Royal College of Physicians and Surgeons of Canada

Health Advocate

Excerpt from the CanMEDS 2015 Physician Competency Framework[a]

DEFINITION

As Health Advocates, physicians contribute their expertise and influence as they work with communities or patient populations to improve health. They work with those they serve to determine and understand needs, speak on behalf of others when required, and support the mobilization of resources to effect change.

DESCRIPTION

Physicians are accountable to society and recognize their duty to contribute to efforts to improve the health and well-being of their patients, their communities, and the broader populations they serve.[b] Physicians possess medical knowledge and abilities that provide unique perspectives on health. Physicians also have privileged access to patients' accounts of their experience with illness and the health care system.

Improving health is not limited to mitigating illness or trauma, but also involves disease prevention, health promotion, and health protection. Improving health also includes promoting health equity, whereby individuals and populations reach their full health potential without being disadvantaged by, for example, race, ethnicity, religion, gender, sexual orientation, age, social class, economic status, or level of education.

Physicians leverage their position to support patients in navigating the health care system and to advocate with them to access appropriate resources in a timely manner. Physicians seek to improve the quality of both their clinical practice and associated organizations by addressing the health needs of the patients, communities, or populations they serve. Physicians promote healthy communities and populations by influencing the system (or by supporting others who influence the system), both within and outside of their work environments.

Advocacy requires action. Physicians contribute their knowledge of the determinants of health to positively influence the health of the patients, communities, or populations they serve. Physicians gather information and perceptions about issues, working with patients and their families[c] to develop an understanding of needs and potential mechanisms to address these needs. Physicians support patients, communities, or populations to call for change, and they speak on behalf of others when needed. Physicians increase awareness about important health issues at the patient, community, or population level. They support or lead the mobilization of resources (e.g. financial, material, or human resources) on small or large scales.

Physician advocacy occurs within complex systems and thus requires the development of partnerships with patients, their families and support networks, or community agencies and organizations to influence health determinants. Advocacy often requires engaging other health care professionals, community agencies, administrators, and policy-makers.

KEY COMPETENCIES

Physicians are able to:

1. Respond to an individual patient's health needs by advocating with the patient within and beyond the clinical environment.

2. Respond to the needs of the communities or populations they serve by advocating with them for system-level change in a socially accountable manner.

---

a Sherbino J, Bonnycastle D, Côté B, Flynn L, Hunter A, Ince-Cushman D, Konkin J, Oandasan I, Regehr G, Richardson D, Zigby J. *Health Advocate*.
b In the *CanMEDS 2015 Physician Competency Framework*, a "community" is a group of people and/or patients connected to one's practice, and a "population" is a group of people and/or patients with a shared issue or characteristic.
c Throughout the *CanMEDS 2015 Physician Competency Framework and Milestones Guide*, references to the patient's family are intended to include all those who are personally significant to the patient and are concerned with his or her care, including, according to the patient's circumstances, family members, partners, caregivers, legal guardians, and substitute decision-makers.

KEY TERMS OF THE HEALTH ADVOCATE ROLE

Determinants of health are the social and physical factors that impact the health outcomes of people and populations (e.g. the conditions in which we live and work).[2,3] Learners who understand the determinants of health understand that the health of individuals is closely related to the broader community and environmental context in which they live.[4]

The U.S. Office of Disease Prevention and Health Promotion and the Social Determinants of Health: The Canadian Facts website provide the following examples:[2,3]

Examples of *social determinants of health* include:

- Availability of resources to meet daily needs, such as educational and job opportunities, living wages, or healthful foods;

- Social norms and attitudes, such as discrimination;

- Exposure to crime, violence, and social disorder, such as the presence of trash;

- Social support and social interactions;

- Exposure to mass media and emerging technologies, such as the Internet or cell phones;

- Socio-economic conditions, such as concentrated poverty;

- Quality schools;

- Transportation options;

- Public safety;

- Residential segregation.

Examples of *physical determinants of health* include:

- Natural environment, such as plants, weather, or climate change;

- Built environment, such as buildings or transportation;

- Work sites, schools, and recreational settings;

- Housing, homes, and neighbourhoods;

- Exposure to toxic substances and other physical hazards;

- Physical barriers, especially for people with disabilities;

- Aesthetic elements, such as good lighting, trees, or benches.

3. Preparing to teach the Health Advocate Role

The Health Advocate Role is one of the CanMEDS Roles where learners (and teachers) struggle to understand how it applies to their day-to-day practice, because the word 'advocate' conjures the notion of valiant individual social action working against some injustice or charity work. Here we review common misconceptions about the Role and suggest how to integrate the content and process of health advocacy into practice.

3.1 Common misconceptions to address with learners

There are three misconceptions about the Role that you may need to clear up with your learners. First, your learners may need guidance in understanding the Health Advocate Role as advocacy **with** the patient,[5] rather than **for** the patient. **Advocacy is not an action of an individual physician; rather, it is a shared process done in collaboration with the patient and with other health care providers or individuals.** Although physicians hold a privileged position in society that allows them to uniquely champion the needs of their patients, it is important to remember that it is the patient who determines those needs.[6] The perspective of a physician should be "How can I help?"

Second, learners may define the Health Advocate Role through too narrow a lens. At the start, learners may associate advocacy with activism (i.e. efforts to change the system via large-scale or population-level initiatives, such as initiatives to prevent head injuries in sports). While advocacy at the population level is an essential role for the profession to undertake, the prospect of incorporating such activism into regular, everyday practice may be daunting for clinicians and learners. **Many clinicians will identify more readily with "agency," which entails working within the system day to day to meet the health needs of a specific patient or community** (e.g. ensuring that a child from an impoverished neighbourhood gets access to speech therapy).

Finally, learners may need advice on how to balance their role as health advocates with their responsibility to steward the resources of the health care system wisely (i.e. in their role as leaders). All of the CanMEDS Roles have areas of overlap. However, **an explicit discussion using discipline-specific examples will help learners navigate the overlap in interests between the competencies of the Health Advocate Role and the stewardship competencies of the Leader Role.**

© 2015 Royal College of Physicians and Surgeons of Canada

Health Advocate

3.2 Health advocacy: integrating content and process

Health Advocate competencies will benefit from purposeful use of a structured approach. Introduce your learners to a process for health advocacy by discussing the steps they can work through with their patients or with a community or population.

KEY PROCESS STEPS THAT WILL HELP LEARNERS ADVOCATE:

1. Establish an understanding of the patient's (or community/population's) preferences, needs, strengths, and values for health care.

2. Collaborate with the patient, other health care professionals, and/or health promotion organizations.

3. Develop the action plan with the patient, other health care professionals, and/or health promotion organizations to help the patient achieve his or her self-identified goals.

4. Implement (i.e. by supporting, following, or on occasion leading, as appropriate) the agreed-to plan.

5. Maintain open communication with the patient, other health care professionals, and/or health promotion organizations.

Help your learners understand the content that may arise in day-to-day health advocacy scenarios and the activities related to the Health Advocate competencies. Table HA-2 provides examples of day-to-day situations in which advocacy with patients might be needed. Learners should watch for opportunities to:

- work with patients to address determinants of health that affect them and their access to needed health care services or resources;

- work with patients and their families to increase opportunities to adopt healthy behaviours; and

- incorporate disease prevention, health promotion, and health surveillance activities into interactions with individual patients.

4. Hints, tips and tools for *teaching* the Health Advocate Role

As a teacher your goal is to deliver the right content and in a way that helps your residents learn. Sometimes you will teach directly. Other times you will facilitate and support the teaching of others or self-directed activities by learners. There are parts of the Health Advocate Role that can be especially difficult for learners to relate to and understand in the context of their work. For this reason this section of the Tools Guide includes a short menu of tips and tricks that are highly effective for teaching the Health Advocate Role. You can treat the list as a buffet: pick and choose the tips that resonate most and that will work for you, your program and your learners.

Teaching Tip 1.
Provide explicit orientation information and resources about the most frequent health advocacy needs of the patients, the community, or populations your learners serve

Teach the basics of the top three (or five) most common health advocacy needs and prevention/promotion/surveillance activities for your discipline in your specific clinical context. For efficiency, formalize the content related to these needs and activities as you teach a new group of learners. You can quickly orient learners to effective options by assembling key resources for them and introducing them to key individuals (e.g. bed planners, social workers, nurse managers, community outreach workers) and organizations. Using case examples, alert learners to the "signs and symptoms" that indicate advocacy needs.

Some obvious examples of advocacy at the bedside are facilitating timely access to a test or medication, ensuring appropriate consultation, and facilitating understanding of specific approaches or protocols for a given rotation, clinical setting, or organization. Other examples of advocacy are ensuring adequate housing for a patient, evaluating with a patient the benefits and harms of health screening, identifying patients or populations not being optimally served in clinical practice, and working with a community or population to address the determinants of health that affect them.

© 2015 Royal College of Physicians and Surgeons of Canada

Health Advocate

TABLE HA-2. HEALTH ADVOCACY IN COMMON CLINICAL SCENARIOS

Scenario	Health Advocate Activity		
	Work with patients to address determinants of health that affect them and their access to needed health care services or resources.	Work with patients and their families to increase opportunities to adopt healthy behaviours.	Incorporate disease prevention, health promotion, and health surveillance activities into interactions with individual patients.
An elderly woman is admitted to hospital with a stroke.	At the time of discharge you work with the patient and the community social worker to ensure the patient has a personal support worker who will assist her during a transitional period of convalescence to achieve her goals for independent daily living.	It becomes apparent that the patient is taking her blood pressure medications irregularly. The patient says medication side effects affect their ability to take medications, but she is also concerned that her medication compliance may have contributed to her stroke. You ask a family member to reconcile all of the medications the patient has at home and you flag any medication interactions for side effects. With the patient, you develop an appropriate ongoing medication schedule. During successive conversations with the patient and her family, you develop a shared commitment to the consistent use of medications.	During the standardized discharge planning process the patient is identified as being at high risk for falls on the basis of her age and medical history. Before discharge you arrange physiotherapy and occupational therapy consultations to assess the patient for fall risk, and you offer suggestions to mitigate any risk.
A patient with long-standing mental illness has a new diagnosis of diabetes and requires assistance with foot care.	When you talk with the patient about the care plan, he indicates that he cannot access a chiropodist (podiatrist). You arrange an appointment at a wound care clinic that provides chiropody. You recommend in your consultation letter to his family doctor that an application for medical transport services be made.	You work with the patient, his partner, and his social worker to come up with solutions to his identified concern that his limited financial resources make it difficult for him to afford both his prescribed medications and a healthy, balanced diet. Support via agency funding and access to a local food bank is arranged.	As a result of your interaction with the patient, you incorporate into your medical record template a question about financial resources. This question assists in the early identification of patients who may not be able to afford all treatment recommendations and more broadly those patients whose financial status (or lack of income) affect their health.

Teaching Tip 2.
Help learners start a conversation about health advocacy

Effective communication skills are essential to advocating with (or, when necessary, on behalf of) a patient. Physicians must be able to make their patients comfortable enough to reveal their concerns; they must be able to inspire and support their patients to act; and they must be able to convince others to contribute to resolving problems that impact their patients.

Remind your learners to ask the patient if they need advocacy. For example, the physician could say, "We've talked about what your options are and you've decided that you want to do A, B, and then C. Is there anything that could slow you down in getting A, B, and then C done that we need to sort out before we move forward?" It is possible that the patient will identify barriers that need the physician's consideration and assistance to resolve — in other words, items that will take additional time or will require the assistance of other professionals or organizations. However, it is more effective to know and manage the barriers at the beginning of care than to assume that no barriers exist and then have to deal with them later.

Health behaviour change can be a particularly challenging context for communication. Learners may be reluctant to talk to patients about adopting healthy behaviours for fear of sounding paternalistic. One effective approach to introducing this conversation is to ask the patient to identify a health behaviour he or she wants to address. However, the physician must explore whether there are physical and socio-economic factors that might hinder a potential change in health behaviour. For example, the patient may identify high serum cholesterol as the health issue to be addressed, but poverty and limited access to nutritious food may be the root cause of the unhealthy diet that led to this issue.

© 2015 Royal College of Physicians and Surgeons of Canada

Teaching Tip 3.
Model health advocacy

Learners watch faculty and try to model what faculty do well and avoid what they do not do well. Help learners deconstruct when faculty are successful at supportive, educative, non-judgmental health advocacy activities. Acknowledge that much health advocacy occurs without direct input from faculty. Cue learners to the advocacy work of other health care professionals as they work with patients. Remember, the hidden curriculum (i.e. the implicit messages of action or inaction) has a powerful influence on your learners.

Teaching Tip 4.
Be explicit and acknowledge out loud — in other words, signpost — when you start to act as an advocate in the patient's journey through the health care system

Health advocacy is best learned in the clinical setting in real time. The concepts of health advocacy (e.g. determinants of health) can be taught around a seminar table, but health advocacy is best modelled, observed, and practised in day-to-day clinical activities.

Learners benefit from witnessing the "inside the head," back-and-forth tensions and dilemmas of health advocacy, being exposed to various points of view, and seeing that there is usually no perfect answer, just the best answer for this patient with these needs and strengths at this time and place.

During case rounds or at the bedside, make learners aware when you are moving from being a Medical Expert problem solver to being a Health Advocate. Advocacy is about physicians providing a unique biomedical perspective (among many other perspectives) on an issue and then working collaboratively to help a patient (or community or population) reach their goal.

Be explicit in telling learners how and where you make choices as an experienced clinician in balancing the need to advocate with one patient with the need to manage many patients in a health care system with finite resources. This is the most effective way for learners to get to know what drives the choices made about an individual patient and when it is appropriate to engage or refer to broader systems solutions (e.g. committees and groups).

Sometimes faculty will try to shield trainees from the messiness of advocacy: the phone calls, discussions, and back and forth that are part of supporting a patient who is navigating the health care system. However, learners need to be exposed to these things and coached to become progressively more active in appropriate advocacy activities (e.g. filling in funding forms, problem-solving patient priorities for diagnostic tests).

Teaching Tip 5.
Help learners recognize the advocacy needs of a community or population

Sometimes learners notice patterns of disease or need among patients on their own. At other times they need to participate in purposeful activities that help them recognize or explore patterns so they can identify a "systems" issue that would benefit from action to improve the health of a community or population. This could be done during a semi-annual meeting with a program or clinical director in the course of a high-level discussion about their inventory of patients, problems, interventions, and outcomes. Sources of information might include case logs, practice analysis information, or electronic medical record summaries, with appropriate safeguards to ensure patient privacy. Examples might include a pattern of adverse events with care, or delays to an aspect of treatment.

Teaching Tip 6.
Create conditions for learners to act as an advocate with a community or population

When a pattern of the same or similar health advocacy needs emerges among a number of patients, you can work with your trainees to explore if, how, when, and where health challenges or barriers to care might be generally improved. Caution learners about rushing in to solve a problem without consulting the community or population or without understanding the other individuals or organizations already working to address the issue. Learners will benefit from opportunities you can facilitate for them to contribute their expertise and energy to local health organizations, communities, or populations. Examples include reviewing hospital patient-education resources, guest speaking to patient groups, and becoming involved in policy development related to health promotion, prevention, and surveillance. Learners could also complete electives with vulnerable patient populations or work with leaders in health advocacy or with health promotion organizations.

Health Advocate

Sample teaching tools

You can use the sample *Teaching Tools for Health Advocate* at the end of this section as is, or you can modify or use them in various combinations to suit your objectives, time allocated, sequence within your residency program, and so on.

Easy-to-customize electronic versions of the *Teaching Tools for Health Advocate* (in .doc, .ppt and .pdf formats) are found at: canmeds.royalcollege.ca

The tools provided are:

- T1 Lecture or Large Group Session: Foundations of the Health Advocate Role

- T2 Presentation: Teaching the Health Advocate Role

- T3 Guided Reflection and Discussion: Recognizing health advocacy

- T4 Small Group Learning: Inventorying and evaluating your health advocacy

- T5 Guided Reflection and Discussion: Health advocacy resources

- T6 Case Report: Preparing a case report on health advocacy habits

- T7 Tools and Strategies: Summary sheet for the Health Advocate Role

5. Hints, tips and tools for *assessing* the Health Advocate Role

Assessment for learning is a major theme in this CanMEDS Tools Guide and a growing emphasis in medical education. You can and should use assessment as a strategy to inform a resident's learning plan (e.g. to alert or signpost to learners what is important to learn as well as what and how they will be assessed). This section of the Health Advocate chapter offers a number of hints to help you develop a program of assessment that will ensure that both teachers and learners have a clear understanding of their performance and what needs improvement.

Assessment Tip 1.

Assess the Role in the clinical setting with the help of other health care professionals

Health advocacy involves the physician, patient, and many health care professionals. Much of the patient advocacy with which learners are involved is not performed under the direct observation of faculty, however. To accurately assess the process and outcomes of learners' health advocacy, elicit input and feedback from team members using multisource feedback (MSF) forms or daily encounter forms[d], or by asking for input for the interim or end-of-session in-training evaluation (ITER) form.

Assessment Tip 2.

Include health advocacy in case presentations, case reports, and rounds

In day-to-day cases, provide feedback, coaching, and formative assessments to learners about met or missed opportunities to advocate for resources; work with patients and families on adopting healthy behaviours; and incorporate prevention, promotion, and surveillance appropriate to your specific clinical practice. Prompt learners to think about how they might deal with issues that recur in a series of patients.

Assessment Tip 3.

Assess how well your learners are balancing the need for health advocacy with the reality of finite resources and the need to provide equitable access to health care

Health advocacy is contextual and requires reflection. Advocacy is challenging because the correct answer is "it depends."

Learners benefit from taking time to order their thoughts, values, and views as they briefly describe the elements influencing their advocacy with a patient, community, or population. They can ask themselves such questions as: What was the issue? Why was advocacy needed? Who was involved? Whose goals are we working toward? How did the patient identify his or her goals? How successful was the advocacy? What could be better done next time? What are the broader systems solutions or resources required? Did the advocacy for this patient mean that I had less time to spend with another patient? Was the advocacy a wise use of resources and time given other patients' needs?

This reflection about advocacy can be captured during a formative discussion in the clinical environment, submitted as a report for marking against a standard rubric, or integrated into a practice oral exam.

---

d For a sample MSF or daily encounter form, see the Assessment Tool at the end of the Health Advocate section.

© 2015 Royal College of Physicians and Surgeons of Canada

Sample assessment tools

You can use the sample *Assessment Tools for Health Advocate* found at the end of this section as is, or you can modify or use them in various combinations depending on your objectives, time allocated, sequence within your residency program, and so on.

Easy-to-customize electronic versions of the *Assessment Tools for Health Advocate* (in .doc, .ppt and .pdf formats) are found at: canmeds.royalcollege.ca

The tools provided are:

- A1 Multisource Feedback: Health Advocate multi-source feedback

- A2 Written Questions and Answers: Short-answer and essay questions for the Health Advocate Role

- A3 Objective Structured Clinical Exam (OSCE): for the Health Advocate Role

- A4 Essay Assignment: Health Advocate essay assignment on clinical experiences

6. Suggested resources

- **Dobson S, Voyer S, Hubinette M, Regehr G. From the clinic to the community: the activities and abilities of effective health advocates. *Acad Med.* 2015;90(2):214–20.** This study describes a range of health advocacy activities that can be regularly incorporated into the clinical practice of most physicians. It suggests additional activities that might be achieved by physicians with additional training or interest in advocacy.

- **Dobson S, Voyer S, Regehr G. Perspective: agency and activism: rethinking health advocacy in the medical profession. *Acad Med.* 2012;87(9):1161–4.** This commentary suggests that there are two distinct elements to advocacy: agency (i.e. "working the system") and activism (i.e. "changing the system").

- **Hubinette M, Dobson S, Voyer S, Regehr G. 'We' not 'I': health advocacy is a team sport. *Med Educ.* 2014;48(9):895–901.** This study suggests that effective health advocates are not stand-alone experts; rather, they work in collaboration with other individuals and organizations.

- **Stafford S, Sedlak T, Foc MC, Wong RY. Evaluation of resident attitudes and self-reported competencies in health advocacy. *BMC Med Educ.* 2010;10:82.** This study describes a decrease in involvement in health advocacy activities among residents after they begin residency training and identifies barriers that limit their active participation.

VIDEOS ON THE DETERMINANTS OF HEALTH:

- "'If you want to help me, prescribe me money': toward a radical rethinking of social issues in medical care." Dr. Gary Bloch presents poverty as a disease and shares how to work with patients to manage poverty and improve their health. https://www.youtube.com/watch?v=FLRT0bvaz98

- "A healthy society." Dr. Ryan Meili discusses the connection between determinants of health and health outcomes and makes the case for our social agenda to be driven by the determinants of health. https://www.youtube.com/watch?v=c78GnlSHKvM

- "What makes us get sick? Look upstream." Dr. Rishi Manchanda discusses how living and working conditions impact a patient's health and how attending to upstream issues like a poor diet, a stressful job, and a lack of fresh air can improve health. http://www.ted.com/talks/rishi_manchanda_what_makes_us_get_sick_look_upstream

7. Other resources

- Dharamsi S, Ho A, Spadafora SM, Woollard R. The physician as health advocate: translating the quest for social responsibility into medical education and practice. *Acad Med.* 2011; 86(9):1108–13.

- Flynn L, Verma S. Fundamental components of a curriculum for residents in health advocacy. *Med Teach.* 2008;30(7):e178–83.

- Hubinette M, Ajjawi R, Dharamsi S. Family physician preceptors' conceptualizations of health advocacy: implications for medical education. *Acad Med.* 2014;89(11):1502–9.

Health Advocate

8. HEALTH ADVOCATE ROLE DIRECTORY OF TEACHING AND ASSESSMENT TOOLS

You can use the sample ***teaching and assessment tools for the Health Advocate Role*** found in this section as is, or you can modify or use them in various combinations to suit your objectives, the time allocated, the sequence within your residency program, and so on. Tools are listed by number (e.g. T1), type (e.g. Lecture), and title (e.g. Foundations of the Health Advocate Role).

Easy-to-customize electronic versions of the sample ***teaching and assessment tools for the Health Advocate Role*** in .doc, .ppt and .pdf formats are found at: <u>canmeds.royalcollege.ca</u>

TEACHING TOOLS

ASSESSMENT TOOLS

Health Advocate

© 2015 Royal College of Physicians and Surgeons of Canada

T1. FOUNDATIONS OF THE HEALTH ADVOCATE ROLE

Created for the *CanMEDS Teaching and Assessment Tools Guide* by S. Glover Takahashi. Reproduced with permission of the Royal College.

This learning activity includes

- Presentation: Foundations of health advocacy

Instructions for Teacher:
Sample learning objectives

- Guided reflection and discussion: Recognizing health advocacy in day-to-day practice (T3)

- Small group learning: Inventorying and evaluating your health advocacy in day-to-day practice (T4)

- Guided reflection and discussion: Health advocacy resources for use in day-to-day practice (T5)

Instructions for Teacher:
Sample learning objectives:

1. Recognize common words related to the process and content of health advocacy.

2. Apply key health advocacy steps to examples from day-to-day practice.

3. Develop a personal health advocacy resource for common patient needs.

Audience: All learners.

How to adapt:

- Consider whether your session's objectives match the sample ones. Select from, modify, or add to the sample objectives as required.

- The sample PowerPoint presentation is generic and foundational and tied to simple objectives. Consider whether you'll need additional slides to meet your objectives. Modify, add or delete questions as appropriate to include specific information related to your discipline and context.

- Depending on whether you are using these materials in one session (e.g. Health Advocacy basics workshop) or a series of two to four academic half days will determine which teaching activities you select and in what sequence.

- You may wish to review and customize the Health Advocate Summary Sheet (e.g. most frequent health advocacy needs in different locations or among different patient populations) with your learners as an additional activity.

Logistics:

- Select one or two teaching activities for each teaching session.

- Plan for about 20 minutes for each activity: this time will be used for you to explain the activity and for your learners to complete the worksheet individually, share their answers with their small group, discuss, prepare to report back to the whole group, and then deliver their small group's report to the whole group.

- Allow individuals to read the worksheet and spend about five minutes working on the answers on their own before starting to work in groups. This allows each person to develop his or her own understanding of topic.

- Depending on the group and time available, you may wish to assign one or more worksheets as homework to be completed before the session or as a follow-up assignment.

- Depending on the group and time available, you may also wish to explore the Specialty Training Requirements (STRs) or work through applying the teaching tips and/or the assessment tips to the specialty or program. See the Royal College website for STRs.

Setting:

- This information is best done in a small-group format (i.e. less than 30 learners) if possible. It can also be effectively done with a larger group if the room allows for learners to be at tables in groups of five or six. With larger groups, it is helpful to have additional teachers or facilitators available to answer questions arising from the worksheet activities.

Health Advocate

© 2015 Royal College of Physicians and Surgeons of Canada

T2. TEACHING THE HEALTH ADVOCATE ROLE

Created for the *CanMEDS Teaching and Assessment Tools Guide* by S. Glover Takahashi. Reproduced with permission of the Royal College.

Instructions for Teacher:

- Setting and Audience: Faculty and/or all learners
- How to use: Use as an orientation to the Role
- How to adapt:
  - Select only those slides that apply to your teaching objectives
  - Slides can be modified to match the specialty or the learners' practice context
- Logistics: Equipment — laptop, projector, screen

Slide #	Words on slide	Notes to teachers
1.	**Health advocacy**	• Add information about presenters. • Modify title as necessary.
2.	**Objectives and agenda** 1. Recognize common words related to the process and content of health advocacy. 2. Apply key health advocacy steps to examples from day-to-day practice. 3. Develop a personal health advocacy resource for common patient needs.	Sample goals and objectives of the session – revise as required. • Consider doing a warm-up activity before or after slide 2. • Review/revise goals and objectives. • Insert agenda slide if desired.
3.	**Why the Health Advocate Role matters** 1. Advocacy happens all the time. 2. Health advocacy is a team sport 3. Effective medical care requires disease prevention, health promotion, health protections and promotion of health equity.	• Reasons why this Role is important
4.	**The details: What is the Health Advocate Role?**[a] As Health Advocates, physicians contribute their expertise and influence as they work with communities or patient populations to improve health. They work with those they serve to determine and understand needs, speak on behalf of others when required, and support the mobilization of resources to effect change.	Definition from the CanMEDS 2015 Physician Competency Framework. • Avoid including competencies for learners. • If you are giving this presentation to teachers or planners, you may want to add the key and enabling competencies (provided as slides 18-20 below).
5.	**Determinants of health** • Determinants of health are the social and physical factors that impact the health outcomes of people and populations. • Learners who understand the determinants of health understand that the health of individuals is closely related to the broader community and environmental context in which they live.	• Insert definitions, descriptions, and URL • Determinants of health are the conditions in which we live and work that impact the health outcomes of people and populations. • Provide examples of social and physical determinants of health.
6.	**Recognizing health advocacy** **Processes** • Advise • Justify • Assist • Liaise • Empower • Navigate • Encourage • Negotiate • Facilitate • Recommend • Influence • Support	• Trigger words relating to the process of health advocacy

a   Sherbino J, Bonnycastle D, Côté B, Flynn L, Hunter A, Ince-Cushman D, Konkin J, Oandasan I, Regehr G, Richardson D, Zigby J. *Health Advocate*. In: Frank JR, Snell L, Sherbino J, editors. *CanMEDS 2015 Physician Competency Framework*. Ottawa: Royal College of Physicians and Surgeons of Canada; 2015. Reproduced with permission.

© 2015 Royal College of Physicians and Surgeons of Canada

Health Advocate

T2. TEACHING THE HEALTH ADVOCATE ROLE (continued)

Slide #	Words on slide	Notes to teachers
7.	**Recognizing health advocacy** **Content** • Access • Barriers • Competing needs • Health behaviours • Health promotion • Health literacy • Literacy • Policy • Poverty • Prevention • Risk factor modification • Safety • Social environment • Surveillance	• Trigger words relating to the content of health advocacy
8.	**What Health Advocacy is** • Advocacy is not an action of an individual physician; rather, it is a shared process done in collaboration with the patient and with other health care providers or individuals. • Many clinicians will identify with advocacy as "agency," which entails working within the system day to day to meet the health needs of a specific patient or community. • An explicit discussion using discipline-specific examples will help learners navigate the overlap in interests between the competencies of the Health Advocate Role and the stewardship competencies of the Leader Role.	• These are the 'answers' to the misconceptions
9.	**Guided reflection and discussion**	• T3: Guided Reflection and Discussion: Recognizing health advocacy in day-to-day practice
10.	**Key process steps in health advocacy** 1. Establish an understanding of the patient's preferences, needs, strengths, and values for health care. 2. Collaborate with the patient, other health care professionals, and/or health promotion organizations. 3. Develop the action plan with the patient, other health care professionals, and/or health promotion organizations to help the patient achieve their self-identified goals. 4. Implement the agreed-to plan (i.e. by supporting, following, or on occasion leading, as appropriate). 5. Maintain open communication with the patient, other health care professionals, and/or health promotion organizations.	Insert the five steps. • Explore each of the steps with the whole group. • Explore how to prepare for, act on, and evaluate each step in your specialty, based on experience — you can draw on either learners' or teachers' experience.
11.	**Putting health advocacy into action** 1. Advocacy for services or resources. 2. Advocacy for healthy behaviours. 3. Advocacy for prevention, promotion, surveillance.	• Consider focusing each session on one or two of the topics. • Consider focusing each session on one or a small number of patient issues. • Orient learners to these issues and explore them with the whole group.
12.	**Small group learning**	• T4: Small group learning: Inventorying and evaluating your health advocacy in day-to-day practice.
13.	**Health advocacy in day-to-day practice**	• Provide a personal example of when, where, and how to do health advocacy in day-to-day practice. • Offer hints and tips for success from your personal experience based on situations that went well for you, or offer personal lessons you learned from your missteps.
14.	**Guided reflection and discussion**	• T5: Guided Reflection and Discussion: Health advocacy resources for use in day-to-day practice

Health Advocate

© 2015 Royal College of Physicians and Surgeons of Canada

T2. TEACHING THE HEALTH ADVOCATE ROLE (continued)

Slide #	Words on slide	Notes to teachers
15.	**Tips for teaching health advocacy** 1. Provide resources about health advocacy needs of the communities and populations you serve. 2. Start a conversation about health advocacy. 3. Model health advocacy. 4. Signpost when you start to act as an advocate. 5. Help learners recognize advocacy needs. 6. Create opportunities for learners to act as advocates.	• Explore each of the hints with the whole group. • Explore how to prepare for, act on, and evaluate each hint in your specialty, based on experience.
16.	**Tips for assessing health advocacy** 1. Assess in a clinical setting with the help of other health professionals. 2. Include health advocacy in case presentations, case reports and rounds. 3. Assess how your learners are balancing the needs for health advocacy.	
17.	**Recap, revisiting objectives, and next steps**	• Revisit workshop goals and objectives
OTHER SLIDES		
18.	**Health Advocate Key Competencies**[a] ***Physicians are able to:*** 1. Respond to an individual patient's health needs by advocating with the patient within and beyond the clinical environment. 2. Respond to the needs of the communities or populations they serve by advocating with them for system-level change in a socially accountable manner.	Insert from *CanMEDS 2015 Physician Competency Framework*. • Avoid including competencies for learners. • You may wish to use this slide if you are giving the presentation to teachers or planners.
19.	**Health Advocate Key Competency**[a] ***Physicians are able to:*** 1. Respond to an individual patient's health needs by advocating with the patient within and beyond the clinical environment. 1.1 Work with patients to address determinants of health that affect them and their access to needed health services or resources. 1.2 Work with patients and their families to increase opportunities to adopt healthy behaviours. 1.3 Incorporate disease prevention, health promotion, and health surveillance into interactions with individual patients.	Insert from *CanMEDS 2015 Physician Competency Framework*. • Use one slide for each key competency and associated enabling competencies.
20.	**Health Advocate Key Competency**[a] ***Physicians are able to:*** 2. Respond to the needs of the communities or populations they serve by advocating with them for system-level change in a socially accountable manner. 2.1 Work with a community or population to identify the determinants of health that affect them. 2.2 Improve clinical practice by applying a process of continuous quality improvement to disease prevention, health promotion, and health surveillance activities. 2.3 Contribute to a process to improve health in the community or population they serve.	
21.	**Health advocacy for a community or population(s)**	• Consider focusing on one or a small number of examples if doing this with the whole group. • Offer hints and tips on success from your personal experience based on situations that went well, or offer personal lessons you learned from your missteps as a health advocate for a community or population. • Consider assigning this topic as a project that learners report back on. • Invite other community advocates or health care professionals to participate in the session.

Health Advocate *(sidebar)*

© 2015 Royal College of Physicians and Surgeons of Canada

T3. RECOGNIZING HEALTH ADVOCACY

Created for the *CanMEDS Teaching and Assessment Tools Guide* by S. Glover Takahashi.
Reproduced with permission of the Royal College.

See Health Advocacy Role teacher tips appendix for this teaching tool

Completed by:_____

1. Complete the table below, providing specific details from your clinical practice over the past month.

Clinical location (include details about when, where, how long, type of service)	**Community details about patients in this clinical location** (e.g. determinants of health)	**Common, frequent problems** (experienced by YOUR patients during this clinical experience)
1.		
2. (complete this second row if you practise at two different clinical locations)		

© 2015 Royal College of Physicians and Surgeons of Canada

Health Advocate

T3. RECOGNIZING HEALTH ADVOCACY (continued)

2. Think back to one or two specific patients from a clinical location from the table above and describe features of their need for health advocacy and/or your health advocacy actions. You may find the table of trigger words below useful.

Patient	Describe the **health needs** that this patient in this community or clinical location identified in collaboration with you	Describe the **health advocacy action(s)** that you and the health care team completed with this patient in this community or clinical location	What was the purpose of the action(s)?		
			To advocate for health care services or resources	To advocate for healthy behaviours	To incorporate disease prevention, health promotion, or health surveillance into the patient's care
"X"					
"Y"					

RECOGNIZE health advocacy when you are doing these actions		RECOGNIZE health advocacy when you are discussing these topics	
• Advise • Assist • Empower • Encourage • Facilitate • Influence	• Justify • Liaise • Navigate • Negotiate • Recommend • Support	• Access • Barriers • Competing needs • Health behaviours • Health literacy • Health promotion • Literacy	• Policy • Poverty • Prevention • Risk factor modification • Safety • Social environment • Surveillance

Health Advocate

© 2015 Royal College of Physicians and Surgeons of Canada

T4. INVENTORYING AND EVALUATING YOUR HEALTH ADVOCACY

Created for the *CanMEDS Teaching and Assessment Tools Guide* by S. Glover Takahashi.
Reproduced with permission of the Royal College.

See Health Advocacy Role teacher tips appendix for this teaching tool

Completed by:_____

1. Thinking back to your clinical experiences over the past two or three months, and using the table below, estimate the frequency, type, and appropriateness of your health advocacy activities.

PURPOSE of your health advocacy	Frequency of this type of health advocacy						Examples of this type of advocacy	Resources used for this type of advocacy	Rate the frequency of your advocacy on a scale of 1–5	Are there barriers to your advocating more often? If yes, how can you manage or overcome them?
	Many times a day	At least daily	Several times a week	Several times a month	Once or twice per month	Less than once per month			1 = can do better 3 = good enough 5 = terrific advocacy	
To advocate for health care services or resources										
To advocate for healthy behaviours										
To incorporate disease prevention, health promotion, or health surveillance into the patient's care										

Health Advocate

T4. INVENTORYING AND EVALUATING YOUR HEALTH ADVOCACY (continued)

2. In what areas of advocacy with patients are you most skilled?

_____

_____

_____

_____

_____

_____

_____

3. In what areas of advocacy with patients are you most comfortable?

_____

_____

_____

_____

_____

_____

_____

4. In what areas of advocacy with patients do you require improvement?

_____

_____

_____

_____

_____

_____

_____

© 2015 Royal College of Physicians and Surgeons of Canada

Health Advocate

T4. INVENTORYING AND EVALUATING YOUR HEALTH ADVOCACY (continued)

5. Rate your approach to health advocacy and provide examples using the table below.

Key steps to HEALTH ADVOCACY	In general, on a scale of 1–5, how well do you do this step?			Example(s) of when you did this well over the past few months	Example(s) of when you could have been more effective in doing this
	1 Can do better	3 Good enough	5 Strong at this step		
1. Establish an understanding of the patient's (or community or population's) preferences, needs, strengths, and values for health care.					
2. Collaborate with the patient, other health care professionals, and/ or health promotion organizations.					
3. Develop the action plan with the patient, other health care professionals, and/ or health promotion organizations to help the patient achieve their self-identified goals.					
4. Implement (i.e. by supporting, following, or on occasion leading, as appropriate) the agreed-to plan.					
5. Maintain open communication with the patient, other health care professionals, and/ or health promotion organizations.					

Health Advocate

© 2015 Royal College of Physicians and Surgeons of Canada

T4. INVENTORYING AND EVALUATING YOUR HEALTH ADVOCACY (continued)

6. Which step(s) of advocacy with patients are you most skilled at?

_____

_____

_____

_____

7. Which step(s) of advocacy with patients are you most comfortable with?

_____

_____

_____

_____

8. How did you balance your patient's health, preferences, needs, and values with the reality of finite resources and the need to ensure equitable access to health care?

_____

_____

_____

_____

9. How can you improve your skills at balancing health advocacy with a wise management of resources?

_____

_____

_____

_____

10. Do you have other observations or comments about health advocacy?

_____

_____

_____

_____

Health Advocate

© 2015 Royal College of Physicians and Surgeons of Canada

T5. HEALTH ADVOCACY RESOURCES

Created for the *CanMEDS Teaching and Assessment Tools Guide* by S. Glover Takahashi.
Reproduced with permission of the Royal College.

See Health Advocacy Role teacher tips appendix for this teaching tool

Completed by:_____

Information about and features of the clinical practice context

_____

_____

Features of the patient populations within this clinical practice environment

_____

_____

Most frequent and/or important health needs for this location/patient population	Resources for this location/patient population			
	Health team members who can help with this need (include contact information)	Organizations in community who can help with this need (include contact information)	Information resources (list brochures, handouts, websites, etc., and indicate where to find them)	Other resources

Other notes:

© 2015 Royal College of Physicians and Surgeons of Canada

Health Advocate

T6. PREPARING A CASE REPORT ON HEALTH ADVOCACY HABITS

Created for the *CanMEDS Teaching and Assessment Tools Guide* by S. Glover Takahashi.
Reproduced with permission of the Royal College.

See Health Advocacy Role teacher tips appendix for this teaching tool

Instructions for Learner:

- Observe and take (non-identifying) notes on your health advocacy activities in day-to-day practice.

- Remember to be cautious about privacy when taking notes.

- Review with faculty as arranged or initiate a review of your case reports to get feedback.

Completed by:_____

1. Descriptors of this clinical practice environment (e.g. clinical context, location, common health advocacy issues):

_____

_____

_____

2. Notes about observed cases at this location (MRP = most responsible physician)

#	Non-identifying description of patient	MRP for this case	Purpose(s) of health advocacy in this case	Which step(s) of health advocacy were done? How well was each step done?	Areas of strength for health advocacy in this case	Areas for improvement for health advocacy in this case	Other notes about health advocacy in this case
1.							
2.							

© 2015 Royal College of Physicians and Surgeons of Canada

T6. PREPARING A CASE REPORT ON HEALTH ADVOCACY HABITS (continued)

3. In this clinical environment, which individuals are part of the patient's team and are working with the patient and the MRP in health advocacy?

_____

_____

_____

_____

4. In this clinical environment, what are the resources for health advocacy?

_____

_____

_____

_____

5. Did you observe the need to balance the patient's health, preferences, needs, and values with the reality of finite resources and the need to provide equitable access to health care? If yes, describe briefly the choices you made to find that balance.

_____

_____

_____

_____

6. Did you notice any systems issues that would improve health outcomes with some effort or action? If yes, describe briefly how the improvement could be achieved.

_____

_____

_____

_____

7. Do you have any other observations or comments?

_____

_____

_____

_____

Health Advocate

T7. SUMMARY SHEET FOR THE HEALTH ADVOCATE ROLE

Created for the *CanMEDS Teaching and Assessment Tools Guide* by S. Glover Takahashi. Reproduced with permission of the Royal College.

See Health Advocate Role teacher tips appendix for this teaching tool

HEALTH ADVOCATE

- Advocacy is not an action of an individual physician; rather, it is a shared process done in collaboration with the patient and with other health care providers or individuals and often other organizations (eg community organizations).

- Many clinicians will identify with advocacy as "agency," which entails working within the system day to day to meet the health needs of a specific patient or community.

- An explicit discussion using discipline-specific examples will help learners navigate the overlap in interests between the competencies of the Health Advocate Role and the stewardship competencies of the Leader Role.

RECOGNIZE that you are moving to health advocacy when you are doing these actions

- Advise
- Assist
- Empower
- Encourage
- Facilitate
- Influence
- Justify
- Liaise
- Navigate
- Negotiate
- Recommend
- Support

RECOGNIZE that you are moving to health advocacy when you are discussing these topics

- Access
- Barriers
- Competing needs
- Health behaviours
- Health promotion
- Health literacy
- Literacy
- Policy
- Poverty
- Prevention
- Risk factor modification
- Safety
- Social environment
- Surveillance

KEY STEPS TO HEALTH ADVOCACY

1. Establish an understanding of the patient's (or community or population's) preferences, needs, strengths, and values for health care.

2. Collaborate with the patient, other health care professionals, and/or health promotion organizations.

3. Develop an action plan with the patient, other health care professionals, and/or health promotion organizations to help the patient achieve their self-identified goals.

4. Implement the agreed-to plan (i.e. by supporting, following, or on occasion leading as appropriate).

5. Maintain open communication with the patient, other health care professionals, and/or health promotion organizations.

HINTS ABOUT HEALTH ADVOCACY

1. Advocate with the patient, rather than for the patient.

2. Ask the patient if there are barriers to moving forward. Determine if/how you can assist.

3. Demonstrate interest in your patient's health, preferences, needs, values and strengths.

4. Balance your patient's health, preferences, needs, and values with the reality of finite resources and the need to provide equitable access to health care.

5. Watch for patterns among patients that might indicate "systems" issues that could benefit from your advocacy.

Health Advocate

© 2015 Royal College of Physicians and Surgeons of Canada

T7. SUMMARY SHEET FOR THE HEALTH ADVOCATE ROLE (continued)

HEALTH ADVOCATE RESOURCES

Location _____

Notes about this patient population

_____

_____

_____

Advocacy planning for this location

_____

_____

_____

Most frequent **advocacy needs** for this clinical location and/or patient population	**Resources** for this location and/or patient population (people, phone #, URL, etc.)
1.	1.
2.	2.
3.	3.
4.	4.
5.	5.

© 2015 Royal College of Physicians and Surgeons of Canada

Health Advocate

A1. HEALTH ADVOCATE MULTISOURCE FEEDBACK

Created for the *CanMEDS Teaching and Assessment Tools Guide* by S. Glover Takahashi. Reproduced with permission of the Royal College.

See Health Advocacy Role teacher tips appendix for this assessment tool

Instructions for Assessor:

- As Health Advocates, physicians contribute their expertise and influence as they work with communities or patient populations to improve health. They work with those they serve to determine and understand needs, speak on behalf of others when required, and support the mobilization of resources to effect change.

- The competencies of the Health Advocate Role can be developed with practice and feedback. Using the form below, please help this resident physician gain insight into his/her skills by providing valuable confidential feedback.

- Rest assured this information will be shared with the physician in aggregate form and for the purposes of helping the physician improve his/her leadership competencies.

- Please return this form in a sealed envelope marked confidential to the attention of:

_____

RESIDENT Name: _____

Postgraduate year (PGY): _____

Indicate ☑ all that apply. I am a:
- ☐ Health professional team member
- ☐ Resident
- ☐ Medical student (including clerk)
- ☐ Faculty
- ☐ Other _____

Degree of Interaction
- ☐ Considerable teaching from this resident
- ☐ ***Occasional or one time teaching*** from this resident

The resident...	1 Very poor	2 Needs improvement	3 Competent	4 Skilful	5 Exemplary	Not able to comment
A. Identifies health needs in a timely and appropriate manner (including advocacy for health services or resources, advocacy for healthy behaviours, and advocacy for prevention, promotion, or surveillance)						
B. Focuses on patient's health care needs, preferences, and values						
C. Collaborates with other health care professionals and/or health promotion organizations						
D. Works with patient (and their family)						
E. Balances health advocacy with stewardship of health care resources						

Comments:

Health Advocate

© 2015 Royal College of Physicians and Surgeons of Canada

A1. HEALTH ADVOCATE MULTISOURCE FEEDBACK (continued)

RESIDENT'S OVERALL PERFORMANCE[a]	1	2	3	4	5
	NEEDS SIGNIFICANT IMPROVEMENT	BELOW EXPECTATIONS	SOLID, COMPETENT PERFORMANCE	EXCEEDS EXPECTATIONS	SUPERB

Areas of strength	Areas for improvement
1.	1.
2.	2.
3.	3.

Comments:

---

a Programs that have moved to Competence by Design may want to modify the performance levels to the four parts of the resident competence continuum.

Health Advocate

A1. HEALTH ADVOCATE MULTISOURCE FEEDBACK (continued)

ASSESSOR SCORING NOTES

A. Identifies health advocacy needs in a timely and appropriate manner

1. Does not recognize the need for advocacy or the impact of barriers on current/future health status of the patient.

3. Addresses or responds to requests for intervention or action to manage barriers in a timely and appropriate manner. Will respond to patient's preferences and values when prompted.

5. Anticipates needs for advocacy through active dialogue with patient and team. Efficiently and sensitively identifies patient's needs, preferences, and values.

B. Focuses on patient's health needs, preferences, and values

1. Focuses on physician and or system needs and priorities. Alternatively, lets patient drive agenda regardless of appropriateness of expressed wants and preferences.

3. Attends to patient. Provides workman-like responses to patient's questions. Demonstrates care and attention to patient's needs, preferences, and values.

5. Skilfully anticipates patient's needs and questions. Responds with efficiency to patient's needs, preferences, and values. Negotiates, manages, and clarifies differences.

C. Collaborates with other health care professionals and/or health promotion organizations

1. Borders on rude or authoritarian or is overly deferential in approach.

3. Polite. Conveys information. Recognizes need for assistance. Communicates thoroughly, clearly, and in a timely fashion. Responsive to others' requests and feedback.

5. Synthesizes and prioritizes information. Provides comprehensive verbal and written communication. Leads, follows, coordinates, and delegates appropriately and respectfully. Negotiates and manages conflicts and differences.

D. Works with patient (and their family)

1. Does not inform patient/family of plans. Does not elicit patient/family wishes. Provides misinformation.

3. Elicits patient/family perspectives. Is respectful, establishes rapport, conveys patient/family concerns to team.

5. Consistently able to effectively communicate with patients/families. Skilled at sharing decision-making. Provides clear patient information. Confidently negotiates differences.

E. Balances health advocacy with stewardship of health care resources

1. Only focuses on one role or the other, losing perspective and not achieving best solution(s). Does not work with others to find solutions that balance competing issues.

3. Recognizes the need for balance. Seeks advice and assistance. With effort of self and others, implements solutions that balance competing issues.

5. Consistently able to efficiently and collaboratively balance competing issues, perspectives, and priorities so that parties come to consensus and/or accept solutions.

Health Advocate

© 2015 Royal College of Physicians and Surgeons of Canada

A2. SHORT-ANSWER AND ESSAY QUESTIONS FOR THE HEALTH ADVOCATE ROLE

Created for the *CanMEDS Teaching and Assessment Tools Guide* by J. Sherbino and S. Glover Takahashi. Reproduced with permission of the Royal College.

See Health Advocacy Role teacher tips appendix for this assessment tool

Name:_____

Date:_____

1. List five determinants of health.

_____

_____

_____

_____

_____

2. What are three main purposes (i.e. areas of influence) for health advocacy in day-to-day practice?

Purpose
1.
2.
3.

© 2015 Royal College of Physicians and Surgeons of Canada

Health Advocate

A2. SHORT-ANSWER AND ESSAY QUESTIONS FOR THE HEALTH ADVOCATE ROLE (continued)

3. Describe two examples from day-to-day practice in our discipline for each of the three purposes of health advocacy.

Purpose	Example of this from our specialty	Example of this from our specialty

4. List five resources (e.g. health care professionals, organizations, educational resources, etc.) that can assist you in advocating with patients in our discipline. Describe the role of each resource.

#	Resource	Role in our discipline
1.		
2.		
3.		
4.		
5.		

Health Advocate

© 2015 Royal College of Physicians and Surgeons of Canada

A2. SHORT-ANSWER AND ESSAY QUESTIONS FOR THE HEALTH ADVOCATE ROLE (continued)

ESSAY QUESTIONS

5. What are three challenges you face when balancing your patients' health, preferences, needs, and values with the reality of finite resources and the need to provide equitable access to health care?

_____

_____

_____

_____

6. Provide one example of a situation where you had to focus yourself or the team on the patient's health, preferences, needs, and values rather than your (i.e. the physician's) preferences, needs, and values, or those of the team.

_____

_____

_____

_____

7. Why do the determinants of health matter to our discipline?

_____

_____

_____

_____

8. Describe an example of the impact of determinants of health in our discipline.

_____

_____

_____

_____

9. Describe potential interventions to influence a determinant of health in our discipline.

_____

_____

_____

_____

Health Advocate

© 2015 Royal College of Physicians and Surgeons of Canada

A2. ANSWER KEY – SHORT ANSWER QUESTIONS

1. List five determinants of health.

   Determinants of health are the social and physical factors that impact the health outcomes of people and populations (e.g. the conditions in which we live and work). The health of individuals is closely related to the broader community and the environmental context in which we live.[a]

   The U.S. Office of Disease Prevention and Health Promotion provides the following examples:[b]

   Examples of **social determinants of health** include:
   - Availability of resources to meet daily needs, such as educational and job opportunities, living wages, or healthful foods;
   - Social norms and attitudes, such as discrimination;
   - Exposure to crime, violence, and social disorder, such as the presence of trash;
   - Social support and social interactions;
   - Exposure to mass media and emerging technologies, such as the Internet or cell phones;
   - Socio-economic conditions, such as concentrated poverty;
   - Quality schools;
   - Transportation options;
   - Public safety;
   - Residential segregation.

   Examples of **physical determinants of health** include:
   - Natural environment, such as plants, weather, or climate change;
   - Built environment, such as buildings or transportation;
   - Work sites, schools, and recreational settings;
   - Housing, homes, and neighbourhoods;
   - Exposure to toxic substances and other physical hazards;
   - Physical barriers, especially for people with disabilities;
   - Aesthetic elements, such as good lighting, trees, or benches.

2. What are three main purposes (i.e. areas of influence) for health advocacy in day-to-day practice?

   1. Advocate for health care services or resources.
   2. Advocate for healthy behaviours.
   3. Incorporate disease prevention, health promotion, or health surveillance into the patient's care.

3. Describe two examples from day-to-day practice in our discipline for each of the three purposes of health advocacy.

Purpose	Example of this in our specialty	Example of this in our specialty
1. Advocate for health care services or resources.		
2. Advocate for healthy behaviours.		
3. Incorporate disease prevention, health promotion, or health surveillance into the patient's care.		

Resources at each institution, site or program may be different than those at others. For this reason, teachers will need to identify appropriate answers and scoring for questions 4-9.

a   Raphael D. 2009. Social determinants of health: Canadian perspectives. 2nd ed. Toronto: Canadian Scholars' Press.
b   U.S. Office of Disease Prevention and Health Promotion. Determinants of health. Last retrieved May 4, 2015, from www.healthypeople.gov/2020/about/foundation-health-measures/Determinants-of-Health

Health Advocate

© 2015 Royal College of Physicians and Surgeons of Canada

A3. OBJECTIVE STRUCTURED CLINICAL EXAM (OSCE) FOR THE HEALTH ADVOCATE ROLE

Created for the *CanMEDS Teaching and Assessment Tools Guide* by S. Glover Takahashi and J Sherbino. Reproduced with permission of the Royal College.

Instructions for Assessor:

- *Learning objectives:* OSCE assessments are an effective way to assess if all of your learners are at, above or below a common standard. They will also provide insight as to who is meeting or exceeding in their understanding and application of Health Advocacy competencies, as well as who is falling behind.

- *How to use adapt:*

  - Select from, modify, or add to the sample OSCE cases. Each case is designed as a ten-minute scenario.

  - Modify these cases to be seven or eight minutes with the standardized patient (SP) and have two to three minutes of probing questions from faculty. The two to four probing questions within the scenario provide considerable additional insight into competence in the area.

  - Combine a variety of different Roles into the same exam.

  - Four to six cases is a reasonable number of cases for an in training program OSCE.

  - Consider using one scenario at a teaching session. Residents or SPs could do a demonstration.

  - Consider using a video recorded scenario for teaching purposes.

Scenario 1:

- A 39-year-old male Portuguese immigrant visits you <psychiatrist, family physician, physiatrist, neurologist, occupational health> for assessment and management of <depression OR pain management>.

- The patient does not have a strong command of English.

- About 18 months ago he sustained a work-related injury resulting in a complex regional pain syndrome in his non-dominant left arm. His application for disability insurance was recently denied.

- *You have <<XX (e.g. eight or ten minutes)>> for health advocacy with this patient.*

Scenario 2:

- A 17-year-old girl presents to the <emergency department, ambulatory pediatric clinic, family medicine clinic> with a soft tissue injury and abrasion to her forearm suffered when she fell off her bike.

- During your assessment it becomes apparent that she was not wearing her helmet because "helmets aren't cool."

- *You have <<XX (e.g. five or seven minutes)>> for health advocacy with this patient.*

Scenario 3:

- As a senior resident you have finished your first day running a busy <<internal medicine, orthopedics, family medicine>> ambulatory clinic.

- Over the course of seeing <<X>> patients it has become apparent that there is a surprising number of lower-extremity diabetic ulcers in the patient group. The ulcers are always an incidental or secondary complaint of patients.

- You are attending team rounds the next day, and the <<unit manager, risk management team, chief resident, physician lead>> asks if anyone has noted opportunities to improve patient care.

- *You have <<XX (e.g. eight or ten minutes)>> to discuss what you observed during your first day running the ambulatory clinic with the unit and the health advocacy considerations that arose from your experience.*

Health Advocate

A3. OSCE: SCENARIO 1 AND 2 SCORING SHEET

Learner's name: _____

Learner's program: _____

Learner's level: _____

HEALTH ADVOCATE: Identifies health needs in a timely and appropriate manner (including advocacy for health care services or resources, advocacy for healthy behaviours, and advocacy for prevention, promotion, or surveillance).

1	2	3	4	5
Does not accurately or appropriately recognize the need for advocacy or the impact of barriers on current/future health status of the patient.		Addresses and responds to need for intervention or action to manage barriers. Responsive to patient's noted preferences and values.		Demonstrates plans for active dialogue with patient and team. Efficiently and sensitively identifies patient's needs, preferences, and values.

HEALTH ADVOCATE: Focuses on patient's health care needs, preferences, and values.

1	2	3	4	5
Focuses on physician and/or system needs and priorities. Alternatively, lets patient drive agenda regardless of appropriateness of expressed wants and preferences.		Attends to patient. Provides workman-like response to questions. Demonstrates care and attention to patient's needs, preferences, and values.		Skilfully anticipates patient needs and questions. Responds with efficiency to patient's needs, preferences, and values. Negotiates, manages, and clarifies differences.

HEALTH ADVOCATE: Works with patient (and their family).

1	2	3	4	5
Does not inform patient/family of plans. Does not elicit patient/family wishes. Provides misinformation.		Elicits patient/family perspectives. Respectful. Establishes rapport.		Able to effectively communicate with patient/family. Skilled at sharing decision-making. Provides clear patient information. Confidently negotiates differences.

HEALTH ADVOCATE: Balances health advocacy with stewardship of health care resources.

1	2	3	4	5
Loses perspective and does not achieve best solution(s). Doesn't work to find solutions that balance competing issues.		Recognizes the need for balanced approach to stewardship and health advocacy. Seeks advice and input.		Generates effective solutions to balance competing issues, perspectives, and priorities so parties come to a consensus and/or accept solutions.

OVERALL PERFORMANCE IN THIS SCENARIO

1	2	3	4	5
Needs significant improvement	Below expectations	Solid, competent performance	Exceeds expectations	Sophisticated, expert performance

PGY LEVEL OF PERFORMANCE[a] – At what level of training was this performance?

B	1	2	3	4	5+
Below PGY1	Mid-PGY1	Mid-PGY2	Mid-PGY3	Mid-PGY4	Mid-PGY5 or above

---

a Programs that have moved to Competence By Design may want to modify these levels to the four parts of the resident competence continuum.

© 2015 Royal College of Physicians and Surgeons of Canada

Health Advocate

A3. OSCE: SCENARIO 1 AND 2 SCORING SHEET (continued)

Areas of strength	Areas for improvement
1.	
2.	
3.	

Comments:

_____

_____

_____

_____

_____

_____

_____

_____

Completed by: _____

Date: _____

© 2015 Royal College of Physicians and Surgeons of Canada

Health Advocate

A3. OSCE: SCENARIO 3 SCORING SHEET (continued)

Learner's name: _____

Learner's program: _____

Learner's level: _____

HEALTH ADVOCATE: Identifies community/population health needs in a timely and appropriate manner (includes advocacy for health care services or resources, advocacy for healthy behaviours, and advocacy for prevention, promotion, or surveillance).

1	2	3	4	5
Does not accurately or appropriately recognize the need for advocacy or the impact of barriers on current/future health status of patients. Seems unaware of determinants of health or their possible role.		Takes determinants of health approach. Initiates inventory of determinants. Provides good description of community/ population, including possible barriers and resources.		Has an effective and sophisticated understanding of determinants, this community, barriers, and resources.

HEALTH ADVOCATE: Collaborates with other health care professionals and/or health promotion organizations.

1	2	3	4	5
Borders on rude, authoritarian or is overly deferential in approach.		Polite. Conveys information. Recognizes need for assistance. Provides thorough, clear communication. Is responsive to requests for information. Integrates views of others.		Demonstrates an effective and sophisticated approach to joint problem-solving. Embraces alternate views and the contribution of others. Negotiates and manages conflicts and differences.

HEALTH ADVOCATE: Balances health advocacy with stewardship of health care resources.

1	2	3	4	5
Only focuses on one role or the other, losing perspective and not achieving best solution(s). Doesn't work to find solutions that balance competing issues.		Approach seems to recognize the need for balance. Seeks advice and assistance. Demonstrates understanding of competing issues.		Able to efficiently and collaboratively balance competing issues, perspectives, and priorities so parties come to consensus and/or accept solutions.

OVERALL PERFORMANCE IN THIS SCENARIO

1 Needs significant improvement	2 Below expectations	3 Solid, competent performance	4 Exceeds expectations	5 Sophisticated, expert performance

PGY LEVEL OF PERFORMANCE[a] – At what level of training was this performance?

B Below PGY1	1 Mid-PGY1	2 Mid-PGY2	3 Mid-PGY3	4 Mid-PGY4	5+ Mid-PGY5 or above

a Programs that have moved to Competence By Design may want to modify these levels to the four parts of the resident competence continuum.

Health Advocate

© 2015 Royal College of Physicians and Surgeons of Canada

A3. OSCE: SCENARIO 3 SCORING SHEET (continued)

Areas of strength	Areas for improvement
1.	
2.	
3.	

Comments:

_____

_____

_____

_____

_____

_____

_____

Completed by: _____

Date: _____

© 2015 Royal College of Physicians and Surgeons of Canada

Health Advocate

A4. HEALTH ADVOCATE ESSAY ASSIGNMENT ON CLINICAL EXPERIENCES

Created for the *CanMEDS Teaching and Assessment Tools Guide* by S. Glover Takahashi and J Sherbino. Reproduced with permission of the Royal College.

See Health Advocacy Role teacher tips appendix for this assessment tool

Prepare a 1,500-word report describing your health advocacy practice during your clinical experiences over the past two or three months. Focus on one or two specific cases of advocacy with a patient, or give one example of advocacy with a community or patient population.

Consider the following points:

- Describe your clinical experience, including details about the clinical context and type(s) of service.

- Describe the determinants of health influencing a patient or community you worked with.

- Describe common or frequent patient issues you encountered during this clinical experience.

- Describe how you participated as an advocate. Consider:
  1. Purpose
  2. Process
  3. Outcomes
  4. Areas for improvement

- **Scoring rubrica**[a]
  - 20% creativity
  - 20% evidence
  - 20% structure
  - 20% clarity
  - 20% mechanics

Deadlines

- A 250-word abstract outlining your paper is due by

  _____

  (one month before the final deadline)

- The paper is due via email by/before

  _____

---

a   Adapted from Appendix C: What are rubrics and how can we use them? In Ambrose SA, Bridges MW, DiPietro M, Lovett MC, Norman MK., eds. 2010. *How learning works: seven research-based principles for smart teaching.* San Francisco: Jossey-Bass;2010 231–43. Reproduced with permission.

© 2015 Royal College of Physicians and Surgeons of Canada

A4. HEALTH ADVOCATE ESSAY ASSIGNMENT: SCORING RUBRIC (continued)

Learner's name: _____

SCORING	Excellent	Competent	Not yet competent	Poor	YOUR PAPER Score and comments
Creativity (20%)	You exceed the parameters of the assignment, with original insights or a particularly engaging style.	You meet all the parameters of the assignment.	You meet most of the parameters of the assignment.	You do not meet the parameters of the assignment.	
Evidence (20%)	The evidence or theory you use to support your viewpoint or approach is specific, rich, and varied, and it unambiguously supports your claims. Quotations and illustrations are framed effectively and explicated appropriately in the text.	The evidence or theory you use to support your viewpoint or approach generally supports your claims. Quotations and illustrations are framed reasonably effectively and explicated appropriately in the text.	The evidence or theory you use to support claims is incomplete or conflicts with your viewpoint or approach. Some of the quotations and illustrations are not framed effectively or explicated appropriately in the text.	Little evidence or theory is used to support the viewpoint or approach outlined in your claims. Few of the quotations and illustrations are framed effectively or explicated appropriately in the text.	
Structure (20%)	Your ideas are presented in a logical and coherent manner throughout the paper, with strong topic sentences to guide the reader. The reader can effortlessly follow the structure of your argument.	The reader can follow the structure of your argument with very little effort.	The reader cannot always follow the structure of your argument.	The reader cannot follow the structure of your argument.	
Clarity (20%)	Your sentences are concise and well crafted, and the vocabulary is precise; the reader can effortlessly discern your meaning.	The reader can discern your meaning with very little effort.	The reader cannot always discern your meaning.	The reader cannot discern your meaning.	
Mechanics (20%)	There are no distracting spelling, punctuation, or grammatical errors, and all quotations are properly cited.	There are few distracting spelling, punctuations, and/or grammatical errors, and all quotations are properly cited.	There are some distracting spelling, punctuation, and/or grammatical errors, and/or some of the quotations are not properly cited.	There are significant and distracting spelling, punctuation, or grammatical errors, and/or the quotations are improperly cited.	
TOTAL					

Other comments:

© 2015 Royal College of Physicians and Surgeons of Canada

Health Advocate

HEALTH ADVOCATE ROLE TEACHER TIPS APPENDIX

T3 RECOGNIZING HEALTH ADVOCACY

Instructions for Teacher:

- Setting and Audience: All learners.
- How to use: Plan for about 20 minutes for the activity.
  - Allow individuals to read the questions and spend about five minutes working on the answers.
  - Compare and discuss answers in small groups.
  - Reporting back by group.
  - Summary of key points by faculty.
- How to adapt:
  - You may wish to assign the activity as homework to be completed before the session or as a follow-up assignment.
  - Select only those questions that apply to your teaching. Modify questions as appropriate to match the specialty or the learners' practice context.
- Logistics:
  - Copies of question sheets, flip chart paper.
  - Extra pens for learners.

T4 INVENTORYING AND EVALUATING YOUR HEALTH ADVOCACY

Instructions for Teacher:

- Setting and Audience: All learners.
- How to use: Plan for about 20 minutes for the worksheet.
  - Allow individuals to read the worksheet and spend about five minutes working on the answers.
  - Compare and discuss answers in small groups.
  - Reporting back by group.
  - Summary of key points by faculty.
- How to adapt:
  - You may wish to assign the worksheet as homework to be completed before the session or as a follow-up assignment.
  - Select only those questions that apply to your teaching. Modify questions as appropriate to match the specialty or the learners' practice context.
- Logistics:
  - Copies of worksheets, flip chart paper. Extra pens for learners.

T5 HEALTH ADVOCACY RESOURCES

Instructions for Teacher:

- Setting and Audience: All learners.
- How to use: Plan for about 20 minutes for the worksheet.
  - Allow individuals to read the worksheet and spend about five minutes working on the answers.
  - Compare and discuss answers in small groups.
  - Reporting back by group.
  - Summary of key points by faculty.
- How to adapt:
  - You may wish to assign the worksheet as homework to be completed before the session or as a follow-up assignment.
  - Select only those questions that apply to your teaching. Modify questions as appropriate to match the specialty or the learners' practice context.
- Logistics:
  - Copies of worksheets, flip chart paper. Extra pens for learners.

T6 PREPARING A CASE REPORT ON HEALTH ADVOCACY HABITS

Instructions for Teacher:

- This tool can be assigned for completion during a clinical experience, such as on one or more days or during a rotation.
- This tool could also be used as a portfolio submission.
- Indicate the number of case reports to be completed and if the case reports are to be done in the same location or during the same rotation.
- The deadline for completion should be established and circulated (e.g. posted in resident physical or virtual bulletin board).
- Reminders are helpful to ensure completion.
- The 'Summary Sheet' information would be important background materials to complete this assignment.
- After the case reports are completed and submitted, it is important to review and debrief, reinforce learning, focus areas for clarification or improvement
- Trainees can do a case report about faculty health advocacy and/or on their own case(s).

© 2015 Royal College of Physicians and Surgeons of Canada

HEALTH ADVOCATE ROLE TEACHER TIPS APPENDIX (continued)

T7 SUMMARY SHEET FOR THE HEALTH ADVOCATE ROLE

Instructions for Teacher:

- The summary sheet is intended to be a cheat sheet for the teacher as well as the learner. It is a one page resource on key concepts, frameworks and approaches.

A1 HEALTH ADVOCATE MULTISOURCE FEEDBACK

Instructions for Teacher:

- Modify the form by adding or removing criteria that do/do not apply.

- To optimize learning and to protect the identity of those who provide feedback, be mindful of the size and composition of your data sample.

- Be sure to provide your 'assessors' with clear instructions and provide guidance on your rating scale.

- It is a good idea to notify your learners of your intention and rationale for collecting feedback on their CanMEDS Health Advocate Role skills. Be clear about the timeframe when you will collect the data, how you will maintain confidentiality and how and when you will present the data back to the learner.

- Plan to share the summary of feedback with your learner in written format and in a face to face meeting. A face to face meeting will allow valuable coaching around areas of strength and areas for improvement.

A2 WRITTEN QUESTIONS AND ANSWERS: HEALTH ADVOCATE

Instructions for Teacher:

- *Learning objectives:* Written questions are an efficient way to assess if all of your learners are at, above or below a common standard. They will also provide insight as to who is meeting or exceeding expectations in their understanding and application of Health Advocacy concepts as well as who is falling behind.

- *Audience:* All learners.

- *How to use:* Select from, modify, or add to the sample questions as appropriate. If selecting all of these questions, we suggest that you allow 30-45 minutes to complete.

- *How to adapt:* Add these or similar questions to a written test (e.g. on own or include in semi-annual program written exam). You may wish to assign as homework to be completed before the session or as a follow-up assignment.

- *Logistics:* Suggest you provide in similar format to specialty exam (i.e. if specialty exam is paper and pencil, suggest you use same. This will allow for some orientation/training for specialty exam)

- *Setting:* Classroom.

A4 HEALTH ADVOCATE ESSAY ASSIGNMENT

Instructions for Assessor:

- *Learning objectives:* Essays allow learners to reflect and document their deep understanding on an important topic. It allows you to have an understanding of the learners' competencies in such areas as reflection skills, deep understanding of Health Advocacy, persuasive writing skills, and organizational skills. You will gain an understanding about which of your learners are at/above/below a common standard at the same point. You will also gain insight into who is meeting or exceeding in understanding and being able to apply Health Advocacy competencies, and who is behind or unclear.

- *Audience:* All learners.

- *How to use:* Select from, modify, or add to the essay assignment as appropriate.

- *How to adapt:* Could be project done in pairs or small groups (e.g. three learners). Add a ten minute presentation of their abstract with focused discussion at a teaching session so all learners can benefit from the diversity of assignments and topics.

- *Logistics:* Provide instructions and rubric in writing. Orient learners to the assignment. Allow eight weeks to complete, with abstract due in four weeks. This will allow for sufficient time to organize and complete high quality assignment. Completion of the abstract/preview of paper is an important opportunity for feedback and focusing of learners. Also provides insight to who may need additional support (e.g. second draft of abstract) to ensure they are on track.

- *Setting:* Classroom. Can be done via phone meetings or video classroom.

Health Advocate

© 2015 Royal College of Physicians and Surgeons of Canada

REFERENCES

1. Hubinette M, Dobson S, Voyer S, Regehr G. 'We' not 'I': health advocacy is a team sport. *Med Educ*. 2014;48(9):895–901. doi: 10.1111/medu.12523.

2. U.S. Office of Disease Prevention and Health Promotion. Determinants of health. Last retrieved May 4, 2015, from www.healthypeople.gov/2020/about/foundation-health-measures/Determinants-of-Health

3. *Social Determinants of Health: The Canadian Facts*. Last retrieved August 20, 2015, from http://www.thecanadianfacts.org

4. Raphael D. 2009. *Social determinants of health: Canadian perspectives*. 2nd ed. Toronto: Canadian Scholars' Press.

5. Hubinette M, Dobson S, Regehr G. Not just 'with' but 'for': health advocacy as a partnership process. *Med Educ*. In press.

6. Dobson S, Voyer S, Regehr G. Perspective: agency and activism: rethinking health advocacy in the medical profession. *Acad Med*. 2012;87(9):1161–4.

Health Advocate

© 2015 Royal College of Physicians and Surgeons of Canada

COACHING

Critical appraisal

Mentoring

FEEDBACK RESEARCHING

Monitoring **Learning plan**

EVIDENCE-INFORMED DECISION-MAKING

SCHOLAR

LIFELONG Scholarship

LEARNING

Assessing **Teaching**

Guided self-assessment

COMMUNITY OF PRACTICE

Continuing professional
development

Anna Oswald

Denyse Richardson

Susan Glover Takahashi

1. Why the Scholar Role matters

The Scholar Role is important to the CanMEDS Framework because of the critical importance of having up-to-date medical knowledge to inform a physician's practice decisions and delivery of care. Physician knowledge and expertise, which is central to the Scholar Role, underpin a physician's ability to provide advice and treatment for the care of patients who are unwell.

Orientation to the Scholar Role may take effort for some of your learners, particularly because the Scholar Role has multiple components. In fact, many learners tend to overlook parts of the Role because the competencies are not explicitly labeled as such during their learning. When introducing your learners to the Scholar Role, be sure to emphasize these five-overarching themes:

- Learning does not end (nor should it) for physicians. Learning is an active process during training and throughout practice. Strategies for effective learning, developing and maintaining competence are essential to one's practice, as are practical strategies for keeping up-to-date on the latest developments in one's practice.

- Teaching others is not only beneficial for the learners; it helps consolidate the information for the teacher – whether that teaching is to students, other residents, the public, health professionals or staff.[a]

- Medical education uses a practice-based education model where practitioners support the learning and mastery of learners. All residents and most physicians have some responsibilities for education, so they need specific support to be effective teachers and assessors.

- Being able to determine the validity of the 'evidence' is critical to a physician's expertise, as is being able to discern how and when to apply evidence to day-to-day clinical decisions. The pace of information growth means searching, sorting and selection skills are key for timely and effectively interpreted application of knowledge to day-to-day clinical decisions.

- Using new knowledge depends on the ability to understand and/or interpret research, which can be used to solve the problems and address the issues that are important to physicians, their patients and the health care system.

2. What the Scholar Role looks like in daily practice

Sometimes learners have trouble breaking down the behaviours and competencies of a physician into its component CanMEDS parts. Learners often find it helpful when a teacher takes the time to 'tag' the Roles for them. This tagging allows the learner to associate certain activities with particular CanMEDS Roles. This section provides a 'top line' look at how the Scholar Role functions and what learners would see in the Scholar Role in daily practice.

The Scholar Role is organized around the various responsibilities the physician has related to knowledge – enhancing, sharing and utilizing – that are done in the service of a patient and the health care system. In this Role there are four distinct parts:

- Enhancing professional activities throughout one's career through lifelong learning

- The sharing of knowledge through teaching and assessment

- The use of knowledge in evidence-informed decision-making

- Assisting in the application and production of knowledge through research or scholarly inquiry

In day-to-day practice, Scholar is linked to many Roles, but has connections to three Roles in particular:

- Scholar is intertwined with Medical Expert when making clinical decisions in day-to-day practice.

- Scholar competencies for lifelong learner and teacher are connected to Leader competencies; both emphasize self-awareness skills and the giving/receiving of feedback.

- Scholar overlaps with Collaborator, given that lifelong learning, teaching, critical appraisal and research are activities enhanced by collaboration.

When learners are able to identify physicians who are using Scholar competencies in their day-to-day practice they may notice that only some have official designations such as 'Educator', 'Scientist', 'Scholar' or 'Researcher'. If your learners are struggling to identify the concepts of the Scholar Role, encourage them to listen for some of the trigger words in Table S-1. This is a quick and easy trick for them to start to make the connection between daily activities and being a Scholar as described in the CanMEDS Framework.

---

a Teaching patients is found in Communicator

© 2015 Royal College of Physicians and Surgeons of Canada

TABLE S-1. TRIGGER WORDS RELATING TO THE PROCESS AND CONTENT OF THE SCHOLAR ROLE

Trigger words relating to the PROCESS of the Scholar Role:		Trigger words relating to the CONTENT of the Scholar Role:	
• Assessing	• Motivating	• Community of practice	• Lifelong learning
• Coaching	• Orienting	• Continuing competence	• Objectives
• Enhancing	• Providing feedback	• Critical appraisal	• Performance assessment
• Evaluating	• Researching	• Evidence	• Portfolio
• Maintaining	• Supervising	• Evidence-informed	• Scholarly inquiry
• Mentoring	• Teaching	• Goals	• Scholarship
• Monitoring		• Learning climate	• Scientific principles
		• Learning environment	• Self-directed learning/ guided self-directed learning
		• Learning plan	

Excerpt from the CanMEDS 2015 Physician Competency Framework[b]

DEFINITION

As Scholars, physicians demonstrate a lifelong commitment to excellence in practice through continuous learning and by teaching others, evaluating evidence, and contributing to scholarship.

DESCRIPTION

Physicians acquire scholarly abilities to enhance practice and advance health care. Physicians pursue excellence by continually evaluating the processes and outcomes of their daily work, sharing and comparing their work with that of others, and actively seeking feedback in the interest of quality and patient safety. Using multiple ways of learning, they strive to meet the needs of individual patients and their families[c] and of the health care system.

Physicians strive to master their domains of expertise and to share their knowledge. As lifelong learners, they implement a planned approach to learning in order to improve in each CanMEDS Role. They recognize the need to continually learn and to model the practice of lifelong learning for others. As teachers they facilitate, individually and through teams, the education of students and physicians in training, colleagues, co-workers, the public, and others.

Physicians are able to identify pertinent evidence, evaluate it using specific criteria, and apply it in their practice and scholarly activities. Through their engagement in evidence-informed and shared decision-making, they recognize uncertainty in practice and formulate questions to address knowledge gaps. Using skills in navigating information resources, they identify evidence syntheses that are relevant to these questions and arrive at clinical decisions that are informed by evidence while taking patient values and preferences into account.

Finally, physicians' scholarly abilities allow them to contribute to the application, dissemination, translation, and creation of knowledge and practices applicable to health and health care.

KEY COMPETENCIES

Physicians are able to:

1. Engage in the continuous enhancement of their professional activities through ongoing learning

2. Teach students, residents, the public, and other health care professionals

3. Integrate best available evidence into practice

4. Contribute to the creation and dissemination of knowledge and practices applicable to health

b Richardson D, Oswald A, Chan M-K, Lang ES, Harvey BJ. Scholar. In: Frank JR, Snell L, Sherbino J, editors. *CanMEDS 2015 Physician Competency Framework.* Ottawa: Royal College of Physicians and Surgeons of Canada; 2015. Reproduced with permission.
c Throughout the CanMEDS 2015 Physician Competency Framework and Milestone Guide, references to the patient's family are intended to include all those who are personally significant to the patient and are concerned with his or her care, including, according to the patient's circumstances, family members, partners, caregivers, legal guardian, and substitute decision-makers.

Scholar

KEY TERMS OF THE SCHOLAR ROLE

One way to help your learners familiarize themselves with the Scholar Role is to have them review key words that are important to the Scholar Role.

Continuing professional development[1] refers to physicians' professional obligation to engage in learning activities that address their identified needs, enhance knowledge, skills, and competencies across all dimensions of professional practice, and continuously improve their performance and healthcare outcomes within their scope of practice.

Lifelong learning includes three areas of focus:

1. **continuing health professions education** focuses on lifelong learning in all CanMEDS competencies.

2. **faculty development** focuses on lifelong learning for physicians with roles in teaching/education, leadership/administration and research/scholarship.

3. **quality improvement** focuses on lifelong learning that maintains and promotes patient safety and quality in health systems to achieve excellence in patient care.

Feedback involves giving specific information about how well (or not) the learner's performance met the established criteria; feedback also points to priority actions for improvement.

Formative assessment refers to assessment that is used to guide and inform progress where the results of the assessment 'do not count'.

Summative feedback refers to assessment which is designed to both guide and inform progress and where the results of the assessment 'count'.

Critical appraisal is the process of carefully and systematically examining literature to judge its trustworthiness, as well as its value and relevance in a particular context.[2]

Evidence-informed decision-making (EIDM) is the process of identifying, distilling and evaluating the best available evidence from research, practice and experience and using that evidence to inform health care decisions.[3]

Information literacy means the ability to find, master and critically analyze information resources in one's professional domain.[4]

3. Preparing to teach the Scholar Role

The skills within the Scholar Role are integral to the CanMEDS Framework and the delivery of quality patient care. The Scholar Role sets an expectation that your learners:

- actively engage in maintaining and enhancing their competence;

- contribute by supporting the 'next generation' of practitioners via teaching, assessing and mentoring others;

- integrate evidence to serve their patients in daily practice; and

- use and contribute to research.

In this section, we review common misconceptions about the Role, and suggest ways to integrate the content and process of the Scholar Role into practice and lifelong learning.

3.1 Common misconceptions to address with learners

The good news is that learners generally appreciate the value of developing their competence in the Scholar Role – it's unlikely to be a hard sell with your learners. Nonetheless, there are a few common misconceptions about the Role that you might wish to address with your learners.

First, you may find that your learners have too narrow a view of the Scholar Role and that they associate it almost exclusively with one aspect such as research or teaching. It is important to ensure that your learners know each of the **four distinct 'parts' of the Scholar Role**:

- ***maintenance and acquisition of new knowledge*** throughout one's career through lifelong learning;

- ***sharing of knowledge*** through teaching and assessment;

- ***use of knowledge*** in evidence-informed decision-making; and

- ***creation of knowledge*** through research and scholarly inquiry.

Scholar

© 2015 Royal College of Physicians and Surgeons of Canada

A second misconception is the idea that the Scholar Role is only applicable to those who work in academic centres and research institutes. While a research career is the career path of some physicians, **the responsibilities in the Scholar Role are shared by all practising physicians vis-à-vis teaching, the use of evidence to inform practice, and through life-long learning.**

Finally, some learners believe that skilful practice in one part of the Scholar Role is generalizable across the other three parts of the Role. Your learners may need you to help them see that the skilful ability to effectively use evidence and knowledge in day-to-day clinical practice requires purposeful learning and mastery of content and processes that are quite different to those skills required for the production of new knowledge through scholarship and innovation. Likewise, the skills for the effective sharing of knowledge and expertise as a teacher are very different from those needed to be motivated, organized and purposeful in maintaining competence throughout one's career. **Encourage learners to pursue focused opportunities for learning and skill development in each of the four parts** of the Scholar Role.

3.2 Help learners embrace learning as a lifelong process for improvement and maintenance

Your residents need to appreciate the value of developing skills[5] that will allow them to continue to develop and maintain their competence throughout their careers. During residency (if not sooner) your learners will need to take 'firm control' of their learning and this responsibility will continue after their residency is completed. It is important that your learners understand that there is no 'end' to learning: to stay competent, all physicians must stay current and connected.

USING SELF-ASSESSMENT AND FEEDBACK TO INFORM LEARNING

Residency is a good time to help your learners appreciate the value of self-awareness about their strengths and weaknesses and the need to actively gather information (feedback) about their performance. Your learners will benefit from knowing that many physicians receive regular information to guide and inform their performance throughout their career. The information that practising physicians might receive is wide-ranging and includes patient demographics, patient care outcomes, chart reviews or performance reviews from the health organization; and possibly multi-source feedback (MSF) or practice audits required by the provincial regulator. Your learners will benefit from knowing how their teachers use this same type of information to help identify their own learning needs and inform their learning plan and future development.

PITFALLS OF SELF-ASSESSMENT

Self-assessment refers to the monitoring of one's own performance. Much research suggests that we do this poorly when we rely on internal assessment alone and that guided self-assessment is better. Guided self-assessment is most effective using established criteria or metrics and with feedback or information collected from others,[6] especially mentors. Help your residents understand that self-assessment is inherently difficult and that they need a 'mirror' or feedback from others to have an accurate self-assessment.

Residents need a good handle on their strengths and weaknesses, so encourage your learners to make a point of regularly soliciting feedback and taking measures to learn from the feedback. Share with them the research which shows that people who seek feedback, especially feedback that is corrective or instructive, are perceived to be more competent, settle into new responsibilities more quickly, and get better performance reviews.[7] Help them understand that they should rely on a full picture of their practice (including strengths and areas for improvement) to inform their day-to-day practice as well as to inform their learning plans. The habit of developing learning plans based on their needs will bode well for their skills as a lifelong learner.

USING FEEDBACK TO INFORM LEARNING

Feedback allows trainees to learn about themselves from people and experiences. Recent work on feedback says that how someone asks for, receives, and integrates feedback is more important than how the feedback is given. To get the most from feedback, the receiver needs to see himself or herself as the key player in the feedback exchange. Help your learners understand that if they want to improve at anything, they need to take charge of the learning opportunity.

Teach your learners to be feedback seeking. Asking for feedback is a good way for learners to gather information, but learners will need to be coached on techniques for obtaining such feedback. Since people tend to focus only on corrective components or to resist what they hear (and become defensive), you can help your learners listen for what they are doing well in addition to what they should change with the following tips (see Table S-2).

Encourage your learners to build and sustain a support team of people (personal and professional) who can provide affirmation, advice, and perspective to your learners. Encourage your learners to empower 'their team' so that the team can and will point out when/if the learner needs to make a course correction.[8] Their own support team (e.g. supervisors, mentors, coaches, peers, friends and family) can also help them broaden their perspective on the feedback they receive.

Scholar

TABLE S-2. TIPS TO HELP LEARNERS PRACTICE ASKING FOR FEEDBACK[7,d]

1. Ask someone who is willing and constructive.

- Be sure to ask them whether they have *time and interest* to provide feedback.

- *Ask someone who has perspective.* Ask someone who sees you work. Even if you like someone and they like you, if they don't see you work, then they cannot help you improve. Ask a peer when you need peer feedback ("What more can I do, to better organize our study group's sessions?"), and a supervisor when you need a supervisor's feedback ("How could I have improved the flow of this patient from the emergency to the inpatient unit?").

- *Ask someone who is known to be direct* (or you might even consider asking someone with whom you have differences of opinion). You want feedback that is instructive and constructive. Ask this person to tell you one thing you are doing that is either helping or getting in the way of the performance you are interested in.

2. Ask for specific feedback.

- *Avoid phrases like* "Do you have any feedback for me?" This question is too general for the assessor to formulate an actionable answer, and you leave yourself open to feedback that is not useful.

- *Use prompts like*, "What is one thing you see me doing — or failing to do — that is getting in the way of my being more efficient at leading ward rounds?" This question directs the focus, asks for specific and constructive feedback, and gives the feedback provider permission to be honest.

3. Listen and focus on what is helpful and specific.

- *Pay attention and avoid interrupting*, even if you feel defensive.

- *Focus on feedback that is given in a helpful way.* If feedback does not make sense to you or is contrary to previous feedback in the same setting, then seek additional external perspectives and discuss further.

- *Focus on what is helpful* in the feedback (i.e. behaviours to continue and behaviours to change).

4. Thank your feedback providers for their input/help.
Remember: Those who get curious and ask for feedback can really accelerate their own learning

---

Learners watch faculty and supervisors and try to model what they do, so being open to feedback and demonstrating an enthusiasm for new ideas and information is a powerful positive influence on learners. This modelling will also help learners to develop their skills in giving feedback when they take on the teaching aspects of the Scholar Role (see Section 3.4 on giving feedback).

3.3 Nurture your learners to move from active learners to skilled teachers

Teaching is one of the cornerstones of the physician role. In fact, the word doctor is derived from the Latin verb 'docēre' which means 'to teach'.[9] Teaching is an important activity in the Scholar Role, with learners responsible for teaching peers, more junior learners and others. Many learners may already have experience with the content and process of learning, teaching and assessment; they may be coaching in sports or teaching music lessons, for example. You can build on this rich teaching and coaching experience because it may help them understand that:

- Skills practice is different than performance of skills with patients in a clinical setting.

- A lot of skill building practice is necessary to be a satisfactory/good/great performer — practice leads to improvement.

- Improving skills and performance requires individual effort, accepting assistance from others and plenty of specific feedback.

- Winning, success or excellence is celebrated but it doesn't always occur. For this reason, people need to know how to learn from losses, disappointment or poor performance.

- Analysis of both victories and losses or poor performance are viewed as an opportunity to understand what needs improvement for next time.

With some orientation (or refreshing) of your learners' experience to the teaching or coaching process you can help them make the link between those processes, and being an active learner or a teacher of their peers or others (see Table S-3).

---

d This chart is based on material in Stone D, Heen S. Thanks for the feedback, the science and art of receiving feedback well (Penguin, 2015) New York: Viking, 2014. Used with permission.

© 2015 Royal College of Physicians and Surgeons of Canada

Scholar

TABLE S-3. COACHING PROCESSES REFLECTED IN COMPETENCY BASED MEDICAL EDUCATION (CBME)[10]

COACHING STEPS[e]	Examples of coaching processes	What this means to resident as LEARNER	What this means to resident as TEACHER
1. GOALS	Identifying areas needing improvement that will impact performance.	*Attend to* • Needed competencies, • Entrustable Professional Activities or EPAs), • Goals and objectives	*Attend to* • Purpose of the teaching • Goals and objectives
2. PRACTICE OF KNOWLEDGE, SKILLS, ABILITIES	Regular skill building practice is necessary to be a satisfactory/ good/ great performer.	*Learn* • The parts (i.e. knowledge, skills, attitudes = competencies) • Usual sequence (i.e. milestones) • Demo in patient care (i.e. EPAs)	Learner centred teaching *Assess* • Inventory starting point • Assessment for learning = formative
3. FEEDBACK	Improving skills and performance requires individual effort, accepting assistance from others and ongoing specific feedback.	• Learners need internal motivation • Learn from many people (mentors, teachers, team, community of practice) • Ask for and accept assistance of others (self-directed) • Ask for specific feedback	• Support learner engagement and motivation (e.g. motivating learners, monitoring progress, summative assessments) • Support a positive environment (e.g. learning climate) • Provide timely and focused feedback: Relationship, Reaction, Content, Coaching (R2C2)
4. REFLECTION ON PERFORMANCE	Winning, success or excellence is celebrated and tips are gathered to ensure future success Losses, disappointment or poor performance also provides great lessons learnt which will always be remembered.	• Accept losses, disappointment or poor performance as part of learning and life (e.g. resilience, motivation).	• Teachers need to support a positive learning environment where mistakes are disclosed, discussed and learned from (e.g. learning climate, safety culture, wellness).
5. SETTING GOALS	Analysis of both victories and losses or poor performance are viewed an opportunity to understand what needs to be changed next time and setting priorities for improvement or moving forward.	• Revisit the focus for learning re: drills to develop abilities • Analyze available data to guided self-awareness of what did/did not work; where on/off usual milestones; what are/are not strengths; what are/are not in need of improvement	• Collect, organize and discuss analysed data re: learner's assessments and performance to sort out what did/did not work; where on/off usual milestones; what are/are not trends over time; what are/are not current strengths; what are/are not in need of current improvement.
6. PLANNING FOR IMPROVEMENT	Plan for skill practice; future performance checks; consider changes to individuals, groups, systems, and processes.	• What are the next steps/plan for improvement (self-directed, motivated, feedback, milestones, learning planning, competency based medical education).	• Next steps/plan re: content and process for improvement (e.g. learner centred, motivating learners, monitoring progress, summative assessments, feedback, milestones, learning planning, CBME education).

e   Glover Takahashi, S. 2015. Created for the *CanMEDS Teaching and Assessment Tools Guide*. Royal College.

Scholar

USING TEACHING SCRIPTS

The timing of how quickly learners need to function as teachers will depend on your organization and specialty. Before you expect learners to assume a teaching role, you will need to equip your learners with the basics of teaching. The most common approaches for building this foundation in teaching include directed reading, workshops, courses or online modules. You may also wish to develop teaching scripts (see Table S-4).

Teaching scripts are a key component to in-the-moment teaching. Usually based on your expertise in your area and in your observations of trainee learning gaps, these mini-lectures are meant to be delivered in a very short period of time. They are usually done for Medical Expert but can be effective for roles such as the Scholar Role or Communicator Role. Teaching scripts are perceived by learners to be a reflection of high quality teaching.

SETTING EXPECTATIONS OF YOUR LEARNERS TO FUNCTION AS TEACHERS

Let your learners know when and where they will have formal or informal roles as teachers, including if they will need to provide feedback or complete assessment forms for their peers or other learners. Also, if their performance as a teacher will be assessed, provide them with a sample of the assessment forms so they can prepare accordingly.

Provide your learners with some grounding in educational principles with special emphasis on current competency based medical education practices and how they relate to your organization and specialty. Your learners will need to understand both the content and processes related to:

- teaching in clinical settings and in structured/formal settings;

- assessing learners using local tools for demonstration of competencies and performance in practice;

- providing effective feedback that accounts for their relationship with and response from the learner; and

- they need to understand the value of focusing feedback on content of performance and coaching for improvement.[11]

3.4 Help your learners develop the art of giving quality feedback

Giving feedback is a particularly important skill to develop with your learners. In their role as teacher, your learners need to understand the importance of giving good feedback that a learner will recognize as feedback. Medical educators often express frustration that they frequently provide feedback to learners, but the same learners perceive that they rarely receive feedback. Which perception is accurate? This debate is less likely to happen when teachers label the feedback by using the word (repeatedly) to signpost what they are doing.

The well-known 'sandwich' approach to giving feedback has fallen out of favour given its many limitations.[12] A recent approach called R2C2[11] builds on much of the recent research about giving feedback about professional performance in medical education. In this approach, feedback involves giving personalized specific information about how well (or not) the performance met the established criteria and some hints or tips on the priority actions for improvement (see Table S-5). Another complementary model is the six-step approach by Brown and Hodges.[13]

3.5 Guide your learners as they are sourcing, selecting, interpreting and applying evidence in the service of patients' problems – integrating best evidence

The need for and the principles of critical appraisal are fairly well established[4] so working on these competencies with your learners should be straightforward for you and your faculty. In contrast, the art of accessing available information resources is a moving target. This field evolves so quickly that you may wish to recruit the help of your colleagues in health informatics and library science.

Information management is now a broad field where experts in health informatics and library or information science focus on how to assist in managing and using information to inform health care and health care practitioners. Knowing who to talk to and where to access available information resources is essential to your learners. Help them connect with people who specialize in this area so that they develop an understanding of the complexity of this important competency.

Scholar

© 2015 Royal College of Physicians and Surgeons of Canada

TABLE S-4. HOW DO YOU CREATE AND USE TEACHING SCRIPTS?

#	Step	HINTS
1.	Inventory very common, frequent teaching interactions that you teach repeatedly OR the challenging ones that need 'extra accuracy'	• Interactions may be skills, procedures, content knowledge.
2.	Outline the core content	• Include some key phrases that you find particularly helpful.
3.	PICK and choose what parts of the content you will emphasize in the 'script'	• Do you want to highlight one task? Two? Whole process? • Highlight the key content and process needed.
4.	Recruit 'script writers'	• Faculty are the obvious choice, but consider making the drafting a learning/teaching activity. • Consider having residents develop scripts – on their own or in groups. • Consider combining junior residents and senior residents in the same group so they can learn from each other as they develop the scripts.
5.	Develop scripts (i.e. draft, review, revise, finalize)	• Residents can 'draft' their script and work with other more senior members of their team to make revisions (if needed). • Revisions could be done in real time or online (e.g. email, wiki, etc.)
6.	Use scripts to teach and assess	• The best timing to refer to a script is in the clinical setting – immediately after a patient interaction so that learning is solidified. • Allow for feedback and coaching conversations to be geared toward the level of competence of the learner. • Also share scripts with learners

TABLE S-5. R2C2 FEEDBACK FOR CBME[11,f]

R2C2 has four phases: 2R phases, 2C phases	Approaches
Relationship building: Goal: to engage the learner, build the relationship and mutual respect and trust. e.g. How has your rotation gone for you? **R**eactions exploration about feedback: Goal: for learner to feel understood and that their views are heard and respected. e.g. Did anything surprise you in the feedback? **C**ontent exploration: Goal: for the learner to be clear about what the assessment data mean and opportunities suggested for change. e.g. What strikes you as something to focus on? **C**oaching for performance change: Goal: for the learner to identify areas for change and develop an achievable learning/change plan. e.g. What do you see as the priority?	The **R2C2** feedback model is informed by three theoretical and evidence-based approaches for facilitating acceptance and use of assessment data and feedback: Humanism and person-centredness: (build relationships, engage the learner, foster ownership of the data) Informed or guided self-assessment: (recognize that feedback that is inconsistent with one's own perceptions may be difficult to accept; recognize resistance) Behaviour change and domains influencing change: (coach for learning and change and integrate factors which influence one's ability to change).

Scholar

f   Sargeant J, Lockyer J, Mann K, Holmboe E, Silver I, Armson H, Driessen E, MacLeod T, Yen W, Ross K, Power M. Facilitated reflective performance feedback: Developing an evidence and theory-based model. Acad Med (In Press). First published online doi: 10.1097/ACM.0000000000000809.

© 2015 Royal College of Physicians and Surgeons of Canada

USING DIGITAL LITERACY, DIGITAL COMPETENCY AND DIGITAL PROFESSIONALISM TO SOLVE PATIENTS' PROBLEMS

It is not reasonable to think that your learners can meaningfully undertake a formal critical appraisal process 'in real time' to inform decisions on current patient problems when there are so many reviews, guidelines and algorithms than can be analyzed. Much of information literacy is about knowing how to identify and navigate widely available pre-appraised resources – both public and proprietary.

One of your tasks as a teacher is to help your learners establish an appropriate level of information literacy (e.g. the ability to navigate large volumes of information and assess the accuracy of online resources), digital competency (e.g. knowledge on how to use hardware and software) and digital professionalism (e.g. maintaining confidentiality).[14] Given the explosion of information and the numerous public and proprietary resources that are online or mobile, your learners may need your help to discern what your specialty, program and organization consider as trusted sources for information and other resources.

USING ELECTRONIC TOOLS AND AIDS APPROPRIATELY

It is important to orient your learners to specific resources that are helpful for different patient problems, and to cover topics like when to use the resources and when not to use them and what the limitations of the resources are. It is also important to advise learners about the kinds of information that must be learned versus retrieved.

At times there can be tension between residents and faculty about the risk of being overly reliant on electronic forms of information, which are often very easy to use. Your advice will likely be informed by such things as how frequently the learner will need to 'access' the information to make a decision and how critical it might be to the outcome of a situation if the data isn't available temporarily (i.e. would it negatively impact an outcome of connectivity were down temporarily). Some parts of clinical practice do require residents to be able to efficiently interpret and apply large amounts of knowledge with and without electronic assistance. As such, your learners will benefit from your insight on when it is appropriate (or not) to count on their electronic resources in day-to-day practice.

3.6 Help your learners understand the process of evidence-informed decision-making by collaborating with specialists in health informatics and library science

Your learners may find the art of focusing or narrowing their evidence question is a particularly challenging part of EIDM. It is likely that you and your clinical faculty will need to ask probing questions that allow your learners to refine or focus their question so that both the evidence they find and the solutions they collect are sufficiently 'on topic' to inform the case or questions of interest.

The EIDM process outlines seven steps[15] that need to be done to effectively practise EIDM to solve related patient problems and/or a clinical problem of interest (see Table S-6):

1. **Ask** by framing a focused question (aka PICO question, P = population, I = intervention, C = comparison, O = outcomes);

2. **Acquire** the evidence in an efficient manner

3. **Appraise** the evidence for quality and applicability

4. **Integrate** the evidence

5. **Adapt** the evidence for your clinical problem

6. **Apply** the evidence in your clinical plan.

7. **Analyze** if the plan worked.

Once the question is identified, your learner needs to decide what type of search is applicable. Can the question be answered by looking in a pre-appraised resource or is a search of primary publications needed? What is a reasonable trusted guideline or online resource that can help navigate a timely solution to a clinical problem in 'real time'? If the answer is satisfactory and 'done', then the resident can move along, but if the answer needs further exploration, more information may be needed.

When needed and if time allows for a more thorough look at the literature, your learners may identify a 'personal learning project' or 'clinical evidence question'. In this case, if available, you can encourage them to work with colleagues in health informatics and library science to complete a search followed by collection, extraction and synthesis of evidence. Ensure your learners consult with clinical faculty when they are ready to interpret and adapt evidence to this patient or problem. Lastly, with information gathered on their own or with the help of informatics colleagues, the learner and clinical faculty can plan, implement and evaluate the selected solutions for this patient or problem.

© 2015 Royal College of Physicians and Surgeons of Canada

TABLE S-6. SEVEN STEPS FOR EVIDENCE-INFORMED DECISION-MAKING[15]

EIDM process step	Who might help the resident develop this skill (as appropriate)
1. **Ask** by framing a focused question	Clinical Faculty
2. **Acquire** the evidence in efficient manner	Colleagues from health informatics and info science
3. **Appraise** the evidence for quality and applicability	Colleagues from health informatics and info science, Clinical Faculty
4. **Integrate** the evidence	Colleagues from health informatics and info science
5. **Adapt** the evidence for your clinical problem	Clinical Faculty
6. **Apply** the evidence in your clinical plan	Clinical Faculty
7. **Analyze** if the plan worked	Clinical Faculty

When it comes to organizing EIDM learning opportunities for your learners, consider the following factors that are described in the EIDM literature:[16]

1. Assessments for learning and achievement are most important.

2. Short courses are more effective than longer courses.

3. It is important to focus on a small number of topics.

4. Include special sessions devoted to statistical issues.

5. A small group learning approach is preferred.

3.7 Develop the research, scholarship and inquiry abilities of your learners

Learners in most programs often need to learn the fundamentals of research skills for the purpose of being an effective consumer of research. *The Research guide: a primer for residents, other health care trainees, and practitioners*[17] is a key resource for residents to use a self guide and for faculty to mentor or teach residents the key steps to effective research in residency. Advanced research skills and high-level scholarship (e.g. research grants, publication in high impact journal) are not the usual expectation of most learners, however. It is therefore important to set reasonable expectations about research and scholarship for your learners, knowing that not all will pursue a career path in research.

The competencies of the Scholar Role will support the lifelong learning of all physicians, whether they pursue a career path in research or not. Furthermore, acquiring the skills as they relate to the production of knowledge and support of scholarship will help learners to be better equipped to explain the results of research to both patients and colleagues in training and throughout their career.

4. Hints, tips and tools for *teaching* the Scholar Role

As a teacher your goal is to deliver the right content and in a way that helps your residents learn. Sometimes you will teach directly. Other times you will facilitate and support the teaching of others or self-directed activities by learners. There are parts of the Scholar Role that can be especially difficult for learners to relate to and understand in the context of their work. For this reason this section of the Scholar chapter includes a short menu of tips and tricks that are highly effective for teaching the Scholar Role. You can treat the list as a buffet: pick and choose the tips that resonate most and that will work for you, your program and your learners.

Teaching Tip 1.

Help your learners plan their learning by analyzing their assessment data

Your learners need to appreciate the importance of having a learning plan that is aligned with the program but specific to their own learning needs. Their plans should evolve over time to reflect their changing learning needs. To establish a truly robust learning plan, your learners need to seek data about their performance from multiple sources.

By collecting and analyzing performance data on a regular basis, learners and teachers can identify gaps that can be incorporated into the learning plan. Use your regular meetings with learners to check in on both the content and the process of their learning. You may also consider using a structured agenda or encounter assessment tool at these regular meetings so that the information is gathered in a systematic way that allows you to track the learner's progress over time and plan for further improvement.

© 2015 Royal College of Physicians and Surgeons of Canada

Scholar

Teaching Tip 2.
Help learners get the most out of their learning planning meetings

Make the most of your valuable meeting time as well as that of your learners by preparing and circulating material before the meeting.

- Examples of documents or information *you can send in advance* include:

    - An agenda (be sure to cover the length and location of the meeting);

    - Explain how you expect the learner to prepare for the meeting including what documents they should send in advance (be sure to set a deadline);

    - Be clear about what will happen if the documents are not sent on time (e.g. reschedule);

    - If you are talking about their performance, send all of the data that you have so they can confirm whether you have the correct data.

- Examples of documents or information you may expect *your learners to send in advance* include:

    - Elective choices – so you can review at the meeting based on progress and learning needs;

    - Learning progress inventory or learning needs and interests inventory;

    - Research plans (if applicable) – so you can assist with matching them with a supervisor before the meeting

    - Assignments – so you can review in advance and discuss at the meeting.

Teaching Tip 3.
Provide explicit practice that will enable your learners to run through teaching skills for effective workplace teaching and assessment

Your learners need plenty of opportunities to teach in the clinical setting. The teaching that happens around case presentations is an easy and natural setting for your learners to watch others as they role model good and bad teaching skills. Teach them to appraise the performance of others and to reflect on what teaching, assessment and feedback works and what aspects of the person's performance need improvement. Providing a structured reflection tool to your learners in advance may help them organize their analysis in the early days. After they've had some practice using a structured tool, you can encourage your learners to practise providing feedback to others on teaching, thus reinforcing the notion that teaching (about teaching) will help reinforce the content for your learners.

An important preliminary step when working on a learning plan with your learners is to establish expectations by clarifying which assessments are formative (i.e. to guide and inform progress) and which assessments are summative (i.e. 'counts' with specific expectations for performance or achievement). Given that assessment tools can be used either for formative or summative purposes, it is important that the purpose of each assessment tool be spelled out.

For example, case logs function well as a formative assessment tool. They are used to monitor activities and to provide feedback to your resident and faculty by providing detailed data about the number, types and variety of cases that a learner experiences. From this data, it is easy to identify gaps in a learner's experience so that needed learning opportunities can be provided to the trainee.

Alternately, case logs also function well as summative assessment tools. In these situations, the program sets specific requirements about the number, types and variety of cases that learners must fulfill. When reviewing the case logs you might have a similar conversation to identify gaps so that needed learning opportunities but the consequences of 'not completing' the requirements need to be clear.

Teaching Tip 4.
Develop an information literacy resource for your learners

Help your learners by providing them with a tip sheet that inventories trusted sources of information and information resources as it relates to your specialty, organization and program. This tip sheet can include general information literacy about the trustworthiness of different resources; guidelines, reviews, case reports and decision algorithms; and knowing when to use them (or not) and what the limits of each resource are. Remember to indicate if these should be 'hard wired' into their memories for ease or importance and which ones make sense to keep with their electronic resources. If you don't already have one, consider having the program prepare a tip sheet for review at orientation. Alternatively, you could turn the development of a tip sheet into a learning activity led by senior learners for new learners early in residence.

Scholar

© 2015 Royal College of Physicians and Surgeons of Canada

Teaching Tip 5.
Decide how scholarship and research fits best in your program

Clarifying the role and structure of research early on in residency will help your learners understand how to meet the program requirements and their interests in this regard.

You will need to clarify for your learners whether the program focus is on how best to be a 'consumer' of research or if the program has expectations about production of scholarship or research participation or production. If a research project is expected, provide guidance on the types of research projects that are appropriate. Be sure learners know whether the scholarship or research project for your program is a capstone activity — that is, something done near or at the end of training that consolidates or builds on clinical practice — or a core activity that starts at the beginning of the program with expectations for progress along the way. If there are many options depending on learners' interests and abilities, be sure they know this and be prepared to give them guidance on what options are available.

Sample teaching tools

You can use the sample *Teaching Tools for Scholar* at the end of this chapter as is, or you can modify or use them in various combinations to suit your objectives, time allocated, sequence within your residency program, and so on.

Easy-to-customize electronic versions of the *Teaching Tools for Scholar* (in .doc, .ppt and .pdf formats) are found at: canmeds.royalcollege.ca

The tools provided are:

- T1 Lecture or Large Group Session: Foundations of the Scholar Role

- T2 Presentation: Teaching the Scholar Role

- T3 Guided Reflection: Planning for learning

- T4 Coaching: Coaching learners to give and receive feedback

- T5 Teaching Scripts: Teaching script sample and template for evidence-informed decision-making

- T6 Case Report: Teaching report for the Scholar Role

- T7 Guided Reflection: Evidence-informed decision-making in day-to-day practice

- T8 Research Planning: Sample timetable for a two-year study

- T9 Tools and Strategies: Summary sheet for the Scholar Role

5. Hints, tips and tools for *assessing* the Scholar Role

Assessment for learning is a major theme in this CanMEDS Tools Guide and a growing emphasis in medical education. You can and should use assessment as a strategy to inform a resident's learning plan (i.e. to alert or signpost to learners what is important to learn as well as what and how they will be assessed). This section of the Tools Guide offers a number of hints to help you develop a program of assessment that will ensure that both teachers and learners have a clear understanding of their performance and what needs improvement.

Assessment Tip 1.
Assess the learners' ability to focus on 'the' question(s) that arise in the clinical setting and solutions for answering

Look for opportunities to observe your learners as they ask and answer questions that arise in the clinical setting. How effective were they? Assess their ability to navigate large volumes of information and their skill at appraising the accuracy of online resources in a timely way. Be sure to give them feedback on what you observe. Try to focus on the answer(s) they came up with, their knowledge of how to use hardware and software, and their digital professionalism throughout the process (e.g. maintaining confidentiality).

Practise this skill individually or in small groups. Make sure to collect multiple data points over time including assessments done as part of discussions during or after rounds, case presentations given by your learner, and/or their answers on a written exam or OSCE.

Assessment Tip 2.
Assess teaching skills in the clinical setting

To assess your learners' teaching skills effectively, your assessments need to consider how they perform when teaching in both clinical settings and in structured, formal teaching. Many residency programs have mandatory teaching expectations of their learners and collect performance data on the resident by way of 'feedback' forms for structured teaching sessions. These forms should be designed to include the important features of teaching,[18] including how available the resident teacher is to support learners' needs, how often and well the teacher provides feedback to learners, how respectful the teacher is to learners and others, how well the teacher stimulated learning, how effectively the teacher serves as a role model, and an overall rating.

Scholar

Additionally, it is important to assess your learners' abilities to teach skills in the clinical setting. That means that you should collect data on actual supervision of clinical teaching and be sure to gather input from the learners about how the resident functions as a teacher.

Assessment Tip 3.
Use formal meetings as an additional surveillance and feedback of your learners' learning plans

Your learners need to practise taking responsibility for their lifelong learning at the start of residency and demonstrate growth and ability in

- self-awareness of personal and professional strengths and limits,

- experience asking for, accepting and including feedback to improve self-awareness, and

- ability to work with others to modify learning plans.

Formal meetings that are scheduled on a regular basis (e.g. semi-annually with the Program Director) can be used to monitor your learners learning plans and the progression of their skills. For example, you may wish to use this 'naturally occurring' event to provide more structure that builds additional skills in guided self-awareness and active management of learning. The implications of the plans for electives, promotion etc. would also need to be discussed.

Assessment Tip 4.
Assess EIDM content and process using structured tools or tests

Validated tools exist for the assessment of EIDM such as the Fresno[19, 20] and Berlin[21] questionnaires. To employ EIDM effectively, learners need to acquire the ability to apply EIDM processes to problems, using statistical analysis skills, for example. Reviews of journal clubs say they don't work for teaching EIDM and critical appraisal skills. It is recommended that tools that track and assess mastery of the skills be used instead. As stated earlier, consider these five factors[16] when organizing EIDM learning opportunities for your learners:

1. Assessments for learning and achievement are most important.

2. Short courses are more effective than longer courses.

3. It is important to focus on a small number of topics.

4. Include special sessions devoted to statistical issues.

5. A small groups learning approach is preferred.

Sample assessment tools

You can use the sample *Assessment Tools for Scholar* at the end of this chapter as is or you can modify or use them in various combinations to suit your objectives, time allocated, sequence within your residency program, and so on.

Easy-to-customize electronic versions of the *Assessment Tools for Scholar* (in .doc, .ppt and .pdf formats) are found at: canmeds.royalcollege.ca

The tools provided are:

- A1 Multisource Feedback: Resident as teacher multisource feedback

- A2 Multisource Feedback: Giving and receiving feedback

- A3 Homework: Evidence-informed decision-making homework assignment

- A4 Monitoring Form: Research project high-level checklist

- A5 One-to-one Teaching: Research project meeting monitoring

6. Suggested resources

- **Miflin BM, Campbell CB, Price DA. A conceptual framework to guide the development of self-directed, lifelong learning in problem-based medical curricula. *Med Educ.* 2000 Apr;34(4):299-306.** Medical schools are increasingly focusing on problem-based curricula to develop the capacity of learners to self-direct further learning. This paper describes the framework that one medical school has developed which may be useful for other institutions that are experiencing difficulties implementing problem-base curricula.

- **Post RE, Quattlebaum RG, Benich JJ 3rd. Residents-as-Teachers Curricula: A Critical Review. *Acad Med.* 2009; Mar;84(3);374–380.** After conducting a systematic review of residents-as-teachers curricula the authors determined that curricula did make a significant improvement in resident's teaching skills. The authors also make recommendations on the most evidence-based curricula and evaluation strategies.

Scholar

© 2015 Royal College of Physicians and Surgeons of Canada

- **Sargeant J, Lockyer J, Mann K, Holmboe E, Silver I, Armson H, Driessen E, MacLeod T, Yen W, Ross K, Power M. Facilitated reflective performance feedback: Developing an evidence and theory-based model. *Acad Med.* (in press).** This paper describes the R2C2 feedback model developed for CBME and informed by three theoretical and evidence-based approaches for facilitating acceptance and uptake of assessment data: humanism and person-centredness (build relationships, engage the learner, foster ownership of the data); informed or guided self-assessment (recognize that feedback inconsistent with one's own perceptions may be difficult to accept); behaviour change and domains influencing change (coach for learning and change and integrate factors which influence one's ability to change).

- **Online resources on evidence-informed decision-making** http://cbpp-pcpe.phac-aspc.gc.ca/resources/evidence-informed-decision-making/ **last retrieved July 4, 2015.** Accessible information from the Public Health Agency Canadian Best Practices Portal includes information and tools on evidence-informed decision-making (EIDM).

- **Harvey BJ, Lang ES, Frank JR, editors. *The Research Guide: a primer for learners, other health care trainees, and practitioners.* Ottawa: Royal College of Physicians and Surgeons of Canada; 2011.** http://www.royalcollege.ca/portal/page/portal/rc/canmeds/resources/publications#The_Research_Guide

7. Other resources

- Ahmadi N, McKenzie ME, Maclean A, Brown CJ, Mastracci T, McLeod RS; Evidence-Based Reviews in Surgery Steering Group. Teaching evidence based medicine to surgery learners — is journal club the best format? a systematic review of the literature. *J Surg Educ.* 2012;69(1):91-100.

- Horsley T, Hyde C, Santesso N, Parkes J, Milne R, Stewart R. Teaching critical appraisal skills in healthcare settings. *Cochrane Database Syst Rev.* 2011;(11):1270.

- Norman GR, Shannon SI. Effectiveness of instruction in critical appraisal (evidence-based medicine) skills: a critical appraisal. *CMAJ.* 1998;158(2):177-81.

- Torre DM, Simpson D, Sebastian JL, Elnicki DM. Learning/feedback activities and high-quality teaching: perceptions of third-year medical students during an inpatient rotation. *Acad Med.* 2005;80(10):950-4.

- Irby DM. Excellence in clinical teaching: knowledge transformation and development required. *Med Educ.* 2014;48(8):776-84.

- Frank JR, Snell LS, Cate OT, Holmboe ES, Carraccio C, Swing SR, Harris P, Glasgow NJ, Campbell C, Dath D, Harden RM, Iobst W, Long DM, Mungroo R, Richardson DL, Sherbino J, Silver I, Taber S, Talbot M, Harris KA. Competency-based medical education: theory to practice. *Med Teach.* 2010;32(8):638-45.

- Hodges B. A tea-steeping or i-Doc model for medical education? *Acad Med.* 2010;85(9 Suppl):S34-44.

- van de Ridder, J.M., Stokking, K.M., McGaghie, W.C., and ten Cate, O.T. (2008) What is feedback in clinical education? *Med Educ.* 2008;42(2):189-97.

Scholar

8. SCHOLAR ROLE DIRECTORY OF TEACHING AND ASSESSMENT TOOLS

You can use the sample *teaching and assessment tools for the Scholar Role* found in this section as is, or you can modify or use them in various combinations to suit your objectives, the time allocated, the sequence within your residency program, and so on. Tools are listed by number (e.g. T1), type (e.g. Lecture), and title (e.g. Foundations of the Scholar Role).

Easy-to-customize electronic versions of the sample *teaching and assessment tools for the Scholar Role* in .doc, .ppt and .pdf formats are found at: canmeds.royalcollege.ca

TEACHING TOOLS

ASSESSMENT TOOLS

Scholar

© 2015 Royal College of Physicians and Surgeons of Canada

T1. FOUNDATIONS OF THE SCHOLAR ROLE

Created for the *CanMEDS Teaching and Assessment Tools Guide* by S Glover Takahashi. Reproduced with permission of the Royal College.

This Learning activity includes:

- Presentation: Teaching the Scholar Role (T2)

Suggested Worksheets:

- Guided Reflection: Planning for learning (T3)
- Coaching: Coaching learners to give and receive feedback (T4)

Instructions for Teacher:
Sample learning objectives

1. Recognize common words related to the process and content of the four different components of Scholar

2. Apply key Scholar skills to examples from day-to-day practice

3. Develop a personal Scholar resource for day-to-day practice

Audience: All learners

How to adapt:

- Consider whether your session's objectives match the sample ones. Select from, modify, or add to the sample objectives as required.

- The sample PowerPoint presentation and worksheets are generic and foundational and tied to simple objectives. Consider whether you'll need additional slides to meet your objectives. Modify, add or delete content as required. You may want to include specific information related to your discipline and context.

- Depending on whether you are using these materials in one session (i.e. Scholar Basics Workshop) or a series of 2-4 academic half days will determine which worksheet(s) you select and in what sequence.

- You may wish to review and customize the Scholar Role Summary Sheet (i.e. most frequent Scholar needs for your learners).

- Use with your learners as an additional worksheet activity.

Logistics:

- Select one or two worksheets for each teaching session.

- Plan for about 20 minutes for each worksheet/group activity: this time will be used for you to explain the activity and for your learners to complete the worksheet individually, share their answers with their small group, discuss, prepare to report back to the whole group, and then deliver their small group's report to the whole group.

- Allow individuals to read the worksheet and spend about five minutes working on the answers on their own before starting to work in groups. This format allows each person to develop his or her own understanding of the topic.

- Depending on the group and time available, you may wish to assign one or more worksheets as homework to be completed before the session or as a follow-up assignment.

Setting:

- This information is best taught in a small-group format (i.e. less than 30 learners) if possible. It can also be effectively done with a larger group if the room allows for learners to be at tables in groups of five or six. With larger groups, it is helpful to have additional teachers or facilitators available to answer questions arising from the worksheet activities.

© 2015 Royal College of Physicians and Surgeons of Canada

Scholar

T2. TEACHING THE SCHOLAR ROLE

Created for the *CanMEDS Teaching and Assessment Tools Guide* by S Glover Takahashi. Reproduced with permission of the Royal College.

Instructions for Teacher:

- Setting and Audience: Faculty and all learners

- How to use: Use as an orientation to the Role

- How to adapt: Slides can be modified to match the specialty or the learners' practice context

- Logistics: Equipment: You will require a laptop, projector, and screen.

Slide #	Words on slide	Notes to teachers
1.	Scholar	• Add information about presenters and modify title
2.	**Objectives and agenda** 1. Recognize the process and content of the four different components of Scholar 2. Apply key leadership skills to examples from day-to-day practice 3. Develop a personal Leadership resource for day-to-day practice	• SAMPLE goals and objectives of the session – revise as required. • CONSIDER doing a 'warm up activity' • Review/revise goals and objectives. • Insert agenda slide if desired
3.	**Why the Scholar Role matters** 1. Learning does not end 2. Teaching others consolidates the information for the teacher 3. All learners and physicians have responsibilities for education 4. Physicians need to know what information is "evidence" and which evidence is applicable to day-to-day decisions 5. Physicians must understand and interpret research	• Reasons why this Role is important
4.	**The details: What is the Scholar Role**[a] As Scholars, physicians demonstrate a lifelong commitment to excellence in practice through continuous learning and by teaching others, evaluating evidence, and contributing to scholarship.	• Definition from the CanMEDS 2015 Physician Competency Framework
5.	**Recognizing the Scholar Role** • Assessing • Coaching • Enhancing • Evaluating • Maintaining • Mentoring • Monitoring • Motivating • Orienting • Providing feedback • Researching • Supervising • Teaching • Pursuing scholarly activity	• Trigger words relating to the PROCESS of the Scholar Role
6.	**Recognizing the Scholar Role** • Community of practice, • Continuing competence • Critical appraisal • Evidence • Evidence–informed, Evidence-based • Goals • Learning climate, Learning environment • Learning plan • Lifelong learning • Objectives • Performance assessment • Portfolio • Scholarship • Scholarly inquiry • Scientific principles • Self-directed learning/guided self-directed learning	• Trigger words relating to the CONTENT of the Scholar Role

---

a Richardson D, Oswald A, Chan M-K, Lang ES, Harvey BJ. Scholar. In: Frank JR, Snell L, Sherbino J, editors. *CanMEDS 2015 Physician Competency Framework*. Ottawa: Royal College of Physicians and Surgeons of Canada; 2015. Reproduced with permission.

© 2015 Royal College of Physicians and Surgeons of Canada

Scholar

T2. TEACHING THE SCHOLAR ROLE (continued)

Slide #	Words on slide	Notes to teachers

7.	**Four distinct 'parts' of the Scholar Role:**
	1. Maintenance and acquisition of new knowledge throughout one's career through lifelong learning,
	2. Sharing of knowledge through teaching and assessment,
	3. Use of knowledge in evidence-informed decision-making, and
	4. Creation of knowledge through research and scholarly inquiry.
	  - The responsibilities in the Scholar Role are shared by all practising physicians vis-à-vis teaching, the use of evidence to inform practice, and through lifelong learning.
	  - Need to pursue focused opportunities for learning and skill development in each of the four parts of the Scholar Role.
		• Correcting misconceptions about Scholar

8.	**Learning is a lifelong process for improvement and maintenance** 1. Take FIRM control of learning. 2. Competent = skilled + current + connected 3. ASK for, look for, receive, and integrate feedback. Receiver is the key player in the feedback exchange.	
9.	T3 – Planning for learning	• Learning activity
10.	**Tips to practice asking for feedback**[b] 1. Ask someone who is willing and can be constructive 2. Ask for SPECIFIC feedback 3. Listen and focus on what is helpful and specific 4. Thank them for their input.	
11.	**R2C2 Feedback model**[c] • **R**elationship building • **R**eactions exploration about feedback • **C**ontent exploration • **C**oaching for performance change	• **Relationship building;** Is the learner ready for feedback? Is there trust of teacher? Motivation of learner? • **Reactions exploration about feedback** re: Is there consistency between giver and receiver? Areas of agreement? Surprises? • **Content exploration** re: What worked, What didn't, Match and progress in program/personal goals, objectives, needs. • **Coaching for performance change** re: What are hints or tips and priority actions for improvement? What is the plan?
12.	T4 – Giving and receiving feedback	• Learning activity
13.	**Steps to EIDM process**[d] 1. **Ask** by framing a focused question 2. **Acquire** the evidence in efficient manner 3. **Appraise** the evidence for quality and applicability 4. **Integrate** the evidence 5. **Adapt** the evidence for your clinical problem 6. **Apply** the evidence in your clinical plan. 7. **Analyze** if the plan worked.	
14.	**COACHING STEPS**[e] 1. Goals 2. Practice of knowledge, skills and abilities 3. Feedback 4. Reflection on performance 5. Setting goals 6. Planning for improvement	
15.	T3	

b Stone D, Heen S. Thanks for the feedback: the science and art of receiving feedback well. New York: Viking; 2014.
c Sargeant J, Lockyer J, Mann K, Holmboe E, Silver I, Armson H, Driessen E, MacLeod T, Yen W, Ross K, Power M. Facilitated reflective performance feedback: Developing an evidence- and theory-based model that builds relationship, explorse reactions and content, and coaches for performance change. *Acad Med*, 2015. (in press)
d Ciliska, D. Introduction to evidence-informed decision-making. Last retrieved July 31, 2015 http://www.cihr-irsc.gc.ca/e/45245.html
e Glover Takahashi, S. 2015. Created for the *CanMEDS Teaching and Assessment Tools Guide*. Royal College.

Scholar

© 2015 Royal College of Physicians and Surgeons of Canada

T2. TEACHING THE SCHOLAR ROLE (continued)

Slide #	Words on slide	Notes to teachers
OTHER SLIDES		
16.	**Scholar Role key competencies**[a] ***Physicians are able to:*** 1. Engage in the continuous enhancement of their professional activities through ongoing learning 2. Teach students, learners, the public, and other health care professionals 3. Integrate best available evidence into practice 4. Contribute to the creation and dissemination of knowledge and practices applicable to health	• Avoid including competencies for learners

17.	**Scholar Role key competency**[a]
	 Physicians are able to:
	 1. Engage in the continuous enhancement of their professional activities through ongoing learning
	   1.1 Develop, implement, monitor, and revise a personal learning plan to enhance professional practice
	   1.2 Identify opportunities for learning and improvement by regularly reflecting on and assessing their performance using various internal and external data sources
	   1.3 Engage in collaborative learning to continuously improve personal practice and contribute to collective improvements in practice
		Key and Enabling competencies on Lifelong Learning from the *CanMEDS 2015 Framework*
		 • Avoid including competencies for learners
		 • You may wish to use this slide if you are giving the presentation to teachers or planners

18.	**Scholar Role key competency**[a]
	 Physicians are able to:
	 2. Teach students, learners, the public, and other health care professionals
	   2.1 Recognize the influence of role-modelling and the impact of the formal, informal, and hidden curriculum on learners
	   2.2 Promote a safe learning environment
	   2.3 Ensure patient safety is maintained when learners are involved
	   2.4 Plan and deliver a learning activity
	   2.5 Provide feedback to enhance learning and performance
	   2.6 Assess and evaluate learners, teachers, and programs in an educationally appropriate manner
		Key and Enabling competencies on Teaching from the *CanMEDS 2015 Framework*
		 • Use one slide for each key competency and associated enabling competencies

19.	**Scholar Role key competency**[a]
	 Physicians are able to:
	 3. Integrate best available evidence into practice
	   3.1 Recognize practice uncertainty and knowledge gaps in clinical and other professional encounters and generate focused questions that address them
	   3.2 Identify, select, and navigate pre-appraised resources
	   3.3 Critically evaluate the integrity, reliability, and applicability of health-related research and literature
	   3.4 Integrate evidence into decision-making in their practice
		Key and Enabling competencies on evidence-informed decision-making from the *CanMEDS 2015 Framework*
		 • Use one slide for each key competency and associated enabling competencies

20.	**Scholar Role key competency**[a]
	 Physicians are able to:
	 4. Contribute to the creation and dissemination of knowledge and practices applicable to health
	   4.1 Demonstrate an understanding of the scientific principles of research and scholarly inquiry and the role of research evidence in health care
	   4.2 Identify ethical principles for research and incorporate them into obtaining informed consent, considering potential harms and benefits, and considering vulnerable populations
	   4.3 Contribute to the work of a research program
	   4.4 Pose questions amenable to scholarly inquiry and select appropriate methods to address them
	   4.5 Summarize and communicate to professional and lay audiences, including patients and their families, the findings of relevant research and scholarly inquiry
		Key and Enabling competencies on Research from the *CanMEDS 2015 Framework*
		 • Use one slide for each key competency and associated enabling competencies

Scholar

© 2015 Royal College of Physicians and Surgeons of Canada

T3. PLANNING FOR LEARNING

Created for the *CanMEDS Teaching and Assessment Tools Guide* by S Glover Takahashi.
Reproduced with permission of the Royal College.

Completed by:_____

Review the questions below and consider how you would answer them.

Learning

- How do you like to learn?
- How do you know what is expected of you as a learner?
- What motivates you to learn?
- What sorts of things help you improve your performance?
- Describe a supportive/safe learning climate. How important is this to you as a learner?
- Do you find it easy to ask for feedback? Who do you ask for feedback?
- Any top line lessons for you as learner?

Teaching

- Who are your learners?
- Are there types of learners you find easier or more enjoyable to teach? Why do you think that is?
- How do you like to teach in the clinical setting?
- What are some ways you motivate or support your learners?
- How do you improve the performance of your learners?
- How can you be 'learner centred'?
- How do you provide a supportive/safe learning climate for your learners?
- Do you find it easy to provide feedback? If you were to give tips on providing feedback to a colleague, what three things would you tell them?

If working with others discuss your responses as a group.

In the space provided below, write down what you learned from this exercise and describe how it will change how you learn and/or how you teach.

_____

_____

_____

_____

_____

_____

_____

Scholar

T4. COACHING LEARNERS TO GIVE AND RECEIVE FEEDBACK

Created for the *CanMEDS Teaching and Assessment Tools Guide* by S Glover Takahashi.
Reproduced with permission of the Royal College.

See Scholar Role teacher tips appendix for this teaching tool

Learner's name: _____

A. Receiving Feedback

1. Take a minute to recall a specific time/situation recently when you received feedback in a way that was effective at improving your performance.

   _____

   _____

   _____

2. Describe the details of that situation (e.g. what, where etc).

   _____

   _____

   _____

3. Why do you think that your performance was improved by that feedback? (Do you have supporting 'evidence' of improved performance – if so describe the evidence?)

   _____

   _____

   _____

4. Now try to recall a specific time/situation recently when you received feedback in a way that was not effective at improving your performance.

   _____

   _____

   _____

5. Describe the details of that situation (e.g. what, where etc)

   _____

   _____

   _____

© 2015 Royal College of Physicians and Surgeons of Canada

Scholar

T4. COACHING LEARNERS TO GIVE AND RECEIVE FEEDBACK (continued)

6. Why do you think that your performance was not improved by that feedback?

_____

_____

_____

7. Are there differences in the features of the situations (e.g. who, what, where and why)? What are the differences? How do you interpret the impact on your performance?

_____

_____

_____

B. Giving Feedback

8. How might you determine
   - if a learner is ready for feedback?
   - If a learner trusts the teacher?
   - If the learner is motivated to improve?

_____

_____

_____

9. What sorts of things/'**content**' would you explore with a learner when discussing their performance (will vary by case and Roles, e.g. interpretation of results/Medical Expert; use of open ended questions/Communicator)?

_____

_____

_____

10. For monitoring the learner's '**reactions**' to the feedback, what sorts of things would you monitor? (e.g. the areas of agreement)

_____

_____

_____

11. In '**coaching**' for performance change, what sorts of things would you include in your coaching? (e.g. tips, priorities)

_____

_____

_____

Scholar

T5. TEACHING SCRIPT SAMPLE AND TEMPLATE FOR EVIDENCE-INFORMED DECISION-MAKING

Created for the *CanMEDS Teaching and Assessment Tools Guide* by A Oswald.
Reproduced with permission of the Royal College.

1. Provide a brief description of your chosen scenario: (2-3 sentences)

_____

_____

_____

_____

2. Focus of the script for evidence-informed decision-making (EIDM)
   ☐ Identified evidence question
   ☐ Developed search strategy

EIDM skills task	Potential script wording	What CONTENT about EIDM would you like to highlight	What PROCESS skills about EIDM would you like to highlight
1. Identified evidence question			
2. Developed search strategy			

© 2015 Royal College of Physicians and Surgeons of Canada

Scholar

T5. TEACHING SCRIPT SAMPLE AND TEMPLATE FOR EVIDENCE-INFORMED DECISION-MAKING (continued)

3. Provide a brief description of scenario: (2-3 sentences)

_____

_____

_____

_____

SAMPLE Answer

- You've just seen a 58 year old man who presents with widespread pain.

- You note his myalgias are focussed in the hip and shoulder girdle and are associated with predominant morning stiffness.

- You feel the most likely diagnosis is polymyalgia rheumatica.

- However, when you explain this to the patient he says that these symptoms all started three weeks after he returned from a trip to the Caribbean and southern Florida and he asks if he should be tested for Chikungunya as he has heard that it is prevalent in these areas.

4. Focus of the script: (in this example)

☐ Evidence-informed decision-making (EIDM)

EIDM skills task	SAMPLE script wording	What CONTENT about EIDM would you like to highlight	What PROCESS skills about EIDM would you like to highlight
1. Identified evidence question	• Begin by acknowledging to the patient that you need to read a little further about whether that testing would be appropriate in his case. • Consider what your specific knowledge gaps in this topic are. • Now remind yourself of the PICO framework for composing specific searchable questions. • It appears in this setting that you are aware of this disorder but are not sure about the best way to test for it. • The question could be posed as: - In patients who have travelled to south Florida and the Caribbean how accurate is clinical history with or without specific serology for ruling out Chikungunya disease? • Now lets try to practice using this question framework as clinical questions come up through the morning.	The PICO question format: • **P**opulation • **I**ntervention • **C**omparator • **O**utcome	• For a given practice scenario, formulate a well-structured question using a specific framework (Scholar 3.3, Entry to residency milestone) • Generate focused questions that address practice uncertainty and knowledge gaps (Scholar 3.1, Core of discipline milestone)
2. Developed search strategy	• Do you need to search the primary literature or is there a trustworthy pre-appraised source that can provide this answer? • Discuss with the learner what pre-appraised sources they feel are trustworthy and compare to your own list	• Describe the advantages and limitations of pre- appraised resources (Scholar 3.2 Entry to residency milestone)	• Select appropriate sources of knowledge as they relate to addressing focused questions (Scholar 3.2 Entry to residency milestone)

Scholar

© 2015 Royal College of Physicians and Surgeons of Canada

T6. TEACHING REPORT FOR THE SCHOLAR ROLE

Created for the *CanMEDS Teaching and Assessment Tools Guide* by S Glover Takahashi.
Reproduced with permission of the Royal College.

Instructions for learners: It is important to ensure appropriate confidentiality when completing this exercise. Please avoid identifying specific learner(s) or patient(s).

1. **Choose a teaching case** from the past four weeks and describe it in 2-3 sentences

_____

_____

_____

2. **Describe the learners** (e.g. number, level, learning needs, features of learners' styles/motivation)

_____

_____

_____

3. **Describe the teacher** (e.g. was the teaching done on own/or was it team teaching, what teaching strategies/approaches were used)

_____

_____

_____

4. **Describe the content** (e.g. what was taught/learned, goals and objectives, learners' priorities, learners progress, learning climate, feedback to learners, assessment of learners, feedback to teaching/teacher)

_____

_____

_____

5. **Describe the learning/teaching context** (e.g. ambulatory clinic, operating room, laboratory)

_____

_____

_____

© 2015 Royal College of Physicians and Surgeons of Canada

T6. TEACHING REPORT FOR THE SCHOLAR ROLE (continued)

6. Complete the table below about this case. (this table can be a self-report OR completed by the learners for the teacher)

1 Poorly	2 Needs improvement	3 Satisfactorily	4 Skilfully	5 Exemplary

CRITERIA	Rate this case. *Illustrate and explain rating*	Areas or ideas for improvement?
1. Goal setting *Did the resident as teacher:* • Discuss purpose of teaching, goals and objectives for this rotation/day/activity		
2. Skill practice *Did the resident as teacher:* • Use a learner centred approach • Confirm skill level at beginning • Use assessment to support learning		
3. Feedback *Did the resident as teacher:* • Support learner engagement and motivation, monitoring progress, summative assessments, etc. • Support positive learning climate. • Provide timely and focused feedback		
4. Reflection on performance *Did the resident as teacher:* • Support a positive learning environment where mistakes are disclosed, discussed and used for learning (e.g. learning climate, safety culture, wellness)		
5. Revisit goals *Did the resident as teacher:* • Collect, organize and discuss analysed data re: explore learner's assessments and performance to sort out what did/did not work; explore where the learner is on/off milestone trajectory; what are/are not trends over time; what are/are not current strengths; what are/are not in need of current improvement; discuss next steps/plan re: content and process for improvement		

7. SUMMARY of PRIORITIES for improving teaching skills

Review your answers above and your ratings on this case. Based on this data, fill out the table below.

#	Area	Goal including timeframe	I know I will be successful if
SAMPLE	I need to build more rapport before giving feedback	Over the next three weeks, I will watch how others check-in with their learners to ensure the learners are ready to receive the feedback. Based on the good examples I encounter, I will develop some go-to-phrases that I can use	My learners show increased openness to my feedback
1.			
2.			
3.			

Other notes/reflections:

Scholar

© 2015 Royal College of Physicians and Surgeons of Canada

T7. EVIDENCE-INFORMED DECISION-MAKING (EIDM) IN DAY-TO-DAY PRACTICE

Created for the *CanMEDS Teaching and Assessment Tools Guide* by S Glover Takahashi.
Reproduced with permission of the Royal College.

Physicians are expected to integrate best available evidence into their practice. This small group exercise is designed to get you thinking about strategies that you could use to identify, select and navigate pre-appraised resources.

Completed by:_____

Date:_____

1. Take a moment on your own and reflect on your experiences over the past few months to generate a short list of information that you needed or a question that you had when making a clinical decision.

    1.

    2.

    3.

2. Could the information/questions be answered by looking in a pre-appraised resource?
   If yes, what resource? Where did/could you find it?

    1.

    2.

    3.

© 2015 Royal College of Physicians and Surgeons of Canada

Scholar

T7. EVIDENCE-INFORMED DECISION-MAKING (EIDM) IN DAY-TO-DAY PRACTICE (continued)

3. Compare your answers to Questions 1 and 2 with your colleagues. Note the differences and similarities.

_____

_____

_____

4. Take a moment and identify up to three pieces of information or questions that, in your experience, couldn't be answered by a pre-appraised source. What was your solution?

_____

_____

_____

5. Choose one of the situations you identified in question 1 or 3 and complete the table (i.e. via self report OR ask a faculty member to fill it out for you).

1 Unacceptably	2 Poorly	3 Competently	4 Very well	5 Superbly	Not Applicable

I was able to:	Rate your approach IN THIS SITUATION. *Illustrate and explain rating*	Areas or ideas for improvement?
Identify an evidence question		
Develop a search strategy		
Collect, extract and synthesize evidence		
Interpret and adapt evidence		
Plan to implement and evaluate		

6. Based on this exercise, summarize briefly any high-level lessons that you took away from this exercise. What, if any, longer term implications did you identify that you could incorporate into your lifelong learning?

_____

_____

_____

Scholar

T8. SAMPLE TIMETABLE FOR A TWO-YEAR STUDY[a]

Instructions to learner:

- It is very common to run into unanticipated delays in research projects. One strategy to prevent eleventh hour panic is to create a comprehensive timetable for your project early on. This will help you break tasks into manageable parts and to plan around the clinical and educational demands of your training program.

- The table below, reproduced from the Dr. Ackryod-Stolarz' chapter in The Research Guide: A primer for residents, other health care trainees, and practitioners, is a sample timetable for a two-year study. Consider this timetable and ask yourself the following in relation to your own research project planning:

1. What aspects of this timeline could you use as a model for your own planning?

_____

_____

_____

_____

_____

_____

_____

2. What sort of changes would you plan to make to this timetable? Sample timetable for a two-year study

_____

_____

_____

_____

_____

_____

_____

_____

a Ackroyd-Stolarz S. Managing and monitoring a study. In Harvey BJ, Lang ES, Frank JR, editors. The research guide: a primer for residents, other health care trainees, and practitioners. Ottawa: Royal College of Physicians and Surgeons of Canada; 2011. Reproduced with permission.

© 2015 Royal College of Physicians and Surgeons of Canada

Scholar

T8. SAMPLE TIMETABLE FOR A TWO-YEAR STUDY (continued)

YEAR ONE	July	Aug	Sept	Oct	Nov	Dec	Jan	Feb	Mar	Apr	May	June
Pre-study	• Identify topic and preceptor • Develop protocol • Consult with statistician (if applicable) • Identify potential funding sources • Develop study timetable		• Prepare REB submission • Submit to REB • Revisions as per REB			B R E A K	• Meet with study investigators to establish roles and responsibilities • Establish routine study-related communication (format/timing) • Determine specific study procedures					
Start-up								• Hire and train study staff • Set up research account • Start data collection • Develop and initiate monitoring regimen	**Data collection Monitoring:** • recruitment (includes response rate for surveys) • adherence to protocol • data quality • consistency of clinical and lab procedures and/ or assessments by multiple assessors • confidentiality • study budget **Routine contact with:** • study team • preceptor • REB (as needed) • participants (as needed)		

© 2015 Royal College of Physicians and Surgeons of Canada

Scholar

T8. SAMPLE TIMETABLE FOR A TWO-YEAR STUDY (continued)

YEAR TWO	July	Aug	Sept	Oct	Nov	Dec	Jan	Feb	Mar	Apr	May	June
On-going	**Data collection** *Monitoring:* • recruitment (includes response rate for surveys) • adherence to protocol • data quality • consistency of clinical and lab procedures and/or assessments by multiple assessors • confidentiality • study budget *Routine contact with:* • study team • preceptor • REB (as needed) • participants (as needed) • Submit request for annual approval to REB			• Data analysis		B R E A K	• Prepare abstract for presentation in January • Synthesize results and review with preceptor • Start manuscript • Complete follow-up for participants		• Present study • Familiarize preceptor with study documentation • Work with study team to prepare documents for archiving • Revise manuscript and prepare for submission		• Submit study closure to REB and archive documents(or make arrangements to have it done)	

© 2015 Royal College of Physicians and Surgeons of Canada

Scholar

T9. SUMMARY SHEET FOR THE SCHOLAR ROLE

Created for the *CanMEDS Teaching and Assessment Tools Guide* by S Glover Takahashi. Reproduced with permission of the Royal College.

See Scholar Role teacher tips appendix for this teaching tool

- **Four distinct 'parts' of the Scholar Role:**

    1. maintenance and acquisition of new knowledge throughout one's career through lifelong learning;

    2. sharing of knowledge through teaching and assessment;

    3. use of knowledge in evidence-informed decision-making; and

    4. creation of knowledge through research and scholarly inquiry.

- The responsibilities in the Scholar Role are shared by all practising physicians vis-à-vis teaching, the use of evidence to inform practice, and through lifelong learning.

- Need to pursue focused opportunities for learning and skill development in each of the four parts of the Scholar Role.

Learning is a lifelong process for improvement and maintenance:

1. Take FIRM control of learning.

2. Competent = skilled + current + connected

3. ASK for, look for, receive, and integrate feedback. Receiver is the key player in the feedback exchange.

ASKING for feedback[a]:

1. Ask someone who is willing and can be constructive

2. Ask for SPECIFIC feedback.

3. Listen and focus on what is helpful and specific (i.e. Do not interrupt. Watch for resistance and defensiveness)

    (Say thank you for the input.)

PROVIDING feedback:

- Giving personalized specific information about how well (or not) the performance met the established criteria and some hints or tips on the priority actions for improvement.

- R2C2 feedback approach[b] has four phases:

    - Relationship building; Is the learner ready for feedback? Is there trust of teacher? Motivation of learner?

    - Reactions exploration about feedback re: Is there consistency between giver and receiver? Areas of agreement? Surprises?

    - Content exploration re: What worked, What didn't, Match and progress in program/personal goals, objectives, needs.

    - Coaching for performance change re: What are hints or tips and priority actions for improvement? What is the plan?

Criteria for positive teaching experiences:[c]

- ORGANIZATION of teaching (e.g. teaching in clinical setting and or structured teaching)

- EDUCATIONAL DESIGN of teaching (e.g. utility of goals and objectives, effectiveness of formal learning, value of 'on the job' learning)

- SUPPORTS LEARNING (e.g. communication, supervision, graded responsibility, feedback)

- LEARNING CLIMATE of teaching (e.g. respectful, collegial, role models attributes expected of a physician, collaborative inter and intra professional teams)

- EDUCATIONAL EXPERIENCE (e.g. balance of work assignments to formal/informal learning opportunities; case mix)

Evidence-informed decision-making (EIDM). Can the question be answered by looking in a pre-appraised resource?

1. What is a reasonable trusted guideline or online resource that can help navigate a timely solution to a clinical problem in 'real time'?

2. If the answer is satisfactory and 'done', then the resident can move along. If the answer needs further exploration via EIDM, is a search for primary publications needed?

a   Stone D, Heen S. Thanks for the feedback: the science and art of receiving feedback well. New York: Viking; 2014.
b   Sargeant J, Lockyer J, Mann K, Holmboe E, Silver I, Armson H, Driessen E, MacLeod T, Yen W, Ross K, Power M. Facilitated reflective performance feedback: Developing an evidence and theory-based model. *Acad Med*, (in press).
c   Glover Takahashi. 2015. Adapted from PGME, University of Toronto.

Scholar

© 2015 Royal College of Physicians and Surgeons of Canada

T9. SUMMARY SHEET FOR THE SCHOLAR ROLE (continued)

COACHING STEPS[d]	Examples of coaching processes	What this means to resident as LEARNER	What this means to resident as TEACHER
1. GOALS	Identifying areas needing improvement that will impact performance.	**Attend to** • Needed competencies, • Entrustable Professional Activities (EPA) • Goals and objectives	**Attend to** • Purpose of the teaching • Goals and objectives
2. PRACTICE OF KNOWLEDGE, SKILLS, ABILITIES	Regular skill building practice is necessary to be a satisfactory/ good/ great performer.	**Learn** • The parts (i.e. knowledge, skills, attitudes = competencies) • Usual sequence (i.e. milestones) • Demo in patient care (i.e. EPAs)	Learner centred teaching **Assess** • Inventory starting point • Assessment for learning = formative
3. FEEDBACK	Improving skills and performance requires individual effort, accepting assistance from others and ongoing specific feedback.	• Learners need internal motivation • Learn from many people (mentors, teachers, team, community of practice) • Ask for and accept assistance of others (self-directed) • Ask for specific feedback	• Support learner engagement and motivation (e.g. motivating learners, monitoring progress, summative assessments) • Support a positive environment (e.g. learning climate) • Provide timely and focused feedback: Relationship, Reaction, Content, Coaching (R2C2)
4. REFLECTION ON PERFORMANCE	Winning, success or excellence is celebrated and tips are gathered to ensure future success Losses, disappointment or poor performance provides great lessons also.	• Accept losses, disappointment or poor performance as part of learning and life (e.g. resilience, motivation).	• Teachers need to support a positive learning environment where mistakes are disclosed, discussed and learned from (e.g. learning climate, safety culture, wellness).
5. SETTING GOALS	Analysis of both victories and losses or poor performance are viewed an opportunity to understand what needs to be changed next time and setting priorities for improvement or moving forward.	• Revisit the focus for learning re: drills to develop abilities • Analyze available data to guided self-awareness of what did/did not work; where on/off usual milestones; what are/are not strengths; what are/are not in need of improvement	• Collect, organize and discuss analysed data re: learner's assessments and performance to sort out what did/did not work; where on/off usual milestones; what are/are not trends over time; what are/are not current strengths; what are/are not in need of current improvement.
6. PLANNING FOR IMPROVEMENT	Plan for skill practice; future performance checks; consider changes to individuals, groups, systems, and processes.	• What are the next steps/plan for improvement (self-directed, motivated, feedback, milestones, learning planning, competency based medical education).	• Next steps/plan re: content and process for improvement (e.g. learner centred, motivating learners, monitoring progress).

Seven steps to EIDM process[d]

1. **Ask** by framing a focused question
2. **Acquire** the evidence in efficient manner
3. **Appraise** the evidence for quality and applicability
4. **Integrate** the evidence
5. **Adapt** the evidence for your clinical problem
6. **Apply** the evidence in your clinical plan
7. **Analyze** if the plan worked

---

d Glover Takahashi, S. 2015. Created for the *CanMEDS Teaching and Assessment Tools Guide*. Royal College.

Scholar

© 2015 Royal College of Physicians and Surgeons of Canada

A1. RESIDENT AS TEACHER MULTISOURCE FEEDBACK

Created for the *CanMEDS Teaching and Assessment Tools Guide* by S Glover Takahashi. Reproduced with permission of the Royal College.

See Scholar Role teacher tips appendix for this assessment tool

Instructions for Assessor:

- As Scholars, physicians demonstrate a lifelong commitment to excellence in practice through continuous learning and by teaching others, evaluating evidence, and contributing to scholarship.

- The competencies of the Scholar Role can be developed with practice and feedback. Using the form below, please help this resident physician gain insight into his/her teaching skills by providing valuable confidential feedback.

- Rest assured this information will be shared with the physician in aggregate form and for the purposes of helping the physician improve his/her leadership competencies.

- Please return this form in a confidential sealed envelope to the attention of:

RESIDENT Name: _____

Postgraduate year (PGY): _____

Indicate ☑ all that apply. I am a:
- ☐ Health professional team member
- ☐ Resident
- ☐ Medical student (including clerk)
- ☐ Other

Degree of Interaction
- ☐ Considerable teaching from this resident
- ☐ *Occasional or one time teaching* from this resident

#	This teacher...	1 Very poor	2 Needs improvement	3 Competent	4 Skilful	5 Exemplary	Not able to comment
1.	Was organized to teach (ie teaching in the clinical setting and or structured teaching)						
2.	Was available to learners so I had the support needed.						
3.	Ensured we agreed on expectations early and did his/her best to meet the expectations						
4.	Encouraged me to explore my limits safely						
5.	Provided regular, meaningful, prompt feedback to me						
6.	Demonstrated respect for me as a learner and as a person						
7.	Asked for and welcomed my questions						
8.	Asked for and welcomed my feedback						
9.	Had the educational experience to balance the work assignments and the formal learning opportunities						

Scholar

A1. RESIDENT AS TEACHER MULTISOURCE FEEDBACK (continued)

Overall Rating	1 Very poor	2 Needs improvement	3 Competent	4 Skilful	5 Exemplary
	One of the worst learning experiences I have had	I learned very little of significance **or** had an unpleasant experience	Good experience **and** learned something important	Excellent experience **and** learned a great deal	One of the best teachers I have had

Areas of strength	Areas for improvement
1.	1.
2.	2.
3.	3.

Other comments:

_____

_____

_____

_____

_____

_____

_____

_____

Scholar

© 2015 Royal College of Physicians and Surgeons of Canada

A2. GIVING AND RECEIVING FEEDBACK

Created for the *CanMEDS Teaching and Assessment Tools Guide* by S Glover Takahashi. Reproduced with permission of the Royal College.

See Scholar Role teacher tips appendix for this assessment tool

Instructions for Assessor:

- As Scholars, physicians demonstrate a lifelong commitment to excellence in practice through continuous learning and by teaching others, evaluating evidence, and contributing to scholarship. One of the competencies associate with this Role is the ability to provide feedback to enhance learning and performance.

- The competencies of the Scholar Role can be developed with practice and coaching. Using the form below, please help this resident physician gain insight into his/her skills around giving and receiving feedback by providing valuable confidential feedback.

- This information will be shared with the physician in **aggregate** form and for the purposes of helping the learner improve his/her leadership competencies.

- Please return this form in a confidential sealed envelope to the attention of:

_____

RESIDENT Name: _____

Postgraduate year (PGY): _____

Indicate ☑ all that apply. I am a:
- ☐ Health professional team member
- ☐ Resident
- ☐ Medical student (including clerk)
- ☐ Other

Degree of Interaction
- ☐ Considerable teaching from this resident
- ☐ *Occasional or one time teaching* from this resident

#	The resident...	1 Very poor	2 Needs improvement	3 Competent	4 Skilful	5 Exemplary	Not able to comment
1.	Asks for and welcomes my feedback						
2.	Asks for SPECIFIC feedback						
3.	Is open to feedback (i.e. does not interrupt, argue, resist or demonstrate defensiveness)						
4.	Attends to relationship building when providing feedback						
5.	Monitors the learner's reactions by exploring their views on the feedback						
6.	Explores content of feedback and performance, (i.e. what worked, what didn't work, match of progress and program/personal goals, objectives, needs)						
7.	Coaches for performance change (e.g. hints or tips for improvement, priority actions, plan)						

Scholar

© 2015 Royal College of Physicians and Surgeons of Canada

A2. GIVING AND RECEIVING FEEDBACK (continued)

OVERALL rating in relation to asking for and providing feedback	1 Unsatisfactory	3 Competently	5 Superior

Areas of strength	Areas for improvement
1.	1.
2.	2.
3.	3.

Other comments::

_____

_____

_____

_____

_____

_____

_____

_____

© 2015 Royal College of Physicians and Surgeons of Canada

Scholar

A3. EVIDENCE-INFORMED DECISION-MAKING HOMEWORK ASSIGNMENT

Created for the *CanMEDS Teaching and Assessment Tools Guide* by S Glover Takahashi.
Reproduced with permission of the Royal College.

Instructions for Learner:

• Complete questions 1-9 on this worksheet

• Submit completed material for discussion at an upcoming meeting with your academic supervisor

1. Describe your evidence question(s)

_____

_____

_____

_____

2. Describe how you identified the evidence question

_____

_____

_____

_____

3. Describe how you developed your search strategy

_____

_____

_____

_____

4. Describe how you collected evidence

_____

_____

_____

_____

Scholar

A3. EVIDENCE-INFORMED DECISION-MAKING HOMEWORK
ASSIGNMENT (continued)

5. Describe how you used pre-appraised evidence

_____

_____

_____

_____

6. Describe how you extracted important information for this question

_____

_____

_____

_____

7. Describe how you interpreted evidence for this question

_____

_____

_____

_____

8. Describe how you adapted evidence for this question

_____

_____

_____

_____

9. Comment on each of these criteria and identify areas for further work or improvement

_____

_____

_____

_____

Scholar

© 2015 Royal College of Physicians and Surgeons of Canada

A3. EVIDENCE-INFORMED DECISION-MAKING HOMEWORK
ASSIGNMENT (continued)

Criteria	Comment on your performance in THIS SITUATION. Illustrate and explain	Areas, ideas or priority for improvement?
1. Identified evidence question		
2. Developed search strategy		
3. Collected evidence (with assistance) in effective manner		
4. Appropriate use and/or balance of pre-appraised evidence and finding evidence		
5. Extracted important information for this question in an effective manner		
6. Synthesizes evidence for this question in an effective manner		
7. Interpreted evidence for this question in an effective manner		
8. Adapted evidence for this question in an effective manner		

Scholar

© 2015 Royal College of Physicians and Surgeons of Canada

A3. EVIDENCE-INFORMED DECISION-MAKING HOMEWORK ASSIGNMENT (continued)

To be completed by assessor:

This assignment is:

☐ Satisfactory

☐ Incomplete. Revisions requested.

☐ Other:_____

Areas of strength	Areas for improvement
1.	1.
2.	2.
3.	3.

Other comments:

_____

_____

_____

_____

_____

_____

_____

_____

_____

© 2015 Royal College of Physicians and Surgeons of Canada

Scholar

A4. RESEARCH PROJECT HIGH-LEVEL CHECKLIST[a]

Instructions for Teacher:

- Meet with your learner for a one-on-one teaching session to assess his/her progress on these high-level steps of a research project.

- Be prepared to walk the learner through the steps if needed.

- Revisit this checklist with the learner on a regular basis (e.g. quarterly) to explore and support their progress.

Checklist items	Complete	Not yet complete	Comments
1. Meet with your program director or departmental research coordinator as soon as possible			
2. Look for resources that provide an introduction to the basic concepts of research methodology and critical appraisal			
3. Find a research supervisor			
4. Pose a focused and specific research question			
5. Develop a research outline			
6. Meet with methodological (especially biostatistical) specialists with particular expertise in your area of study			
7. Develop a research protocol			
8. As applicable, obtain institutional and research ethics approval			
9. Seek necessary funding			
10. If you are conducting a clinical trial, ensure that it is registered with ClinicalTrials.gov			
11. Collect and analyze the data			
12. Present your findings			
13. Prepare and submit a manuscripts describing the study and its results to a suitable journal			
14. If your manuscript is accepted, revise it according to the editors' and reviewers' comments			
15. Celebrate and thank your coauthors and supervisor			

Scholar

a Hahn PM. A research road map: Fifteen Steps to a successful research project (and ten pitfalls to avoid). In Harvey BJ, Lang ES, Frank JR, editors. *The research guide: a primer for residents, other health care trainees, and practitioners.* Ottawa: Royal College of Physicians and Surgeons of Canada; 2011.Reproduced with permission.

© 2015 Royal College of Physicians and Surgeons of Canada

A5. RESEARCH PROJECT MEETING MONITORING[a]

Instructions for Teacher:

- Meet with your learner for a one-on-one teaching session to review the high-level steps to prepare for a Research meeting.

- Be prepared to walk the learner through the steps if needed.

- After your initial meeting with the learner, revisit this checklist with them on a regular basis (e.g. quarterly) to explore and support their progress.

Questions to prepare a learner for discussion at a research meeting

1. Has a timeline been developed for the research study that includes additional time (at least 25%) for inevitable delays? (refer to teaching tool T8)

2. What strategies have been implemented to deal with unexpected challenges, suggestions for useful research resources at your institution, and time-management?

3. Have you consulted the Program Director, Research Director and the research personnel in your department to learn more about the available resources to help you with your research project at your institution?

Summary checklist for review at a research meeting

- ☐ Pre-study

- ☐ Develop protocol

- ☐ Consult with statistician (if applicable)

- ☐ Develop study procedures (e.g. data collection form, mechanisms for tracking progress, etc.)

- ☐ Identify potential sources of funds

- ☐ Develop study timetable (plan for delays)

- ☐ Ethics submission and approval

  Approval date_____

- ☐ Determine roles and responsibilities of study team

- ☐ Determine method(s) and timing of routine study-related communications (e.g. bi-weekly updates)

Start-up

- ☐ Hire and train study staff (if applicable)

- ☐ Establish research account (if applicable)

  Account number_____

- ☐ Develop and initiate monitoring

Ongoing

Routinely monitor:

- ☐ Recruitment of study participants/response rate for surveys

- ☐ Adherence to protocol

- ☐ Data quality

- ☐ Consistency of clinical and laboratory procedures and/or assessments by multiple assessors

- ☐ Confidentiality

- ☐ Study budget

- ☐ Other

Maintain relevant correspondence with Research Ethics Board regarding:

- ☐ Request for annual approval

- ☐ Amendments to protocol and/or consent forms

- ☐ Reports of serious adverse events

- ☐ Study closure

Schedule routine meetings and/or contact with preceptor and study team

Post-study

- ☐ Complete follow-up for participants (i.e. communicate study results)

- ☐ Perform data analysis (with statistician if applicable)

- ☐ Review study documentation with preceptor

- ☐ Archive all study documents as per institutions requirements

Scholar

---

a Ackroyd-Stolarz S. Managing and monitoring a study. In Harvey BJ, Lang ES, Frank JR, editors. *The research guide: a primer for residents, other health care trainees, and practitioners.* Ottawa: Royal College of Physicians and Surgeons of Canada; 2011. Reproduced with permission.

© 2015 Royal College of Physicians and Surgeons of Canada

SCHOLAR ROLE TEACHER TIPS APPENDIX

T4 COACHING LEARNERS TO GIVE AND RECEIVE FEEDBACK

Instructions for Teacher:

- Meet with your learner for a one-on-one coaching session to review the fundamentals of giving and/or receiving feedback. Be prepared to walk the learner through the steps if needed.

- You may choose to adapt this tool by asking them to complete the form before you meet.

- After your initial meeting with the learner schedule time to touch base on a regular basis (e.g. quarterly) to explore and support their progress.

T9 SUMMARY SHEET FOR THE SCHOLAR ROLE

Instructions for Teacher:

- The summary sheet is intended to be a cheat sheet for the teacher as well as the learner. It is a one page resource on key concepts, frameworks and approaches.

A1 AND A2 MULTISOURCE FEEDBACK – TEACHING

Instructions for Teacher:

- Modify the form by adding or removing criteria that do/not apply.

- To optimize learning and to protect the identity of those who provide feedback, be mindful of the size and composition of your data sample.

- Be sure to provide your 'assessors' with clear instructions and provide guidance on your rating scale. You may plan faculty development to support assessors and improve consistency in completion.

- It is a good idea to notify your learners of your intention and rationale for collecting feedback on their teaching skills. Be clear about the timeframe when you will collect the data, how you will maintain confidentiality and how and when you will present the data back to the learner.

- Plan to share the summary of feedback with your learner in written format and in a face to face meeting. A face meeting will allow valuable coaching around areas of strength and areas for improvement.

Scholar

© 2015 Royal College of Physicians and Surgeons of Canada

REFERENCES

1. Adapted from the definition of continuing professional development developed by Connie LeBlanc, Yvonne Steinert, Craig Campbell for the invitational Summit on the Future of Continuing Medical Education in April 2014.

2. Burls, A. What is critical appraisal? Last retrieved July 4, 2015, from http://www.medicine.ox.ac.uk/bandolier/painres/download/whatis/what_is_critical_appraisal.pdf

3. This definition has been developed on the basis of information found at Public Health Agency of Canada. Accessible information from the Public Health Agency Canadian Best Practices Portal. Last retrieved July 4, 2015 from http://cbpp-pcpe.phac-aspc.gc.ca/resources/evidence-informed-decision-making/eidm3/

4. Lang E. Critical Appraisal: *The CanMEDS 2005 Monograph Series*. Royal College of Physicians and Surgeons of Canada. Unpublished.

5. Bravata DM, Huot SJ, Abernathy HS, Skeff KM, Bravata DM. The development and implementation of a curriculum to improve clinicians' self-directed learning skills: a pilot project. *BMC Med Educ*. 2003;3:7.

6. Eva KW, Regehr G, Gruppen LD. Blinded by "Insight": Self-Assessment and Its Role in Performance Improvement In: Hodges BD, Lingard L, editors. *The question of competence: reconsidering medical education in the twenty-first century*. Ithaca: Cornell University Press. 2014.

7. Stone D, Heen S. Thanks for the feedback: the science and art of receiving feedback well. New York: Viking; 2014.

8. George B, Sims P, McLean AN, Mayer D. Discovering your authentic leadership. *Harv Bus Rev*. 2007; 85(2): 129–30, 132–8, 157.

9. Oswald A, Chan M-K. Scholar-Teacher: *The CanMEDS 2005 Monograph Series*. Royal College of Physicians and Surgeons of Canada. Unpublished.

10. Glover Takahashi, S. Created for the *CanMEDS Teaching and Assessment Tools Guide*. Royal College of Physicians and Surgeons of Canada 2015.

11. Sargeant J, Lockyer J, Mann K, Holmboe E, Silver I, Armson H, Driessen E, MacLeod T, Yen W, Ross K, Power M. Facilitated reflective performance feedback: Developing an evidence and theory-based model. *Acad Med*. (in press).

12. Milan FB, Parish SJ, Reichgott MJ. A Model for Educational Feedback Based on Clinical Communication Skills Strategies: Beyond the Feedback Sandwich. *Teach Learn Med*. 2006;18(1): 42-47.

13. Brown M, Hodges B, Wakefield J. Chapter 1.3 - Points for giving effective feedback. In *Evaluation Methods: a resource handbook*, Norman G (Ed). Hamilton: McMaster University 1995.

14. Glover Takahashi S. 2014. Scoping review of eLearning. Unpublished manuscript.

15. Ciliska, D. Introduction to evidence-informed decision-making. Last retrieved July 31, 2015 http://www.cihr-irsc.gc.ca/e/45245.html

16. Kunz R, Wegscheider K, Fritsche L, Schünemann HJ, Moyer V, Miller D, Boluyt N, Falck-Ytter Y, Griffiths P, Bucher HC, Timmer A, Meyerrose J, Witt K, Dawes M, Greenhalgh T, Guyatt GH. Determinants of knowledge gain in evidence-based medicine short courses: an international assessment. *Open Med*. 2010;4(1):e3-e10.

17. Harvey BJ, Lang ES, Frank JR, editors. *The research guide: a primer for residents, other health care trainees, and practitioners*. Ottawa: Royal College of Physicians and Surgeons of Canada; 2011.

18. Bandiera G, Lee S, Tiberius R. Creating effective learning in today's emergency departments: how accomplished teachers get it done. *Ann Emerg Med*. 2005; 45(3):253-61.

19. Ramos KD, Schafer S. Tracz SM. Validation of the Fresno test of competency in evidence based medicine. *BMJ* 2003. 8;326(7384):319-21.

20. Mohr NM, Stoltze AJ, Harland KK, Van Heukelom JN, Hogrefe CP, Ahmed A. An evidence –based medicine curriculum implemented in journal club improved resident performance on the Fresno test. *J Emerg Med*. 2015;48(2):222-229.

21. Ilic D, HartW, Fiddes P, Misso M, Villanueva E. Adopting a blended learning approach to teaching evidence based medicine: a mixed study. *BMC Med Educ*. 2013;17(13):169.

Scholar

© 2015 Royal College of Physicians and Surgeons of Canada

Balance
RESILIENCE
Accountability Social contract
COMMITMENT
Self-care WELLNESS
Responsibility Honesty
PROFESSIONAL
Identity BOUNDARIES
CONFIDENTIALITY STANDARDS
INTEGRITY Self-regulating
PATIENT Practice
Behaviour Care
ETHICS

Linda Snell

Leslie Flynn

Susan Glover Takahashi

Professional

1. Why the Professional Role matters

The CanMEDS Professional Role sets an expectation and standard that all physicians must develop specific competencies that will allow them to conduct themselves as medical professionals throughout their medical career. The Role itself is often described as having two parts to it: being a professional and demonstrating professional behaviours.

Learning to be a professional refers to the evolution of a person's identity into that of a practising physician in a specific specialty.[1] Professionalism is at the core of the contract between a physician and society.[2] Society has expectations that physicians are individually and collectively committed to patients[a], families, colleagues, the public and themselves.

Demonstrating professionalism refers to the day-to-day practice behaviours that reflect:

- a commitment to ethics of care, clinical integrity, independence, and interdependence;
- the development and maintenance of clinical competence within the boundaries of professional regulations; and
- managing the demands of one's practice while taking care of oneself.[3, 4]

Orienting your learners to the Professional Role can help them appreciate the time and effort required to focus on learning, teaching, and assessing this Role. When introducing your learners to the Role, be sure to cover these points:

- Patients expect their physicians to provide high-quality, safe medical care.[3]
- Being a professional is central to being a physician and requires active effort to evolve into a specialist.[3]
- Professional behaviour is central to patient safety and effectiveness in team-based care.[3]
- The resilience, wellness and self-care of a physician impacts their patients' care, their co-workers and the health system, requiring the need to manage the demands of work/practice while also attending to personal health activities and constructive coping skills.[4, 5]

2. What the Professional Role looks like in daily practice

Sometimes learners have trouble breaking down the behaviours and competencies of a physician into its component CanMEDS parts. Learners often find it helpful when someone takes the time to 'tag' the Roles for them so that they can begin to associate certain activities with particular CanMEDS Roles. This section provides you with a quick overview of how the Professional Role functions and what learners can look for in the Professional Role in their daily practice.

In day-to-day practice, the Professional Role involves being committed to effectively performing all seven CanMEDS Roles. The Professional Role is linked to all the CanMEDS Roles, for example:

- Commitment to patient in the Professional Role links with the Communicator Role's patient-centred communication, the Health Advocate Role's focus on supporting the patient's needs and values, and the Scholar Role's focus on ensuring the best of patient care by maintaining and enhancing personal competence.
- Commitment to society in the Professional Role links with the Health Advocate Role's attention to supporting the needs and values of a patient population and the community.
- Commitment to the profession in the Professional Role links with the Collaborator Role's attention to working effectively in teams and the Scholar Role's focus on building the knowledge that is based on research and scholarly inquiry as well as through the important responsibility of teaching.

If your learners are struggling to grasp some of these concepts, encourage them to listen for some of the trigger words in Table P-1, which can be associated with being a professional and demonstrating professionalism in day-to-day practice. This is a quick and easy trick for them to start to make the connection between daily activities and being a Professional as described in the CanMEDS Framework.

---

a   Throughout the Physician Competency Framework and Milestones Guide, reference to the patients's family are intended to include all those who are personally significant to the patient and are concerned with his or her care, including, according to the patient's circumstances, family members, partners, caregivers, legal guardians, and substitute decision-makers.

© 2015 Royal College of Physicians and Surgeons of Canada

Professional

TABLE P-1. TRIGGER WORDS RELATING TO THE PROCESS AND CONTENT OF THE PROFESSIONAL ROLE

Trigger words relating to the PROCESS of the Professional Role:	Trigger words relating to the CONTENT of the Professional Role:	
• Accountability • Behaving • Fulfilling • Respecting • Self-regulating • Trust	• Balance • Boundaries • Commitment • Confidentiality • Conflicts of interest • Ethics, Ethical issues • Honesty • Identity • Integrity • Medico legal frameworks • Morality • Professional Identity	• Regulatory • Reliable • Resilience • Responsibility • Social contract • Societal need • Society's expectations of physicians • Standards • Trustworthiness • Wellness

Excerpt from the CanMEDS 2015 Physician Competency Framework[b]

DEFINITION

As Professionals, physicians are committed to the health and well-being of individual patients and society through ethical practice, high personal standards of behaviour, accountability to the profession and society, physician-led regulation, and maintenance of personal health.

DESCRIPTION[c]

Physicians serve an essential societal role as professionals dedicated to the health and care of others. Their work requires mastery of the art, science, and practice of medicine. A physician's professional identity is central to this Role. The Professional Role reflects contemporary society's expectations of physicians, which include clinical competence, a commitment to ongoing professional development, promotion of the public good, adherence to ethical standards, and values such as integrity, honesty, altruism, humility, respect for diversity, and transparency with respect to potential conflicts of interest.

It is also recognized that, to provide optimal patient care, physicians must take responsibility for their own health and well-being and that of their colleagues. Professionalism is the basis of the implicit contract between society and the medical profession, granting the privilege of physician-led regulation with the understanding that physicians are accountable to those served, to society, to their profession, and to themselves.

KEY COMPETENCIES

Physicians are able to:

1. Demonstrate a commitment to patients by applying best practices and adhering to high ethical standards

2. Demonstrate a commitment to society by recognizing and responding to societal expectations in health care

3. Demonstrate a commitment to the profession by adhering to standards and participating in physician-led regulation

4. Demonstrate a commitment to physician health and well-being to foster optimal patient care

b Snell L. Flynn L, Pauls M, Kearney R, Warren A, Sternszus R, Cruess R, Cruess S, Hatala R, Dupré M, Bukowskyj M, Edwards S, Cohen J, Chakravarti A, Nickell L, Wright J. Professional. In: Frank JR, Snell L, Sherbino J, editors. *CanMEDS 2015 Physician Competency Framework*. Ottawa: Royal College of Physicians and Surgeons of Canada; 2015. Reproduced with permission.
c The Role description draws from Cruess SR, Johnston S, Cruess RL. "Profession": a working definition for medical educators. Teach Learn Med. 2004; 16(1):74-6 and from Cruess SR, Cruess RL. Professionalism and medicine's social contract with society. Virtual Mentor 2004 6(4).

Professional

KEY TERMS OF THE PROFESSIONAL ROLE

One way to help your learners familiarize themselves with the Professional Role is to have them review key words that are central to the Professional Role.

Professionalism signifies a set of values, behaviours, and relationships that underpins the trust the public has in physicians.[6]

Professional identity[7] is described as a 'way of being' with the focus on becoming a physician by internalizing the values of the profession. In residency, the identity is a representation of self, achieved in stages over time during which the characteristics, values and norms of the specialty are internalized, resulting in an individual thinking, acting and feeling like a specialist in that specialty.[2] Professional identity is distinct from 'professionalism', which is described as a 'way of acting'.[8]

Fiduciary relationship refers to the special relationship of trust between physicians and their patients that requires physicians to always act in their patients' best interests, including providing care, effectively communicating treatment and care options, protecting privacy and confidentiality, and maintaining appropriate boundaries.[3]

It involves maintaining an appropriate professional relationship with patients. Boundaries mean setting limits on the nature of relationships with patients, on accepting gifts, and on treating one's family members and friends. Physicians can be relaxed and cordial but need to keep a work-related distance with patients.[9]

Social contract[10] is the implicit contract between society and the medical profession, granting the privilege of physician-led regulation with the understanding that physicians are accountable to those served and to society. Linking professionalism with the social contract provides a rational basis for the presence of medicine's obligations, both individual and collective.

Hidden curriculum refers to the implicit learning through day-to-day examples that are outside of formal and informal teaching.[11,12] Residents watch what you are doing so you need to role model good professional behaviours.

Resilience is a flexible adaptability demonstrated over time to remain positive and constructive in the face of challenge.[13] The dimensions of resilience include self-efficacy, self-control, planning, ability to engage help and support, learning from difficulties and persistence despite blocks to progress.[14]

Coping mechanisms found in resilient individuals and units (e.g. teams, organizations) include humour, management of negative emotions, reflection for learning, and seeking social support in an effective way. In order to develop coping mechanisms and for resilience to mature, exposure to some risks is necessary.

Wellness means the condition of good physical and mental health necessary to provide high quality care to patients.[15] Physicians should only care for patients when they are well enough to do so.[15]

Physicians have a responsibility to:

- Be aware of their own health, which includes being able to recognize when they are not well enough to provide competent care.

- Obtain help, if necessary, from colleagues, their own physician, or other supports, in order to ensure their own wellness.

- Adjust their practice, as necessary, to ensure that patients can and do receive appropriate care.

- Recognize limits imposed by fatigue, stress or illness, taking care to ensure a healthy work-life balance.

- Avoid self-treatment.[15]

Burnout[16] refers to a syndrome characterized by a loss of enthusiasm for work (emotional exhaustion), feelings of cynicism (de-personalization), and a low sense of personal accomplishment.

Self-care means those activities performed independently by an individual to promote and maintain personal and professional well-being throughout life, including self-reflection and self-awareness, identification and prevention of burnout, and appropriate professional boundaries. Strategies for personal self-care include prioritizing close relationships such as those with family; maintaining a healthy lifestyle by ensuring adequate sleep, regular exercise, and time for vacations; fostering recreational activities and hobbies; practising mindfulness and meditation; and pursuing spiritual development.[17]

Fatigue management means the purposeful activities and actions that an individual resident and program undertake before call, during call, and post call to manage and mitigate the impact of sleepiness on patient care and on the resident.[18] Unfortunately many of the 'usual' sleep hygiene suggestions such as sleeping at the same time every day and getting a

© 2015 Royal College of Physicians and Surgeons of Canada

minimum of six uninterrupted hours of sleep every day may be challenging given the training demands of residency. As such, residents need to focus on relevant strategies to mitigate and manage fatigue, sleepiness and sleep. The Royal College refers to this as fatigue risk management which includes such things as taking a nap before driving home.

Self-efficacy is the extent or strength of one's belief in one's own ability to complete tasks and reach goals.[19]

Self-regulation[d] refers to the profession led responsibility for the licensing and registration of the professional including setting educational, technical and ethical standards (i.e. medical regulatory authority).[20]

Emotional intelligence is a group of skills that professionals use to guide their thinking, behaviour, and outcomes. It includes the following:[21,22]

- **Self-awareness** – knowing one's strengths, weaknesses, drivers, values, and impact on others
- **Self-regulation**[d] – the ability to monitor and control one's own behaviour, emotions or thoughts, altering them in accordance with the demands of the situation. It includes the abilities to exhibit first responses, to resist interference from irrelevant stimulation and to persist on relevant tasks even when we don't enjoy them
- **Motivation** – a strong internal drive to pursue goals and achievement for reasons that are personally meaningful
- **Empathy** – considering others' feelings, values, and preferences
- **Social skill** – building rapport and relationships with others

3. Preparing to teach the Professional Role

The Professional Role, like the other CanMEDS Roles, can be difficult for some learners (and teachers) to understand as it is concurrently 'taken for granted' and viewed as the 'ultimate responsibility'. In this section we review some key concepts that will help you prepare to teach professionalism and physician health by addressing some common misconceptions about the Role and exploring how to integrate the content and process of being a professional.

3.1 Common misconceptions to address with learners

First, some suggest that being a professional is impossible to teach because it is primarily a moral endeavour and that a learner's key traits or personality attributes are 'hard wired'. This view is overly simplistic. **Professionalism has multiple factors that can be taught:**

- *individual factors* (e.g. behaviour and cognitive processes);
- *interpersonal factors* (e.g. process or effect of providing patient care with others); and
- *context factors*[23] (e.g. variations and expectations in interactions within or across individuals, institutions, specialties, cultures, countries).

Second, there is a misconception that 'not being *un*professional' is the same as being 'professional'. While there is a double negative in that sentence, which makes it hard to process, the important thing to understand is that this misconception exists and in your role as teacher you will have to work hard to dispel it. It's relatively easy to point out unprofessional behaviours that you want your learners to avoid, but you will help your residents more if you **focus on actively demonstrating positive professional behaviours.** You can also support your learners' efforts in demonstrating professional knowledge, skills, and attitudes by orienting them to the goals and objectives you have for them as individuals and within the program.

The third misconception is that doctors are somehow immune to the illnesses and afflictions of ordinary people and that they don't need to take care of themselves. The profession of medicine has traditionally prioritized work over self care,[24] but the consequences of the 'good old days' to physicians, their patients or the health care system suggest this past view needs to be permanently reset.[16] This misconception has led to the assumption that heroic levels of performance are expected and valued, and that reasonable bounds of effective performance and healthy habits do not apply to doctors. Help your learners understand as professionals – and later when they are teaching others – that **physicians need to demonstrate the importance of their own personal health, wellness, and resilience** to themselves, their patients, their teams, and the organizations where they work.

---

d **Self-regulation** has two meanings, one related to a component of emotional intelligence and the other related to licensing and registration.

Professional

3.2 Set expectations and create a culture that fosters development of positive professional behaviours

One of the important steps to teach the Professional Role is setting clear expectations through orientation sessions, documented policies and procedures and by employing professional codes and charters.[25] Setting and sharing clear expectations allows both learners and teachers to have a common language to describe professional or unprofessional behaviours that are acceptable and not acceptable within your program, specialty and organizational culture. Regular monitoring of the professionalism of residents is important to ensure that feedback is timely and maladaptive behaviours are discussed promptly and modified.[26]

For example, arriving late to clinic or on an assignment occasionally is human. A pattern of lateness, however, falls below the behaviour expectations. To not follow up on serious incidents or patterns of behaviour (i.e. something that is below the standard professional expectations) sends a message to your learners that their behaviour doesn't matter to the program or the organization.

LABEL THE BEHAVIOUR – AVOID JUDGING THE PERSON

Because professionalism is linked to the identity of the physician as a person (i.e. being a physician is being a professional), we may mistakenly label a person as 'unprofessional' when making an error that is considered to fall within the domain (Role) of professional or within the purview of being professional in nature (e.g. is rude and disruptive), when it is the behaviour that is unprofessional.

Physicians are human, and all humans make mistakes as they learn. The close link between a person's identity as a physician (i.e. as a professional person) and behaviour (e.g. professionalism skills) can heighten a person's negative reaction when an error is being discussed.

It should come as no surprise that learners will sometimes underperform. Learners need to understand that underperformance and errors occur in all Roles, not just the Professional Role. Learners often find it challenging to cope with feedback about underperforming or errors, however, if they interpret the feedback as one where their personal identity is being judged or viewed as unsatisfactory, resistance and defensiveness are likely to follow.

It is important to label the behaviour as a mistake, and to avoid words that label a person or that may be interpreted as a personal attack. Using the words **'positive professional behaviour'** and **'unprofessional behaviour'** will help.

Given the realities of residents and that there are many stressors, there may be times when you or others in your program sometimes elect to turn a blind eye on a resident's or faculty member's negative behaviour. The challenge is to ensure that 'giving the benefit of the doubt' is consistent across the whole program and organization and doesn't encourage a double standard that contrasts what is said (i.e. we want our residents and faculty to be professional at all times) with what is done (i.e. if no one complains about our residents unprofessional behaviour, we will tolerate it even if we won't tolerate similar behaviour from other programs' residents or other co-workers). Like all skills, professionalism behaviours are best practiced often: positive behaviours are commended, unprofessional behaviours are identified, and prompt feedback about expectations and improvement are provided to allow for reflection and improvement.

3.3 Provide your learners with a process to develop their professional identity in your specialty

Your residents need help to develop professional identity in your program so that they think, act and feel like a specialist in your discipline.[2] Recent work by Cruess et al,[1] which helps to describe the development of professional identity, provides a common framework and language for professional identity stages, characteristics and features.

This framework can assist teachers and learners identify if there is a lack of progress in professional identity. For example, in moving from residency into readiness for autonomous practitioner, you may find that a learner is struggling to move from stage three (i.e. view multiple perspectives and concern for how s/he is perceived) to stage four (i.e. manages different values and expectations and self is defined independently of others).

Table P-2 provides a sample framework of concepts related to professional identity that help label stages of identity formation. By understanding a model of the sequence of developing professional identity, you and your learners will have a shared language to discuss professional identity and to identify a lack of progress in it.

© 2015 Royal College of Physicians and Surgeons of Canada

Professional

TABLE P-2. KEGAN'S STAGES:[e] TWO TO FOUR[27,28] OF IDENTITY FORMATION ADAPTED TO DESCRIBE PROFESSIONAL IDENTITY IN MEDICINE

Identity stage #[f]	Identity stage name	Personal characteristics of this stage	Features of this stage in practice that you might see
2.	Imperial	An individual who takes into account the views of others but whose own needs and interests predominate	An individual who can assume professional roles but is primarily motivated to follow rules and to be correct: self-reflection is low. Emotions can overwhelm reason.
3.	Interpersonal	An individual who is able to view multiple perspectives simultaneously and subordinate self-interest; who is concerned about how he or she is perceived by others	An individual who can assume professional roles and is oriented towards sharing obligations; tends to seek out those to emulate; is idealistic and self-reflective. Emotions are generally under control, and he or she generally does the right thing.
4.	Institutional	An individual who can assume a role and enter into relationship while assessing them in terms of self-authored principles and standards; the self is defined independently of others	An individual who is able to understand relationships in terms of different values and expectations. The external values of the professional become internal values. Reason is in full control over needs, desires, and passion.

Residents join their programs and specialties with existing personalities, and through residency they are socialized into their program, specialty and organizations. They become competent physicians in their discipline with an evolved personal and professional identify.[1] Cruess et al offer a schema for medical educators to support the identity development of residents, which highlights key areas of development of professional identity.[1]

Early skills for residents to master in developing their identity as a physician in your specialty are:

- **Learning the language** – e.g. of your program, discipline, organization

- **Learning to live with ambiguity** – e.g. personal, professional

Throughout residency, your residents' identity and competence is developed through socialization in your program, discipline and organization through:

- **Learning to play the role** – i.e. pretend until you become; includes playing the role in your program, discipline, organization

- **Learning the hierarchy and power relationships** – e.g. formal, informal, hidden

Central to supporting the identity formation of residents is offering a high volume and wide variety of opportunities that include reflection, mentorship and feedback from teachers in their discipline. These opportunities are important for your residents as they acquire their identity by practising that role over time.[1] Horizontal curriculums (i.e. longitudinal clinics, clustering learners and teachers and facilities over prolonged periods) are an example of a structural design that helps learners and teachers work together in the identity formation of becoming a specialist in a particular discipline.

3.4 Orient your learners to the application of bioethics and professional standards for their patients, program organization and community

Your residents are likely familiar with general professional codes, policies and procedures, which they have likely reviewed earlier in their training. Help your residents get to the next level by applying specific expectations for professionals in practice — what is expected by patients, programs, organizations (e.g. university, hospital, professional bodies), and provincial or federal regulations.

---

e Adapted from Cruess RL, Cruess SR, Boudreau JD, Snell L, Steinert Y. A schematic representation of the professional identity formation and socialization of medical students and residents: a guide for medical educators. Acad Med. 2015;90(6):718-25. Reproduced with permission.

f As stage 1 is the impulsive mind, it is viewed as well below residents' level. Stage 5, the self-transforming mind is viewed as rare and generally not applicable.

Professional

Learners need to understand the tangible and important local variations in expectations, paying particular attention to bioethics and standards such as boundaries, privacy legislation, health records, duty to report, conflicts of interest, consent, immunization, licensing etc. Help your residents learn what applies to them personally and in daily practice (i.e. whether it is acceptable to email a colleague with patient-related questions when on call, who they need to notify if a needle stick injury comes back positive for hepatitis, knowing the age of majority in the event that a patient doesn't want you to contact his or her parents, and knowing how to manage refusal of treatment).

3.5 Role model positive professional behaviours

A supportive environment should reward positive behaviours that are valued by your program and discourage behaviours that your program views as not compatible with responsible, respectful physicians. You and your faculty need to be effective role models so that there is consistency between the expressed curriculum and what is observed by your learners in day-to-day practice.[29] Residents will notice when the values and virtues of professionalism are demonstrated or not.[2] It is important to be aware of the 'hidden curriculum' around professionalism in your program.

Cruess et al[30] outline how you and your residents can actively use role modelling in the development of their professionalism behaviours:[30]

1. Active observation of role model;

2. Making the unconscious conscious;

3. Reflection and abstraction;

4. Translating insights into principles and action; and

5. Generalization and behaviour change.

The active observation of role modelling can be guided by some documented expectations of positive and negative behaviours. Table P-3 outlines three sample areas that learners could be observing in their role models (e.g. clinical competency, teaching skills, and personal qualities) and includes an inventory of positive and negative role modelling behaviours. This sample table from Cruess et al[30] could be used as is or modified to reflect local culture and codes in your faculty development of your teachers or role models as well by residents. Additionally, it could be adapted to generally clarify positive and negative behaviours.

TABLE P-3. POSITIVE AND NEGATIVE CHARACTERISTICS OF ROLE MODELS[g]

POSITIVE ROLE MODELLING CHARACTERISTICS	NEGATIVE ROLE MODELLING CHARACTERISTICS
A. Clinical competency	
1. Excellent knowledge and skill	1. Deficient knowledge and skill
2. Effective communication	2. Ineffective communication
3. Sound clinical reasoning	3. Poor clinical reasoning
B. Teaching skills	
4. Aware of role	4. Unaware of role
5. Explicit about what is modelled	5. Not explicit about what is modelled
6. Makes time for teaching	6. Does not make time for teaching
7. Shows respect for student needs	7. Does not show respect for student needs
8. Provides timely feedback	8. Does not provide timely feedback
9. Encourages reflection in students	9. Does not encourage reflection in students
C. Personal qualities	
10. Compassionate and caring	10. Insensitive to patients' suffering
11. Honesty and integrity	11. Lapses in honesty and integrity
12. Enthusiastic for the practice of medicine	12. Dissatisfaction with the practice of medicine
13. Effective interpersonal skills	13. Ineffective interpersonal skills
14. Commitment to excellence	14. Acceptance of mediocre results
15. Collegial	15. Lack of collegiality
16. Demonstrates humour	16. Humourless approach

g Adapted by permission from the BMJ from Cruess SR, Cruess RL, Steinert Y. Role modelling—making the most of a powerful teaching strategy. *BMJ.* 2008;336(7646):718-21. Reproduced with permission from BMJ Publishing Group Ltd.

© 2015 Royal College of Physicians and Surgeons of Canada

3.6 Provide opportunities to actively demonstrate professionalism

Teach your learners to recognize professionalism when it is done well (i.e. positive professional behaviours), and not just when it is done poorly (i.e. unprofessional behaviours). Trainees will also gain from knowing that actively attending to professionalism not only benefits their patients, team, and organization, but has also been known to reduce medico-legal risk.[3]

Key elements of professionalism[3] that residents can include as part of their day-to-day practice include:

- **Clinical competence:** Your learners need to be effective at determining what they are competent to perform. Additionally they need to understand that clinical competence is an ongoing, never ending activity. As such, clinical competence requires a commitment to lifelong practice enhancement (see Scholar chapter). They need to ask for supervision and/or assistance when they are doing something they are not confident or competent to do. Asking for, receiving, and using feedback to improve clinical competence is vital. Feedback also improves the accuracy of your learners' estimations of their own clinical skills, so they can better gauge whether they need to ask for supervision and/or assistance. *(See the Leader chapter for information on asking for feedback and developing self-awareness and emotional intelligence.)*

- **Responsiveness:** Your learners need to demonstrate active attention to patients' clinical and emotional needs. In the event of an emergency or safety incident, trainees need to be skilled in its incident management. *(See the Communicator chapter re. patient and see the Leader chapter for information on patient safety and incident management.)*

- **Engagement:** Your learners need to demonstrate engagement with patients and with other members of the health care team in a respectful and collaborative manner. This includes working in partnership, using a patient-centred approach, and employing words and actions that are constructive and courteous. *(See the Communicator chapter re. patient and see the Collaborator chapter re. team.)*

- **Integrity:** Patient well-being is central to your learners acting with integrity. Integrity involves maintaining boundaries, being reliable and supportive of colleagues, acting in accordance with regulations, and being accountable for one's actions.

3.7 Provide your learners with resources to support resilience, wellness and self-care as it relates to your specialty, team and organization

Your residents need to understand the value of resilience to their health and that resiliency can be nurtured into a stronger, more effective attribute.[13] Help your residents develop resilience by involving faculty and experts, who can assist your residents in focusing on:

- **Self management**
  - Demonstrating self-directed learning (e.g. reading around cases for daily rounds)
  - Development of realistic goals (e.g. research project plans)
  - Learning to use feedback to build confidence, self-awareness and strengthen performance (i.e. asks for and builds on received feedback in day to day clinical practice)

- **Persistence and commitment**
  - Setting and working towards longer-term goals (e.g. presentation at annual research day)

Your residents need to know that you value their health and their efforts to balance the demands of the work and caring for others with care for oneself. Help your resident know what are or are not reasonable expectations (e.g. coming to work sick is not OK, how to manage or mitigate fatigue).[31] Remind residents that they will benefit by reducing their stress and vulnerability (see Table P-4) through social support (e.g. program-based social events, journal club), personal control (e.g. electives, timing and focus of supervision or mentorship), and by accepting graded exposure to uncertainty and risk (whereby they are assigned a 'stretch' procedure or patient problem for the day and receive coaching or feedback).

TABLE P-4. Tips for managing and mitigating fatigue[31, h]

Pre-call
• Visit a primary health care provider regularly
• Take time to prepare for on-call i.e. preparing a water bottle and healthy food
• Take a short break between the end of daytime duties and initial on-call handover

On-call
• Nap in a dark, cool, and quiet call room
• Eat appropriately
• Have easy access to water
• Use caffeine wisely
• Take short breaks in natural light

Post-call
• Pre-arrange for transport home or nap prior to travel home
• Rehydrate and have a light meal once home
• Minimize external distractions
• Defer exercise until after sleep

Programs
• Provide formal education in fatigue management
• Create a standardized approach to handover
• Curtail or mindfully reschedule academic activities on post-call day

Provide your residents with information and resources about resilience, wellness and self-care in your specialty, team, and organization. These resources can be web, program or organization based. (See also Leader chapter).

3.8 Encourage your residents to care for themselves and to be watchful for warning signs

Your learners need to care for themselves and while there is no 'magic solution' the research shows[4] that some straightforward personal health activities are associated with lower rates of burnout and improved quality of life. These personal health activities include:

- Weekly aerobic and weight training to recommended levels

- Annual visits to primary care provider (i.e. family physician)

- Routine required health screening practices

It is not clear if these are the cause or effect, but nonetheless these three personal health activities reflect a valuing of personal needs and health.

Constructive skills[4,5] that may decrease the risk for burnout and improved personal and professional quality of life include:

- Positive reframing

- Finding meaning in work

- Focusing on what is important in life

- Maintaining a positive outlook and attitude towards work

- Embracing an approach that stresses work-life balance

Your residents will need support to manage the many demands on their professional and personal lives and to balance availability to others with care for themselves. Residents may need encouragement to take responsibility for this and not count on others to do this for them (e.g. the chief resident, program director, program administrator, partner, parent, or friends). There are many handbooks and resources to assist your residents, including a very practical resource, *The Time Management Guide: a practical handbook for physicians by physicians.*[32] Share your programs' advice with your residents and regularly review key hints that you develop, such as:

h Puddester D. Managing and mitigating fatigue in the era of changing resident duty hours. *BMC Med Educ.* 2014;14(suppl 1):S3. Adapted with permission.

© 2015 Royal College of Physicians and Surgeons of Canada

Professional

HINTS TO MAINTAIN WELLNESS

1. *Have a family doctor.* See your family doctor annually or when you are unwell. Attend your needed personal screening health tests. Do not self medicate.

2. *Sleep right.* Sleep hygiene is important. Learn how to capture sleep opportunities as an investment for self and patients.

3. *Eat well.* Make good choices. Plan to feed your body. Shop for foods that DO work with your lifestyle. Pack your lunch or snacks. Remember to eat well and often. Avoid excess caffeine and sugar. Limit use of alcohol and non-prescription drugs.

4. *Exercise regularly.* This is good for your body and your brain. You will learn more if you exercise.

5. *Stay connected.* Manage the challenge to make time to see your family and friends, exercise, relax, do other important activities like completing your taxes, see your family doctor, or go to the dentist. Schedule important things like these with enough regularity. Keep scheduled appointments and commitments. (The corollary to this is that you also don't have time for regret, guilt, divorce/relationship discord, illness, etc.)

It is also important to orient your residents to look for the warning signs of stress and illness in themselves or co-residents in day-to-day practice, and how and where to get assistance and support and from whom.

SAMPLE WARNING SIGNS OF CONCERN ABOUT WELLNESS

If concerned about these warning signs of concern about wellness, promptly seek assistance and support.

1. Sudden or trend for isolation or absence such as not showing up for work, rounds, meeting, assignments.

2. Mood swings, teary, unusual or easily irritated or frustrated.

3. Often late to work or late with assignments.

4. More absences than is usual or typical.

5. Dishevelled, unkempt or loss of attention to self and grooming.

6. Appearance or suspicion of over consumption of alcohol or other substances.

4. Hints, tips and tools for *teaching* the Professional Role

As a teacher your goal is to deliver the right content and in a way that helps your residents learn. Sometimes you will teach directly. Other times you will facilitate and support the teaching of others or self-directed activities by learners. There are parts of the Professional Role that can be especially difficult for learners to relate to and understand in the context of their work. For this reason this section of the Tools Guide includes a short menu of tips and tricks that are highly effective for teaching the Professional Role. You can treat the list as a buffet: pick and choose the tips that resonate most and that will work for you, your program and your learners.

Teaching Tip 1.
Talk about challenges of professionalism in day-to-day practice

Learning and teaching professionalism is best done in the midst of the messiness of the clinical setting in real time.

You and your faculty need to be candid with your learners about the lived experience of a career in medicine and the day-to-day professionalism challenges of living up to the profession's stated ideals; about the dangers of technological expertise without caring human relationships; about conflicts of interest and the difficult professional challenges of dealing with unprofessional colleagues; and about behaviour that risks patients' safety.

Learners benefit from reflecting and talking about the challenges and learning to make decisions where the answers are 'it depends', where there is a balancing of issues, and where they must sort out the implications of taking responsibility for actions.

During case rounds or at the bedside, encourage your learners to be aware when you are moving to the Professional Role – sorting out the push or pull of challenging issues or behaviours that put at risk quality clinical care, responsiveness, engagement or integrity of you as an individual physician, you within the patient care team, or you within the organization system.

© 2015 Royal College of Physicians and Surgeons of Canada

Teaching Tip 2:
Facilitate and foster professionalism in day-to-day practice

By providing explicit experiences that will enable your learners to reflect on professionalism skills in the clinical setting you will enable them to identify role models, professional behaviours and the hidden curriculum. For example, before rounds, ask the residents to identify and be prepared to do a 'case report' on positive (or negative) professional behaviours, role models, professionalism issues that were well-handled (or not) and how the ideal varies from the hidden curriculum of practice. An alternative is to offer important 'hot topics' from the news.

Depending on the 'case report' or 'hot topic', you can also support guided reflection and exploration of professionalism by

- asking questions about key concepts, frameworks or principles,

- probing their observations of positive or negative behaviours,

- discussing management of professionalism issues, problems and challenges,

- asking about management of personal health, resilience and wellness, and

- providing advice on how to respect patient/case confidentiality in the discussions.

Teaching Tip 3.
Provide information and resources about the most frequent or important ethical issues and professional standards topics encountered in practice

Teach the basics of the most common ethical issues or professional standards issues that are encountered in your patients, community or populations in your specific clinical context. For efficiency, formalize the content about these needs and activities as you teach a new group of learners.

You can quickly orient learners to effective options by assembling key resources for them and introducing them to key individuals who can help them with different topics. For example, refusal for treatment is often related to depression. The local protocol might be to contact the social worker, the psychiatrist or psychologist. But if the issue is one of accepting that the patient is nearing his or her last days and hours, then perhaps the local protocol is to contact the palliative care team, chaplain, or social worker.

Provide learners with information about common ethical issues that include local options to provide efficient, timely assistance to their patients, program, organizations and community. Topics to cover in terms of specific professional expectations might include privacy legislation, health records, duty to report, consent, immunization, licensure, substitute decision making, age of majority, end of life decisions, and refusal of treatment.

Teaching Tip 4:
Use specialty specific resources to teach resilience, wellness, and self-care

Encourage your residents to look for examples of resilience in others (i.e. the use of positive reframing of stressful events or environments; effective problem solving) and to critique how they recognize this quality in themselves. They can unpack their critique by considering 1) self-management (i.e. self-directed, realistic goals, uses feedback), and 2) persistence and commitment (i.e. setting and working towards longer-term goals).[14]

Ensure there is a regular sharing or update of information that reinforces the importance of resilience, wellness, self-care and identification of warning signs for concerns about wellness. Residents need to know where to go if they need help and need to be encouraged to maintain good health habits throughout residence. This encouragement can be part of an annual retreat, a wellness day or program, or via centrally available resources.

Bring in faculty guests to talk to your learners. Include faculty who are skilled at resilience, wellness and self-care as well as people who struggle with it but still make it work. Ideally, the guests should be near peers of your learners.

© 2015 Royal College of Physicians and Surgeons of Canada

Professional

Sample teaching tools

You can use the sample *Teaching Tools for Professional* at the end of this chapter as is, or you can modify or use them in various combinations to suit your objectives, time allocated, sequence within your residency program, and so on.

Easy-to-customize electronic versions of the *Teaching Tools for Professional* (in .doc, .ppt and .pdf formats) are found at: canmeds.royalcollege.ca

The tools provided are:

- T1 Lecture or Large Group Session: Foundations of the Professional Role

- T2 Presentation: Teaching the Professional Role

- T3 Case Report: Professionalism scenarios and case discussion

- T4 Case Report: Learner selected case report and reflection

- T5 Direct Observation: Guided observation and role modelling reflection assignment

- T6 Tools and Strategies: Summary sheet for the Professional Role

5. Hints, tips and tools for *assessing* the Professional Role

Assessment for learning is a major theme in this CanMEDS Tools Guide and a growing emphasis in medical education. You can and should use assessment as a strategy to inform a resident's learning plan (i.e. to alert or signpost to learners what is important to learn as well as what and how they will be assessed). This section of the Tools Guide offers a number of hints to help you develop a program of assessment that will ensure that both teachers and learners have a clear understanding of their performance and what needs improvement.

Assessment Tip 1.
Use a combination of assessment tools and multiple observers over a period of time

Professionalism is multidimensional, so you need to organize a 'program' of assessment tools that are longitudinal, stage appropriate, aligned with learning objectives or desired outcomes, use multiple methods and multiple observers, and have consequences.[8,23]

You should select assessment tools that include recognition, documentation and reinforcement of positive professionalism behaviours. Positive professional behaviours need to be distinctly assessed from the identification and documentation of negative behaviours.[23] Methods you can use to assess progress and performance of professionalism include encounter cards, patient feedback, written exams, objective structured clinical exams (OSCEs), multisource feedback (MSF) and attendance monitoring, assignment tracking, professionalism incident reports.[33]

Try giving your learners a written assessment or assignment where you provide them with a written or video scenario that they can analyze. You can use this to test principles of professionalism including terminology, moral reasoning or decision-making as well as what should be done in that particular situation

If you want to assess a learner's performance in a critical or difficult scenario, you may well choose to use an OSCE, which allows you to recreate difficult scenarios for multiple trainees, which you can not always do in a real clinical setting.

A system of gathering input from co-workers into multisource feedback or professionalism encounter forms (i.e. P-MEX)[34] is important, as positive and negative professionalism behaviours need multiple raters over time and in different contexts (i.e. both away/from and within the view of faculty).

A separate tracking system to monitor incidents of negative professional behaviours is also beneficial. With such a system, negative incidents can come to light outside the circuit of usual assessments (i.e. behaviour at rounds, absence from clinic, missed in training exam).[33] A straightforward incident reporting system[35] would include: reporting/documentation, exploration, feedback conversation, follow up or intervention(s).

Assessment Tip 2.
Establish a culture and practice of appropriate disclosure of learners needs

Your program, teachers and learners will benefit from a culture and practice of appropriate disclosure of learner needs which is also called learner handover.[36] This is particularly so for the Professional Role as these competencies are built over time using both multiple assessment tools, including longitudinal monitoring and assessments.

Providing clarity about the strengths, limits and concerns about your learners to your teachers reflects a culture of transparency, support and improvement. Identifying the areas that your learner needs to develop or the professional behaviours that have been problematic will allow for your faculty to be vigilant in preventing negative behaviours or developing early warning systems that would ensure support is provided early. The appropriate disclosure of strengths and needs in the Professional Role will also provide consistency of coaching and feedback regarding both positive and negative professionalism behaviours.

Assessment Tip 3.

Assess your learners in real time in the clinical setting with the input of multiple people

It is important to have many people's input about your residents' professionalism competencies in day-to-day clinical practice. There are a variety of sources of information about your residents' professionalism such as input from your learners' co-residents, chief residents, faculty, or other colleagues via a feedback forms (i.e. multisource from team members using multisource feedback or (MSF) forms) or session encounter forms, or by asking for their input for the interim or end-of-session in-training evaluation form (ITER) form. Many of these forms exist and can be easily modified for your learners' stage of development.

Collecting input from a broad range of faculty, co-workers and co-residents will help provide information on key elements of professionalism. Things you may ask others to comment about the residents include:

- clinical competence and asking for feedback and supervision;

- responsiveness to patients;

- patient safety;

- engagement with patients and team members;

- being respectful, collaborative, constructive, courteous;

- integrity including maintaining boundaries;

- reliability and being supportive;

- compliance with established guidelines and regulations; and

- taking responsibility for work and actions.

It is also important to specifically ask about and follow up on serious incidents or patterns of behaviour that do not meet your programs' documented expectations and guidelines, as well as the established organizational policies and guidelines.

Assessment Tip 4.

Monitor and provide feedback on resident behaviour, resilience, wellness and self-care

It is important to gather and monitor longitudinally (i.e. frequently enough and over a period of time) to get a sense about your residents' patterns of behaviour. Attendance, timeliness, registration/regulation compliance, absence from academic half day, repeated absence from semi-annual or annual examinations, incomplete assignments, and observed episodes of 'minor' behavioural incidents, are the sorts of issues that need to be monitored longitudinally to see if there are patterns over the past few months or over the residency as a whole. These small indicators could be viewed as risks to professionalism. They also may be indicators that your resident is not coping or is unwell.

It is worth noting that being stressed or unwell is not a suitable reason for negative professional behaviours. If a physician is too stressed or unwell to deliver quality care to patients, the expectation is that it is the responsibility of professionals to either 'step out' until they can meet their professional obligations or to change their conduct to meet the established standard.[37]

At a minimum the explicit check-in with residents about resilience, wellness and self-care should be done semi-annually (i.e. meeting between program director and resident, meeting with mentor). By monitoring and managing these 'signs or symptoms' of a resident's troubling or unprofessional behaviour you have the opportunity to have a candid supportive discussion about the trends you see, the resources available, the expectations for changes and the consequences or actions if the pattern persists. And when you combine any new or emerging patterns of negative professionalism behaviour with the information on wellness, you have a 'surveillance' system for resident wellness.

Sample assessment tools

You can use the sample *Assessment Tools for Professional* at the end of this chapter as is, or you can modify or use them in various combinations to suit your objectives, time allocated, sequence within your residency program, and so on.

Easy-to-customize electronic versions of the *Assessment Tools for Professional* (in .doc, .ppt and .pdf formats) are found at: canmeds.royalcollege.ca

The tools provided are:

- A1 Mini-CEX: Professional mini-evaluation exercise (P-MEX)

- A2 Direct Observation: Professionalism incident report

© 2015 Royal College of Physicians and Surgeons of Canada

6. Suggested resources

- **Cruess RL, Cruess SR, Steinert Y, editors.** *Teaching medical professionalism.* **New York: Cambridge University Press, 2008.** This is an important primer on the teaching of medical professionalism. A second edition is under development.

- **Cruess RL, Cruess SR, Boudreau JD, Snell L, Steinert Y. Reframing medical education to support professional identity formation.** *Acad Med.* **2014;89(11):1446-51.** This article explains and illustrates the importance of identity formation in medical education including post-graduate medical education.

- **Eckleberry-Hunt J, Van Dyke A, Lick D, Tucciarone J. Changing the conversation from burnout to wellness: physician well-being in residency training programs.** *J Grad Med Educ.* **2009:1(2);225-230.** This article provides an important contribution to resident education regarding physician well-being. The authors have developed a toolbox of practical steps to create a culture that emphasizes wellness. They provide the definition of wellness and identify the key components to developing and maintaining wellness. It provides a practical and accessible strategy to implement a curriculum for wellness into a residency program.

- **Puddester D, Flynn L, Cohen J.** *CanMEDS physician health guide: a practical handbook for physician health and well-being.* **Ottawa: Royal College of Physician and Surgeons of Canada. 2009.** This handbook is a resource that was developed for those engaged in medical education. This resource introduces topics on physician health, well-being and sustainability. It can be used to develop a curriculum, to provide resources for case discussion, and to assist teachers and learners to develop strategies to manage their own health and well-being.

- **Royal College of Physicians and Surgeons of Canada. Bioethics Curriculum. http://www.royalcollege.ca/ portal/page/portal/rc/resources/bioethics** The bioethics curriculum aims to raise awareness and understanding of the importance of ethical principles and the value of ethical analysis in guiding behaviour and decision-making in medical practice.

7. Other resources

- Avidan AY. Sleep and fatigue countermeasures for the neurology resident and physician. Continuum *(Minneap Minn)*. 2013;19(1 Sleep Disorders):204-22.

- College of Physicians and Surgeons of Ontario (CPSO). *Guidebook For Managing Disruptive Physician Behaviour.* 2008. Last retrieved July 7, 2015 from: http://www. cpso.on.ca/CPSO/media/uploadedfiles/CPSO_DPBI_ Guidebook1.pdf

- Levinson W, Ginsberg S, Hafferty FW and Lucey CR. *Understanding Medical Professionalism.* Columbus: McGraw-Hill Education. 2014.

- Hebert, PC. Doing Right: *A Practical Guide to Ethics for Medical Trainees and Physicians.* Third Edition. Don Mills: Oxford University Press; 2008.

- Hodges BD, Ginsburg S, Cruess S, Delport R, Hafferty F, Ho MJ, Holmboe E, Holtman M, Ohbu S, Rees C, Ten Cate O, Tsugawa Y, Van Mook W, Wass V, Wilkinson T, Wade W. Assessment of Professionalism: recommendations from the Ottawa 2010 conference. *Med Teach.* 2011;33(5):354-63.

- Johnston D, Montpetit M, Hogue RJ, Geller C, MacDonald CJ, Johnston S. uOttawa: Developing the CanMEDS Professional. [PowerPoint slides] Ottawa: University of Ottawa; 2014. http://www.med.uottawa. ca/postgraduate/eng/pgme_ebooks.html

- Shanafelt TD, Oreskovich MR, Dyrbve LN, Satele DV, Hanks JB, Sloan JA, Balch CM. Avoiding burnout: the personal habits and wellness practices of US surgeons, *Ann Surg.* 2012;255(4):625-33.

- The Canadian Medical Protective Association has many online resources for learners and teachers designed to contribute to safe medical practice and help reduce medico-legal risks. Last retrieved July 7, 2015 from: https:// www.cmpa-acpm.ca/serve/docs/ela/goodpracticesguide/ pages/index/index-e.html

Professional

8. PROFESSIONAL ROLE DIRECTORY OF TEACHING AND ASSESSMENT TOOLS

You can use the sample *teaching and assessment tools for the Professional Role* found in this section as is, or you can modify or use them in various combinations to suit your objectives, the time allocated, the sequence within your residency program, and so on. Tools are listed by number (e.g. T1), type (e.g. Lecture), and title (e.g. Foundations of the Professional Role).

Easy-to-customize electronic versions of the sample *teaching and assessment tools for the Professional Role* in .doc, .ppt and .pdf formats are found at: canmeds.royalcollege.ca

TEACHING TOOLS

ASSESSMENT TOOLS

© 2015 Royal College of Physicians and Surgeons of Canada

Professional

T1. FOUNDATIONS OF THE PROFESSIONAL ROLE

Created for the *CanMEDS Teaching and Assessment Tools Guide* by S Glover Takahashi. Reproduced with permission of the Royal College.

This learning activity includes:

- Presentation: Foundations of the Professional Role (T1)

- Case Presentation: Scenarios and case discussion (T3)

- Case Presentation and Guided Reflection: Case report and reflection (T4)

Instructions for Teacher:

Sample learning objectives

1. Recognize common words related to the process and content of the Professional Role

2. Apply professionalism skills to examples from day-to-day practice

3. Develop a personal professionalism resource for day-to-day practice

Audience: All learners

How to adapt:

- Consider whether your session's objectives match the sample ones. Select from, modify, or add to the sample objectives as required.

- The sample PowerPoint presentation is generic and foundational and tied to simple objectives. Consider whether you will need additional slides to meet your objectives. Modify, add or delete content as appropriate. You may want to include specific information related to your discipline and context.

- Depending on whether you are using these materials in one session (i.e. Professional Basics Workshop) or a series of two to four academic half days will determine which worksheet(s) you select and in what sequence.

- You may wish to review and customize the Professional Summary Sheet with your learners as an additional worksheet activity.

Logistics:

- Select one or two worksheets for each teaching session.

- Plan for about 20 minutes for each worksheet/group activity: this time will be used for you to explain the activity and for your learners to complete the worksheet individually, share their answers with their small group, prepare to report back to the whole group, and then deliver their small group's report to the whole group.

- Allow individuals to read the worksheet and spend about five minutes working on the answers on their own before starting to work in groups. This allows each person to develop his or her own understanding of the topic.

- Depending on the group and time available, you may wish to assign one or more worksheets as homework to be completed before the session or as a follow-up assignment.

Setting:

- This information is best done in a small-group format if possible. It can also be effectively done with a larger group if the room allows for learners to be at tables in groups of five or six. With larger groups, it is helpful to have additional teachers or facilitators available to answer questions arising from the worksheet activities.

T2. TEACHING THE PROFESSIONAL ROLE

Created for the *CanMEDS Teaching and Assessment Tools Guide* by S Glover Takahashi. Reproduced with permission of the Royal College.

Instructions for Teacher:

- Setting and Audience: Faculty and all learners

- How to use: Use as an orientation to the Role.

- How to adapt: Select only those slides that apply to your teaching. Slides can be modified to match the specialty or the learners' practice context

- Logistics: Equipment – laptop, projector, screen

Slide #	Words on slide	Notes to teachers
1.	Professional Role	• Add information about presenters and modify title
2.	**Objectives and agenda** 1. Recognize the process and content of Professional Role. 2. Apply professionalism skills to examples from everyday practice. 3. Develop a personal professionalism resource for everyday practice.	• SAMPLE goals and objectives of the session – revise as required • CONSIDER doing a 'warm up activity' • Review/revise goals and objectives • Insert agenda slide if desired
3.	**Why the Professional Role matters** 1. Patients expect their physicians to provide high-quality, safe medical care.[a] 2. Being a professional is central to being a physician and requires active effort to evolve into a specialist.[b] 3. Professional behaviour is central to patient safety and effectiveness in team-based care.[c] 4. The resilience, wellness and self-care of a physician impacts their patients' care, their co-workers and the health system, requiring the need to manage the demands of work/practice while also attending to personal health activities and constructive coping skills.[d, e]	• Reasons why this Role is important • Provide examples from experience to illustrate
4.	**The details: What is the Professional Role[f]** As Professionals, physicians are committed to the health and well-being of individual patients and society through ethical practice, high personal standards of behaviour, accountability to the profession and society, physician-led regulation, and maintenance of personal health.	• Definition from the *CanMEDS 2015 Physician Competency Framework* • Avoid including competencies for learners
5.	**Recognizing Professional actions** • Behaving • Fulfilling • Trusting • Respecting • Self-regulating **Recognizing Professional topics** • Balance • Boundaries • Commitment • Conflict of interest • Ethics, Ethical Issues • Honesty • Identity • Integrity • Reliable • Resilience • Responsibility • Societal need • Social Contract • Society's expectations • Standards • Trustworthiness • Wellness	• Trigger words about Professional Role
6.	**Key terms for Professional Role** • Boundaries • Fiduciary relationship • Social contract • Hidden curriculum • Emotional intelligence • Self-efficacy • Wellness • Resilience • Burnout • Self-care • Fatigue management	• Important day to day language to know, understand meaning, be able to use • See key terms in chapter for details • Provide examples from experience to illustrate

a The Canadian Medical Protective Association. Physician professionalism – is it still relevant? *CMPA Perspective*, 2012;October special edition;4-6.

b Cruess RL, Cruess SR, Boudreau JD, Snell L, Steinert Y. Reframing medical education to support professional identity formation. *Acad Med.* 2014;89(11):1446-51.

c The Canadian Medical Protective Association. Physician professionalism – is it still relevant? *CMPA Perspective*, 2012;October special edition;4-6.

d Eckleberry-Hunt J, Van Dyke A, Lick D, Tucciarone J. Changing the conversation from burnout to wellness: physician well-being in residency training programs. *J Grad Med Educ.* 2009;1(2):225-30.

e Shanafelt TD, Oreskovich MR, Dyrbve LN, Satele DV, Hanks JB, Sloan JA, Balch CM. Avoiding burnout: the personal habits and wellness practices of US surgeons, *Ann Surg.* 2012;255(4):625-33.

f Snell L, Flynn L, Pauls M, Kearney R, Warren A, Sternszus R, Cruess R, Cruess S, Hatala R, Dupré M, Bukowskyj M, Edwards S, Cohen J, Chakravarti A, Nickell L, Wright J. Professional. In: Frank JR, Snell L, Sherbino J, editors. *CanMEDS 2015 Physician Competency Framework*. Ottawa: Royal College of Physicians and Surgeons of Canada; 2015. Reproduced with permission.

© 2015 Royal College of Physicians and Surgeons of Canada

Professional

T2. TEACHING THE PROFESSIONAL ROLE (continued)

Slide #	Words on slide	Notes to teachers
7.	**Professional means showing commitment to:** • patients • society • profession • self	• Provide examples from experience to illustrate

8.	**Important to know about professionalism**
	1. Professionalism has multiple factors that can be taught:
	  • individual factors (i.e. behaviour and cognitive processes);
	  • interpersonal factors (i.e. process or effect of providing patient care with others); and
	  • context factors[g] (i.e. variations and expectations in interactions within or across individuals, institutions, specialties, cultures, countries).
	2. Focus on actively demonstrating positive professional behaviours.
	3. Physicians need to demonstrate the importance of their own personal health, wellness, and resilience.
		• Alternate to misconceptions
		• Provide examples from experience to illustrate

9.	**Skills for residents to master in developing their identity as a physician in your specialty are:** 1. Learning the language 2. Learning to live with ambiguity 3. Learning to play the role 4. Learning the hierarchy and power relationships	
10.	**Label the BEHAVIOUR** • Avoid judging the person	

11.	**POSITIVE PROFESSIONAL CHARACTERISTICS[b]**
	A. Clinical competency
	  1. Excellent knowledge and skill
	  2. Effective communication
	  3. Sound clinical reasoning
	
	B. Personal qualities
	  4. Compassionate and caring
	  5. Honesty and integrity
	  6. Enthusiastic for the practice of medicine
	  7. Effective interpersonal skills
	  8. Commitment to excellence
	  9. Collegial
	  10. Demonstrates humour
		• Share own experiences and examples

12.	**NEGATIVE PROFESSIONAL CHARACTERISTICS[b]**
	A. Clinical competency
	  1. Deficient knowledge and skill
	  2. Ineffective communication
	  3. Poor clinical reasoning
	
	B. Personal qualities
	  4. Insensitive to patients' suffering
	  5. Lapses in honesty and integrity
	  6. Dissatisfaction with the practice of medicine
	  7. Ineffective interpersonal skills
	  8. Acceptance of mediocre results
	  9. Lack of collegiality
	  10. Humourless approach
		• Share own experiences and examples

g Hodges BD, Ginsburg S, Cruess R, Cruess S, Delport R, Hafferty F, Ho MJ, Holmboe E, Holtman M, Ohbu S, Rees C, Ten Cate O, Tsugawa Y, Van Mook W, Wass V, Wilkinson T, Wade W. Assessment of Professionalism: recommendations from the Ottawa 2010 conference. *Med Teach*. 2011;33(5):354-63.

© 2015 Royal College of Physicians and Surgeons of Canada

Professional

T2. TEACHING THE PROFESSIONAL ROLE (continued)

Slide #	Words on slide	Notes to teachers
13.	T3 – Opportunities to actively demonstrate Professionalism	• Learning activity T3 • Share own experiences and scenarios • See A1 and A2 for types of positive/negative professional characteristics
14.	**Use role modelling to improve professional behaviour**[h] 1. Active observation of role model 2. Making the unconscious conscious 3. Reflection and abstraction 4. Translating insights into principles and action 5. Generalization and behaviour change	
15.	**Constructive coping skills**[i, j] **include:** • Positive reframing • Finding meaning in work • Focusing on what is important in life • Maintaining a positive outlook and attitude towards work • Embracing an approach that stresses work-life balance	• Share own experiences and examples • Identify local resources
16.	**Wellness responsibilities**[a] 1. Only care for patients when well enough to do so 2. Be aware of their own health, including recognizing when not well enough to provide competent care 3. Obtain help in order to ensure their own wellness 4. Adjust their practice to ensure that patients can and do receive appropriate care 5. Recognizing limits imposed by fatigue, stress or illness and taking care to ensure a healthy work-life balance 6. Avoid self-treatment	• Share own experiences and examples
17.	**Personal health activities are associated with lower rates of burnout and improved quality of life** • Weekly aerobic and weight training to recommended levels • Annual visits to primary care provider (i.e. family physician) • Routine required health screening practices	• Share own experiences and examples
18.	**Resilience, wellness and self care** 1. Have a family doctor 2. Sleep right 3. Eat well 4. Exercise regularly 5. Stay connected	• Identify local resources • Share own experiences and examples
19.	**Signs of concern about wellness** • Sudden or trend for isolation or absence such as not showing up for work, rounds, meeting, assignments • Mood swings, teary, unusual or easily irritated or frustrated • Often late to work or late with assignments • More absences than is usual or typical • Dishevelled, unkempt or loss of attention to self and grooming • Appearance or suspicion of over consumption of alcohol or other substances	• Identify local resources • Share own experiences and examples

h Cruess SR, Cruess RL, Steinert Y. Role modelling—making the most of a powerful teaching strategy. *BMJ.* 2008;336(7646):718-21.

i Eckleberry-Hunt J, Van Dyke A, Lick D, Tucciarone J. Changing the conversation from burnout to wellness: physician well-being in residency training programs. *J Grad Med Educ.* 2009:1(2);225-230.

j Shanafelt TD, Oreskovich MR, Dyrbve LN, Satele DV, Hanks JB, Sloan JA, Balch CM. Avoiding burnout: the personal habits and wellness practices of US surgeons, *Ann Surg.* 2012;255(4):625-33.

© 2015 Royal College of Physicians and Surgeons of Canada

Professional

T2. TEACHING THE PROFESSIONAL ROLE (continued)

Slide #	Words on slide	Notes to teachers
OTHER SLIDES		
20.	**Professional Key Competencies[f]** *Physicians are able to:* 1. Demonstrate a commitment to patients by applying best practices and adhering to high ethical standards 2. Demonstrate a commitment to society by recognizing and responding to societal expectations in health care 3. Demonstrate a commitment to the profession by adhering to standards and participating in physician-led regulation 4. Demonstrate a commitment to physician health and well-being to foster optimal patient care	• From the *CanMEDS 2015 Framework* • Avoid including competencies for learners • You may wish to use this slide if you are giving the presentation to teachers or planners

21.	**Professional Key Competency 1**
	Physicians are able to:
	1. Demonstrate a commitment to patients by applying best practices and adhering to high ethical standards[f]
	  1.1 Exhibit appropriate professional behaviours and relationships in all aspects of practice, demonstrating honesty, integrity, humility, commitment, compassion, respect, altruism, respect for diversity, and maintenance of confidentiality
	  1.2 Demonstrate a commitment to excellence in all aspects of practice
	  1.3 Recognize and respond to ethical issues encountered in practice
	  1.4 Recognize and manage conflicts of interest
	  1.5 Exhibit professional behaviours in the use of technology-enabled communication
		• From the *CanMEDS 2015 Framework*

22.	**Professional Key Competency 2**
	Physicians are able to:
	2. Demonstrate a commitment to society by recognizing and responding to societal expectations in health care[f]
	  2.1 Demonstrate accountability to patients, society, and the profession by responding to societal expectations of physicians
	  2.2 Demonstrate a commitment to patient safety and quality improvement
		• From the *CanMEDS 2015 Framework*

23.	**Professional Key Competency 3**
	Physicians are able to:
	3. Demonstrate a commitment to the profession by adhering to standards and participating in physician-led regulation[f]
	  3.1 Fulfill and adhere to the professional and ethical codes, standards of practice, and laws governing practice.
	  3.2 Recognize and respond to unprofessional and unethical behaviours in physicians and other colleagues in the health care profession
	  3.3 Participate in peer assessment and standard-setting
		• From the *CanMEDS 2015 Framework*

24.	**Professional Key Competency 4**
	Physicians are able to:
	4. Demonstrate a commitment to physician health and well-being to foster optimal patient care[f]
	  4.1 Exhibit self-awareness and manage influences on personal well-being and professional performance
	  4.2 Manage personal and professional demands for a sustainable practice throughout the physician life cycle
	  4.3 Promote a culture that recognizes, supports, and responds effectively to colleagues in need
		• From the *CanMEDS 2015 Framework*

f   Snell L. Flynn L, Pauls M, Kearney R, Warren A, Sternszus R, Cruess R, Cruess S, Hatala R, Dupré M, Bukowskyj M, Edwards S, Cohen J, Chakravarti A, Nickell L, Wright J. Professional. In: Frank JR, Snell L, Sherbino J, editors. *CanMEDS 2015 Physician Competency Framework*. Ottawa: Royal College of Physicians and Surgeons of Canada; 2015. Reproduced with permission.

Professional

T3. PROFESSIONALISM SCENARIOS AND CASE DISCUSSION[a]

Created for the *CanMEDS Teaching and Assessment Tools Guide* by S Glover Takahashi.
Reproduced with permission of the Royal College.

See Professional Role teacher tips appendix for this teaching tool

Based on the selected/assigned scenario/case (below), answer the following questions.

1. In this case what are the Professional Role issues/problems?

    _____

    _____

    _____

    _____

    _____

    _____

    _____

2. What was (or should be) the action plan (e.g. who, what, how, when)? What is the desired outcome(s) or solution(s)?

    _____

    _____

    _____

    _____

    _____

    _____

    _____

3. Which elements of the process(s) and outcomes of this case/situation were

    a. Done very well (i.e. little, no improvement needed)

    b. Met expectations (i.e. but would benefit from some improvement)

    c. Need improvement (i.e. need significant change in approach or considerable improvement)

    d. Overall: what is your view about this case?

---

a   Cruess RL, Cruess SR, Steinert Y, editors. *Teaching medical professionalism.* New York: Cambridge University Press, 2008.

© 2015 Royal College of Physicians and Surgeons of Canada

T3. PROFESSIONALISM SCENARIOS AND CASE DISCUSSION (continued)

SAMPLE SCENARIOS AND LONGER CASES

#	SCENARIOS
1.	You are reviewing your recent social media messages and notice that a co-resident has written a highly negative comment about a patient situation. There is no specific patient name, but the hospital initials and case make it easy to figure out the nurses and physicians that are being described.
2.	While you were in a family meeting to sort out patient goals for a family member whose health is declining quickly, another part of the medical team intubated the patient which is against the specific decision made in the family meeting.
3.	A 14-year-old girl asks that you not include her parents in consent for the birth control pill.
4.	You smell alcohol on the breath of the consulting surgeon. He finishes his assessment and you overhear the conversation between the surgeon and their fellow that the plan is to take the patient to surgery as soon as the patient can be transferred.
5.	Your co-resident for the overnight on call shift doesn't help with any of the patient care saying they are busy getting ready for rounds where he is presenting tomorrow. This has happened before where the resident didn't pull their weight.
6.	You are at a large social gathering and realize that one of the residents is there on a date with their supervisor.
7.	You are asked to do a consult on a patient. When you go to see that patient they indicate that they don't want you to take care of them (i.e. because of your race, gender, ethnicity, culture).
8.	You observe a very disruptive patient who lives in a local shelter being cursed at and roughly handled by a senior resident.
	LONGER CASES
9.	Dr. B is a senior resident who has been assigned his first rotation as the lead of a team of three residents on a busy clinical service. You are the Chief Resident and have managed a series of email complaints over the past three days from the residents at that site. You now have a second page from the charge nurse. Dr. B works hard, but the concern is that he is a stickler for details about how orders and consults are to be done. He references policies, guidelines and procedures repeatedly. When you spoke to Dr. B, he said he was proud that he was, "going by the book". When you offered other, more common solutions, at first he was resistant to your intervention and is now aggressive when you ask questions about his assignments. You notice that referrals and patient care is now noticeably slower.
10.	You are working in a community placement for the month with a more senior resident Avery who you have met previously at the quarterly journal club. Avery is a past award winner for the program Leadership award and you know him for his energetic welcoming manner. By the end of the first week you notice that Avery is distracted, irritable and has been late for am clinic twice and pm rounds three times. Yesterday, when Avery didn't answer his pages, they called you even though you weren't on call. The patient problem was straightforward and it was no trouble for you to handle it on your own. You told Avery about taking the call and he said the battery on his pager must be dead, but when he pulls it out of his backpack it clearly is working.
11.	You are working in the Emergency department. Your current case is Stephanie, a 35-year-old woman presenting with pain and bruising in her left wrist and shoulder. X-rays show a simple fracture to her left wrist. You take a history regarding the injury and find the following: • Stephanie is a married, stay at home Mom with two small children who are with a neighbour • Her husband, Kyle, is a corporate lawyer with a substance use problem/history • Verbal abuse started when she was pregnant with her first child. After the birth of the second child he also started becoming physically abusive when under the influence of alcohol (verbally demeaning and belittling, escalating to shoving and pushing) • She is currently in the emergency department after he threw her against a wall three days ago • She is keen to get home and pick up her children • She minimizes husband's behaviour and is sympathetic towards her husband's work problems. She notes he has apologized • Previous injuries were a sprained wrist (1 yr. ago) and some fractured ribs three months ago.
12.	Other

© 2015 Royal College of Physicians and Surgeons of Canada

T4. LEARNER SELECTED CASE REPORT AND REFLECTION

Created for the *CanMEDS Teaching and Assessment Tools Guide* by S Glover Takahashi.
Reproduced with permission of the Royal College.

See Professional Role teacher tips appendix for this teaching tool

CASE REPORT ID:_____

Prepared by: _____

Describe a case situation from your own experience that included issues related to the Professional Role.

_____

_____

_____

1. In this case what are the Professional Role issues/problems?

_____

_____

_____

2. What was (or should be) the action plan (e.g. who, what, how, when)? What is the desired outcome(s) or solution(s)?

_____

_____

_____

3. Which elements of the process(s) and outcomes of this case/situation were
   a. Done very well (i.e. little, no improvement needed)
   b. Met expectations (i.e. but would benefit from some improvement)
   c. Need improvement (i.e. need significant change in approach or considerable improvement)
   d. Overall: what's your view about this case?

4. What are some concrete changes (i.e. what you would start or stop) for action in a similar future case/situation?

_____

_____

_____

© 2015 Royal College of Physicians and Surgeons of Canada

Professional

T4. LEARNER SELECTED CASE REPORT AND REFLECTION (continued)

5. Reflect on your role and document any next steps that would lead to an improvement or development of your professionalism skills?

☐ APPLIES TO PERIOD: FROM _____ TO _____

#	Area (i.e. identity development, professionalism issues management, professionalism behaviours, personal health, resilience and wellness)	Goal(s) or objectives including timeframe	Metrics or criteria for success	Key next steps, resources, supports for success
1.				
2.				
3.				

Other notes:

Professional

T5. GUIDED OBSERVATION AND ROLE MODELLING REFLECTION ASSIGNMENT

Created for the *CanMEDS Teaching and Assessment Tools Guide* by S Glover Takahashi.
Reproduced with permission of the Royal College.

See Professional Role teacher tips appendix for this teaching tool

Instructions for Learners:

Role modelling can be a powerful influence on learners and particularly when it comes to the development of professional behaviours. This exercise is designed to help you reflect on positive role modelling behaviour vs negative role modelling behaviour. This exercise should help you differentiate between the types of behaviours you encounter and encourage you to assume the positive behaviours.

REPORT Prepared by: _____

1. Consider specific role model that you have worked with in the last year. Write a very brief description about this experience, but do not include any names or identifying information. This exercise is designed for your learning and it should not detract from a positive learning climate

   _____

   _____

   _____

   _____

   _____

2. Describe the setting where you were: ***Workplace***

   ☐ Patients present

   ☐ Patients not present

   ☐ Ward

   ☐ Clinic

   ☐ OR

   ☐ ER

   ☐ Other: _____

© 2015 Royal College of Physicians and Surgeons of Canada

T5. GUIDED OBSERVATION AND ROLE MODELLING REFLECTION ASSIGNMENT (continued)

OBSERVATION ON ROLE MODEL

POSITIVE ROLE MODELS POSITIVE CHARACTERISTICS[a]	NEGATIVE ROLE MODELS NEGATIVE CHARACTERISTICS
A. Clinical competency	
• Excellent knowledge and skill	• Deficient knowledge and skill
• Effective communication	• Ineffective communication
• Sound clinical reasoning	• Poor clinical reasoning
B. Teaching skills	
• Aware of role	• Unaware of role
• Explicit about what is modelled	• Not explicit about what is modelled
• Makes time for teaching	• Does not make time for teaching
• Shows respect for student needs	• Does not show respect for student needs
• Provides timely feedback	• Does not provide timely feedback
• Encourages reflection in students	• Dose not encourage reflection in students
C. Personal qualities	
• Compassionate and caring	• Insensitive to patients' suffering
• Honesty and integrity	• Lapses in honesty and integrity
• Enthusiastic for the practice of medicine	• Dissatisfaction with the practice of medicine
• Effective interpersonal skills	• Ineffective interpersonal skills
• Commitment to excellence	• Acceptance of mediocre results
• Collegial	• Lack of collegiality
• Demonstrates humour	• Humourless approach
TOTAL # POSITIVE BEHAVIOURS:	**TOTAL # NEGATIVE BEHAVIOURS:**

Which elements of this role model were

a.   Done very well (i.e. little, no improvement needed)

b.   Met expectations (i.e. but would benefit from some improvement)

c.   Need improvement (i.e. need significant change in approach or considerable improvement)

d.   Overall: What did you learn from working with this role model?

Other comments:

---

a   Adapted by permission from the BMJ from Cruess SR, Cruess RL, Steinert Y. Role modelling—making the most of a powerful teaching strategy. *BMJ.* 2008;336(7646):718-21. Reproduced with permission from BMJ Publishing Group Ltd.

Professional

T6. SUMMARY SHEET FOR THE PROFESSIONAL ROLE

Created for the *CanMEDS Teaching and Assessment Tools Guide* by S Glover Takahashi. Reproduced with permission of the Royal College.

See Professional Role teacher tips appendix for this teaching tool

PROFESSIONAL

1. Professionalism has multiple factors that can be taught:
   - *individual factors* (i.e. behaviour and cognitive processes);
   - *interpersonal factors* (i.e. process or effect of providing patient care with others); and
   - *context factors*[a] (i.e. variations and expectations in interactions within or across individuals, institutions, specialties, cultures, countries).

2. Focus on actively demonstrating positive professional behaviours.

3. Physicians need to demonstrate the importance of their own personal health, wellness, and resilience.

Professional means showing commitment to:
- patients
- society
- profession
- self

Early skills to master in developing an identity:[b]
- Learn the language
- Learn to live with ambiguity
- Learn to play the role/identity
- Learning the hierarchy and power relationships

Boundaries means maintaining appropriate professional relationship with patients including setting limits on the nature of relationships with patients, on accepting gifts, and on treating one's family members and friends. Need to be relaxed and cordial but also keep a work-related distance with patients.[c]

Using role modelling to develop professionalism behaviours:[d]
- Active observation of role model
- Making the unconscious conscious
- Reflection and abstraction
- Translating insights into principles and action
- Generalization and behaviour change

Fiduciary relationship refers to the special relationship of trust between physicians and their patients that requires physicians to always act in their patients' best interests, including providing care, effectively communicating treatment and care options, protecting privacy and confidentiality, and maintaining appropriate boundaries.[c]

RECOGNIZE Professional actions:
- Behaving
- Fulfilling
- Trusting
- Respecting
- Self-regulating

RECOGNIZE Professional topics:
- Balance
- Boundaries
- Commitment
- Conflict of interest
- Ethics, Ethical Issues
- Honesty
- Identity
- Integrity
- Reliable
- Resilience
- Responsibility
- Societal need
- Social Contract
- Society's expectations
- Standards
- Trustworthiness
- Wellness

Wellness means the condition of good physical and mental health necessary to provide high quality care to patients.[f] Wellness responsibilities:[a]
- Only care for patients when well enough to do so;
- Be aware of their own health, including recognizing when not well enough to provide competent care;
- Obtain help in order to ensure their own wellness;
- Adjust their practice to ensure that patients can and do receive appropriate care;
- Recognizing limits imposed by fatigue, stress or illness and taking care to ensure a healthy work-life balance;
- Avoid self-treatment

a Hodges BD, Ginsburg S, Cruess R, Cruess S, Delport R, Hafferty F, Ho MJ, Holmboe E, Holtman M, Ohbu S, Rees C, Ten Cate O, Tsugawa Y, Van Mook W, Wass V, Wilkinson T, Wade W. Assessment of Professionalism: recommendations from the Ottawa 2010 conference. *Med Teach*. 2011;33(5):354-63.

b Cruess RL, Cruess SR, Boudreau JD, Snell L, Steinert Y. A schematic representation of the professional identity formation and socialization of medical students and residents: a guide for medical educators. *Acad Med*. 2015;90(6):718-25.

c The Canadian Medical Protective Association. Building Trust – what are the boundaries with patients? 2011 Sept.

d Adapted by permission from the BMJ from Cruess SR, Cruess RL, Steinert Y. Role modelling – making the most of a powerful teaching strategy. *BMJ*. 2008;336(7646):718-21. Reproduced with permission from BMJ Publishing Group Ltd.

e The Canadian Medical Protective Association. Physician professionalism – is it still relevant? *CMPA Perspective*. 2012;October special edition;4-6.

© 2015 Royal College of Physicians and Surgeons of Canada

Professional

T6. SUMMARY SHEET FOR THE PROFESSIONAL ROLE (continued)

Personal health activities are associated with lower rates of burnout and improved quality of life:
- Weekly aerobic and weight training to recommended levels
- Annual visits to primary care provider (i.e. family physician)
- Routine required health screening practices

Constructive coping skills[g, h] include:
- Positive reframing
- Finding meaning in work
- Focusing on what is important in life
- Maintaining a positive outlook and attitude towards work
- Embracing an approach that stresses work-life balance

IF concerned about these warning signs of concern about wellness, promptly seek assistance and support.
- Sudden or trend for isolation or absence such as not showing up for work, rounds, meeting, assignments.
- Mood swings, teary, unusual or easily irritated or frustrated.
- Often late to work or late with assignments.
- More absences than is usual or typical.
- Dishevelled, unkempt or loss of attention to self and grooming.
- Appearance or suspicion of over consumption of alcohol or other substances.

Hints to maintain wellness
1. *Have a family doctor.* See your family doctor annually or when you are unwell. Attend your needed personal screening health tests. Do not self medicate.
2. *Sleep right.* Sleep hygiene is important. Learn how to capture sleep opportunities as an investment for self and patients.

3. *Eat well.* Make good choices. Plan to feed your body. Shop for foods that DO work with your lifestyle. Pack your lunch or snacks. Remember to eat well and often. Avoid excess caffeine and sugar. Limit use of alcohol and non-prescription drugs.
4. *Exercise regularly.* This is good for your body and your brain. You will learn more if you exercise.
5. *Stay connected.* You will never have enough time to see your family and friends, exercise, relax, or do other important activities like completing your taxes, seeing your family doctor, or going to the dentist. Schedule important things like these with enough regularity. Keep scheduled appointments and commitments. (The corollary to this is that you also don't have time for regret, guilt, divorce/relationship discord, illness, etc.)

Emotional intelligence is a group of skills use to guide their thinking, behaviour, and outcomes:[a]
- Self-awareness: knowing one's strengths, weaknesses, drivers, values, and impact on others.
- Self-regulation: ability to monitor and control own behaviour, emotions or thoughts, altering with the demands of the situation.
- Motivation: strong internal drive to pursue goals and achievement for reasons that are personally meaningful.
- Empathy: able to understand the emotions of others and treating them appropriately.
- Social skill: identifies socials cues to build rapport, establish common ground and build networks.

POSITIVE PROFESSIONAL CHARACTERISTICS[b]	NEGATIVE PROFESSIONAL CHARACTERISTICS
A. Clinical competency	
• Excellent knowledge and skill	• Deficient knowledge and skill
• Effective communication	• Ineffective communication
• Sound clinical reasoning	• Poor clinical reasoning
B. Personal qualities	
• Compassionate and caring	• Insensitive to patients' suffering
• Honesty and integrity	• Lapses in honesty and integrity
• Enthusiastic for the practice of medicine	• Dissatisfaction with the practice of medicine
• Effective interpersonal skills	• Ineffective interpersonal skills
• Commitment to excellence	• Acceptance of mediocre results
• Collegial	• Lack of collegiality
• Demonstrates humour	• Humourless approach

f   The College of Physicians and Surgeons of Ontario. Duties: to themselves and colleagues. Last retrieved July 7, 2015 from: http://www.cpso.on.ca/Policies-Publications/The-Practice-Guide-Medical-Professionalism-and-Col/Principles-of-Practice-and-Duties-of-Physicians/Duties-to-Themselves-and-Others/Duties-To-Themselves-and-Colleagues-Wellness

g   Eckleberry-Hunt J, Van Dyke A, Lick D, Tucciarone J. Changing the conversation from burnout to wellness: physician well-being in residency training programs. *J Grad Med Educ.* 2009:1(2);225-230.

h   Shanafelt TD, Oreskovich MR, Dyrbve LN, Satele DV, Hanks JB, Sloan JA, Balch CM. Avoiding burnout: the personal habits and wellness practices of US surgeons, *Ann Surg.* 2012;255(4):625-33.

Professional

A1. PROFESSIONAL MINI-EVALUATION EXERCISE P-MEX[a]

GUIDELINES FOR USING THE P-MEX

- The Professionalism Mini-Evaluation Exercise (P-MEX) focuses on the healing and professional behaviours that learners demonstrate in various settings during their daily professional activities.

- It is designed to be easily implemented and to encourage early feedback.

- It is to be used following an observation of a minimum of 15-20 minutes of a student/resident activity.

- The P-MEX can also be used for critical events

FORM AND RATING SCALE

- For each encounter, each behaviour should be categorized utilizing the following rating scale.

- Use the N/A (not applicable) category if the behaviour was not observed or if the category is not applicable to the setting.

Rating	Description of behaviour
UNacceptable	• Lapses of professional behaviour that are intentional, are likely to harm, and for which there are no mitigating circumstances.
BELow expectations	• Lapses of professional behaviour that are unintentional, result in minimal to no harm, or for which there may be mitigating circumstances.
MET expectations	• Demonstrated the performance expected for the level of the student/resident.
EXCeeded expectations	• Exceptional performance, demonstrating the behaviours expected of an outstanding physician-to-be.
Not **A**pplicable	• Can include does not apply and behaviour not observed in this encounter or critical incident.
Critical incident	• A concerning breach of professional boundaries or demonstration of unprofessional behaviour. • Documentation of a critical event is sent directly to the appropriate authority for prompt follow up.

RESIDENT Name:_____

Postgraduate year (PGY):_____

Date and time:_____

1. **Type:**

   ☐ Critical event

   ☐ Concerning event/situation

   ☐ Routine assessment report

   ☐ Clinic

2. **About reporter/evaluator:**

   - Health professional team member (i.e. including co-resident) that has worked closely with this resident

   - Health professional (i.e. including co-resident) that has had some interactions with this resident

   - Resident supervisor that has worked closely with this resident

- Resident supervisor that has had some interactions with this resident

- Other, please describe:_____

The period I have worked with this resident is:

_____

3. **SETTING:** *Workplace*

   ☐ Clinic   ☐ Clinic

   ☐ Patient Present   ☐ OR

   ☐ Patient Not Present   ☐ ER

   ☐ Ward   ☐ Other:_____

Non Workplace

   ☐ Structured Teaching

   ☐ Informal/unstructured Teaching

   ☐ Other:_____

a   Cruess RL, McIlroy J, Cruess SR, Ginsberg S, Steinert, Y. The Professionalism Mini-Evaluation Exercise: A preliminary investigation. *Acad Med* 2006;574-8 (Table 1). Permission from Wolters Kluwer Health, Inc.

© 2015 Royal College of Physicians and Surgeons of Canada

A1. PROFESSIONAL MINI-EVALUATION EXERCISE P-MEX (continued)

4. Please rate the behaviour during this event/situation
UNacceptable, BELow expectations, MET expectations, EXCeeded expectations, Not Applicable.

Criteria	N/A	UN	BEL	MET	EXC
Listened actively to patient					
Showed interest in patient as a person					
Recognized and met patient needs					
Extended his/herself to meet patient needs					
Ensured continuity of patient care					
Advocated on behalf of a patient					
Demonstrated awareness of limitations					
Admitted errors/omissions					
Solicited feedback					
Accepted feedback					
Maintained appropriate boundaries					
Maintained composure in a difficult situation					
Maintained appropriate appearance					
Was on time					
Completed tasks in a reliable fashion					
Addressed own gaps in knowledge and skills					
Was available to colleagues					
Demonstrated respect for colleagues					
Avoided derogatory language					
Maintained patient confidentiality					
Used health resources appropriately					

OVERALL RATING for performance during this event/situation:

☐ **Un**acceptable   ☐ **BEL**ow expectations

☐ **MET** expectations   ☐ **EXC**eeded expectations

Comments:

_____

_____

_____

Completed by: _____

Signature: _____

© 2015 Royal College of Physicians and Surgeons of Canada

Professional

A2. PROFESSIONALISM INCIDENT REPORT[a]

Created for the *CanMEDS Teaching and Assessment Tools Guide* by S Glover Takahashi. Reproduced with permission of the Royal College.

See Professional Role teacher tips appendix for this assessment tool

RESIDENT Name: _____

Postgraduate year (PGY): _____

Program: _____

Date and time: _____

1. Type:

☐ Critical event

☐ Concerning event/situation

☐ Clinic

2. About reporter/evaluator:

- Health professional team member (i.e. including co-resident) that has worked closely with this resident

- Health professional (i.e. including co-resident) that has had some interactions with this resident

- Resident supervisor that has worked closely with this resident

- Resident supervisor that has had some interactions with this resident

- Other, please describe: _____

3. Contact name, follow up phone and email:

_____

4. SETTING: Workplace

☐ Clinic   ☐ Clinic

☐ Patient Present   ☐ OR

☐ Patient Not Present   ☐ ER

☐ Ward   ☐ Other: _____

Non Workplace

☐ Structured Teaching

☐ Informal/unstructured Teaching

☐ Other: _____

5. Brief overview of incident or concern:

_____

_____

_____

_____

_____

_____

_____

6. Type of incident or concern:

A. Professional ethics

☐ Behaved in a dishonest manner

☐ Used illicit substances OR alcohol, non-prescription drugs or prescription drugs in a manner that compromises ability to contribute to patient care

☐ Misrepresented self, others, or members of the team to others

☐ Breached patient confidentiality

☐ Acted in disregard for patient welfare (e.g. wilfully reports incomplete or inaccurate patient information)

☐ Took credit for the work of others

☐ Misused equipment, bio hazardous materials or other scientific specimens

B. Reliability and responsibility

☐ Consistently arrives late to scheduled events or assignments

☐ Has unexcused/unexplained absences

☐ Fails to notify appropriate staff in a timely manner of absences

☐ Does not respond to communications (e-mail, pages, phone calls, etc.) in a timely or professional manner. Please specify frequency and duration(s) of delay(s):

☐ Fails to complete required or assigned tasks

☐ Requires constant, repeated reminders from staff/faculty to complete required or assigned tasks

---

a   Additional sample see https://www.umassmed.edu/uploadedfiles/profincidentreport.pdf

© 2015 Royal College of Physicians and Surgeons of Canada

A2. PROFESSIONALISM INCIDENT REPORT[a] (continued)

C. Professional relationships and responsibilities

☐ Has inappropriate demeanour or disruptive behaviour (raises voice, disrespects authority, rude, condescending etc.)

☐ Inappropriate appearance (dirty white coat, wrinkled clothes, un-bathed, etc.) in the classroom or in the health care setting

☐ Fails to accept responsibility for own errors

☐ Fails to recognize limitations and seeking help

☐ Does not accept constructive feedback

☐ Does not incorporate feedback to modify behaviour

☐ Engages in relationships with patients or any other member of the health care team which are disruptive to learning and patient care

☐ Acts disrespectfully toward others

☐ Engages in disruptive behaviour in class or with health care team (situational dependent)

D. Patient, faculty, resident, administrative staff, and other team member interactions

☐ Is unable to establish rapport

☐ Is not sensitive to patient needs

☐ Is disrespectful of the diversity or race, gender, religion, sexual orientation, age, disability or socio-economic status

☐ Struggles with establishing and maintaining appropriate boundaries in work and learning situations

☐ Contributes to an atmosphere that is not conductive to learning

☐ Relating poorly to other learners in a learning environment

☐ Relating poorly to staff in a learning environment

☐ Relating poorly to faculty in a learning environment

E. Other

☐ _____

☐ _____

☐ _____

6. Immediate action taken

☐ Spoke to patient(s)

☐ Spoke to learner(s)

☐ Spoke to supervisor(s)

☐ Contacted supervisor via email

☐ Called police or hospital security

☐ Documented in patient record

☐ Other: _____

Brief summary of action taken:

_____

_____

_____

_____

_____

_____

_____

_____

_____

7. Next steps

☐ Yes, please contact me for further discussion

☐ Contact me at your discretion

☐ Other: _____

© 2015 Royal College of Physicians and Surgeons of Canada

Professional

PROFESSIONAL ROLE TEACHER TIPS APPENDIX

T3 AND T4 CASE REPORT: PROFESSIONAL ROLE

Instructions for Teacher:

- Faculty or residents select real or sample cases/situations to be explored related to one or more of:
  - professional identity,
  - professionalism issues management (i.e. ethics, boundaries, duty to report, disruptive behaviour, privacy)
  - personal health, resilience or wellness

- Pre-teaching or pre-reading on topics would be important prior to the case discussion.

- If real cases are used, participants should be reminded about the need for appropriate confidentiality re: cases and positive learning climate.

- Establish how you will discuss or debrief these cases/situations (e.g. at one to one meeting, in small groups, via academic half day, via portfolio review, based on a summary paper or report).

- The sample cases and table provided can be used to guide discussions. These can be used where they are consistent with the local professional culture, codes and policies. If local approaches are different, then modification of the table is advisable.

T5 GUIDED OBSERVATION AND ROLE MODELLING REFLECTION ASSIGNMENT

Instructions for Teacher:

- Assign residents a number of role modelling reports to complete. For example you may ask them to complete and submit two to four reports by the end of week two of a four-week block. You could then plan to discuss it with the assignment with the learner in week three.

- Faculty to remind all about need for appropriate confidentiality re: cases and positive learning climate.

T6 SUMMARY SHEET FOR THE PROFESSIONAL ROLE

Instructions for Teacher:

- The summary sheet is intended to be a cheat sheet for the teacher as well as the learner. It is a one page resource on key concepts, frameworks and approaches.

A2 PROFESSIONALISM INCIDENT REPORT

Instructions for Teacher:

- It is important to monitor incidents of negative professional behaviours via a dedicated tracking system.

- Explicit lists are useful with patterns of unprofessional behaviour where remediation and clarity of expectations are paramount.

- Modify form and listed behaviours based on local codes, culture and policies.

- Prior to implementation it is important to:
  - Set clear expectations through orientation sessions, documented policies and procedures and employing professional codes and charters.
  - Detail processes in how incidents will be managed including consequences for very serious or repeated incidents.
  - Faculty development to the purpose and processes will also be important.

© 2015 Royal College of Physicians and Surgeons of Canada

Professional

REFERENCES

1. Cruess RL, Cruess SR, Boudrean JD, Snell L, Steinert Y. A Schematic Representation of the Professional Identity Formation and Socialization of Medical Students and Residents: A Guide for Medical Educators. *Acad Med.* 2015 90(6):718-25.

2. Cruess RL, Cruess SR, Boudreau JD, Snell L, Steinert Y. Reframing medical education to support professional identity formation. *Acad Med.* 2014;89(11):1446-51.

3. The Canadian Medical Protective Association. Physician professionalism – is it still relevant? *CMPA Perspective.* 2012;October special edition;4-6.

4. Shanafelt TD, Oreskovich MR, Dyrbye LN, Satele DV, Hanks JB, Sloan JA, Balch CM. Avoiding burnout: the personal habits and wellness practices of US surgeons, *Ann Surg.* 2012;255(4):625-33.

5. Eckleberry-Hunt J, Van Dyke A, Lick D, Tucciarone J. Changing the conversation from burnout to wellness: physician well-being in residency training programs. *J Grad Med Educ.* 2009:1(2);225-230.

6. Royal College of Physicians. Definition of professionalism. Last retrieved July 7, 2015 from: https://www.rcplondon.ac.uk/sites/default/files/documents/doctors_in_society_reportweb.pdf

7. Jarvis-Selinger S, Pratt DD, Regehr G. Competency is not enough: integrating identity formation into the medical education discourse. *Acad Med.* 2012;87(9):1185-90.

8. Snell L, Sherbino J, Dath D, Van Melle E. CanMEDS Professional: Monograph. 2013. Unpublished.

9. The Canadian Medical Protective Association. Building Trust – what are the boundaries with patients? *CMPA Perspective.* 2011;Sept.

10. Cruess RL, Cruess SR. Expectations and obligations: professional and medicine's social contract with society. *Perspect Biol Med.* 2008;51(4):579-98.

11. Hafferty FW, Franks R. The hidden curriculum, ethics teaching, and the structure of medical education. *Acad Med.* 1994;69(11):861-71.

12. Mahood SC. Medical education: beware the hidden curriculum. *Can Fam Physician.* 2011;57(9):983-5.

13. Dyrbye L, Shanafelt T. Nurturing resiliency in medical trainees. *Med Educ.* 2012;46(4):343.

14. Howe A, Smajdor A, Stöcki A. Towards an understanding of resilience and its relevance to medical training. *Med Educ.* 2012;46(4):349-56.

15. The College of Physicians and Surgeons of Ontario. Duties: to themselves and colleagues. Last retrieved July 7, 2015 from: http://www.cpso.on.ca/Policies-Publications/The-Practice-Guide-Medical-Professionalism-and-Col/Principles-of-Practice-and-Duties-of-Physicians/Duties-to-Themselves-and-Others/Duties-To-Themselves-and-Colleagues-Wellness

16. Shanafelt TD, Boone S, Tan L, Dyrbye LN, Sotile W, Satele D, West CP, Sloan J, Oreskovich MR. Burnout and satisfaction with work-life balance among US physicians relative to the general US population. *Arch Intern Med.* 2012;172(18):1377-1385.

17. Sanchez-Reilly S, Morrison LJ, Carey E, Bernacki R, O'Neill L, Kapo J, Periyakoil VS, Thomas Jde L. Caring for oneself to care for others; physicians and their self-care. *J Support Oncol.* 2013;11(2):75–81.

18. Irish LA; Kline CE; Gunn HE; Buysse DJ; Hall MH. The role of sleep hygiene in promoting public health: a review of empirical evidence. *Sleep Med Rev.* 2015;22:23-36.

19. Wikipedia. Definition of self-efficacy. Last retrieved Aug 5, 2015 from: http://en.wikipedia.org/wiki/Self-efficacy

20. Federation of Medical Regulatory Authorities of Canada. Federation of State Medical Boards, Milbank Memorial Fund. Medical Regulatory Authorities and the Quality of Medical Services in Canada and the United States. 2008. Report available from http://www.milbank.org/uploads/documents/0806MedServicesCanada/0806MedServicesCanada.html

21. Goleman D. *What makes a leader?* Harv Bus Rev. 1998;76(6):93-102.

22. Goleman, D. *Emotional intelligence.* New York: Bantam Books; 1995.

23. Hodges BD, Ginsburg S, Cruess R, Cruess S, Delport R, Hafferty F, Ho MJ, Holmboe E, Holtman M, Ohbu S, Rees C, Ten Cate O, Tsugawa Y, Van Mook W, Wass V, Wilkinson T, Wade W. Assessment of Professionalism: recommendations from the Ottawa 2010 conference. *Med Teach.* 2011; 33(5):354-63.

24. Eley DS, Stallman H. Where does medical education stand in nurturing the 3Rs in medical students: responsibility, resilience and resolve? *Med Teach.* 2014 Oct;36(10):835-7.

25. Stern, DT, Papadakis M. The developing physician—becoming a professional. N Engl J Med. 2006;355(17):1794-9.

26. Papadakis MA et al. Disciplinary action by medical boards and prior behaviour in medical school. N Engl J Med. 2005;353(25):2673-2682.

REFERENCES

27. Kegan, R. *In over our heads: the mental demands of modern life.* Cambridge: Harvard University Press. 1994. (reprint edition)

28. Wikepedia. Robert Kegan, Last retrieved August 5, 2015 from: https://en.wikipedia.org/wiki/Robert_Kegan

29. Doukas DJ, Kirch DG, Brigham TP, Barzansky BM, Wear S, Carrese JA, Fins JJ, Lederer SE. Transforming educational accountability in the medical ethics and humanities education toward professionalism. *Acad Med.* 2015;90(6):738-43.

30. Cruess SR, Cruess RL, Steinert Y. Role modelling—making the most of a powerful teaching strategy. *BMJ.* 2008;336(7646):718-21.

31. Puddester D. Managing and mitigating fatigue in the era of changing resident duty hours. *BMC Med Educ.* 2014;14(Suppl 1):S3.

32. Patel H, Puddester D. *The time management guide: a practical handbook for physicians by physicians.* Ottawa: Royal College of Physicians and Surgeons; 2012.

33. Wilkinson TJ, Wade WB, Knock LD. A blueprint to assess professionalism: results of a systematic review. *Acad Med.* 2009;84(5):551-8.

34. Cruess R, McIlroy JH, Cruess S, Ginsberg S, Steinert Y. The professionalism mini-evaluation exercise: a preliminary investigation. *Acad Med.* 2006;81(10 Suppl):S74-8.

35. Papadakis MA, Paauw DS, Hafferty FW, Shapiro J, Byyny RL, Alpha Omega Alpha Honor Medical Society Think Tank. Perspective: the education community must develop best practices informed by evidence-based research to remediate lapses of professionalism. *Acad Med.* 2012;87(12):1694-8.

36. Cleary L. "Forward Feeding" about students' progress: the case for longitudinal, progressive, and shared assessment of medical students." *Acad Med.* 2008:83(9);800.

37. The College of Physicians and Surgeons of Ontario. Guidebook for managing disruptive physician behaviour. 2008. Last retrieved July 7, 2015 from: http://www.cpso.on.ca/CPSO/media/uploadedfiles/policies/policies/Disruptive_Behaviour_Guidebook.pdf

© 2015 Royal College of Physicians and Surgeons of Canada

Professional